THE
STRONG
WOMEN'S
GUIDE TO
TOTAL
HEALTH

THE
STRONG
WOMEN'S
GUIDE TO
TOTAL
HEALTH

MIRIAM E. NELSON, PhD
and Jennifer Ackerman

RODALE

© 2010 by Miriam E. Nelson, PhD, and Jennifer Ackerman

Illustrations © 2010 by Rodale Inc.

Printed in the United States of America

"HEART" acronym on page 205–206 used with permission from Miriam E. Nelson, PhD; Alice H. Lichtenstein, DSc; with Lawrence Linder, MA, *Strong Women, Strong Hearts*, G. P. Putnam's Sons, 2005

Exercise illustrations © Karen Kuchar; medical illustrations © Lisa Clark

Photographs on page 167 © David W. Dempster

Book design by Christina Gaugler

ISBN-13: 978-1-59486-779-8

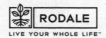

RODALE

LIVE YOUR WHOLE LIFE™

To our colleagues at Tufts University

Contents

Part IV: Standing Strong: Our Living Framework

Part V: Heart Smart and Breathing Easy

Part VI: In Our Defense

Part VII: Sensing: Staying in Touch with the World

Part VIII: Headstrong: Minding Your Emotional and Mental Health

Foreword

What's in This Book for You?

The huge strides we've made recently in understanding human health are truly amazing; much good has come of the new findings, from the development of the HPV vaccine to prevent cervical cancer to the latest strategies for maintaining muscle and bone strength into advanced age. But one aspect of the deluge of discoveries worries me: When some new bit of health information comes to light, we tend to focus on it to the exclusion of all else. Far too often we reduce the great wondrous complexity of our bodies in favor of focusing solely on the effects of this particular diet or that particular vitamin, the value of this new screening tool or that telling "biomarker." In so doing, we lose sight of the bigger picture: By far the most important factor in ensuring our own good health is to live our lives in a healthful way that integrates body and mind. This means knowing every part of yourself, understanding your individual health concerns, and addressing them with good basic self-care.

The *Strong Women's Guide to Total Health* is designed to help you return to this commonsense approach, to take charge of your own health and minimize your risk of disease by making knowledgeable personal health choices.

For more than 2 decades I've been working in the field of women's health as a research scientist and an advocate. I've consulted dozens of colleagues—experts in women's reproduction, weight management, mental health, and many other disciplines—about the key health issues affecting women and what we should do about them. I've served on national health policy committees such as the 2008 Physical Activity Guidelines for Americans and the 2010 Dietary Guidelines for Americans. I've talked with thousands of women in communities across the country about the health issues that most concern them.

This book is the fruit of those discussions. It distills the relentless and often contradictory chatter of popular health claims about everything from diet and exercise to vitamin and hormone regimens, offering a set of basic, reliable guidelines for staying well in body, mind, and spirit. It focuses on the health concerns that matter most to women—from weight gain to infertility, from mental health to sexuality—and provides tools and strategies to tackle them.

I wrote this book with my close friend and colleague Jennifer Ackerman. Jenny has been writing about human biology and health for more than 25 years, first as a staff writer at the National Geographic Society and more recently as an independent author with a special interest in the workings of the human body. We met 12 years ago when we were both fellows at the Bunting Institute at Harvard University and discovered our shared interest in and excitement about women's health. We wanted to write a book together that was factual, practical, and accessible, a book that we ourselves would find useful in sorting out the cacophony of health advice.

This book is not a treatment manual for specific diseases (though it does offer helpful references on treatment and other topics in the Resources section). Rather, it emphasizes health promotion and disease prevention—how you can avoid common medical conditions that affect women—and tells you how to make good decisions about the many important health choices you'll make over your lifetime.

The book begins with a special self-assessment tool for gauging your health status and priorities, which will help you determine where you should direct your energy for self-care.

The rest of the book is organized into nine parts. The first eight parts move through your body, exploring key health issues, including fertility and sexual satisfaction, skin care, eye care, weight control, bone and muscle health, immune system support, and mental health maintenance. Each part offers a set of **S.M.A.R.T.** health strategies. These are **S**pecific, **M**easurable, **A**ctionable, **R**elevant, and **T**imely ways of maintaining health in these areas—a sort of "bottom line" on what you should be doing. Part IX, "Flipping the Switch: An Action Plan for Health," offers detailed, comprehensive programs to enhance your health and help you address your individual concerns, including physical activity plans, techniques for managing stress, and ways to create a healthier food environment.

We offer this book as an indispensable tool to help you take charge of your own good health and happiness.

Here's to Strong Women!

Introduction

What Makes Us Women?

What makes us women? And perhaps more important, what makes us strong women?

Biology, of course, is central—the presence of your potent X chromosome, along with the alchemy of estrogen and other hormones that make your body female. In my view, the female body in all of its various shapes and sizes is nothing short of miraculous: beautiful, efficient, complex, wondrous.

But there's more to your womanhood than your biology. Much of your makeup—your personality, temperament, health, appearance, behavior—is not spelled out in your genes. You are molded by your social and cultural surroundings, where you live, who your friends are, and how you define yourself within your world—from stay-at-home mom to high-powered CEO of a Fortune 500 company (or US secretary of state!); from one who has never worn lipstick to one who won't leave the house without it.

In short, being a woman is biological, cultural, environmental, tribal.

Being a strong woman, in my view, means being assertive, advocating for your own needs, surrounding yourself with positive influences, and being willing to take risks with things outside your comfort zone. Above all, it means taking care of yourself. Whatever your role in society, whatever your style—lipstick or makeup free—strength arises from a sense of well-being in both body and mind. Knowing how to take care of yourself in the best way possible is what this book is all about.

WOMEN ARE DIFFERENT

In the past few decades, society has striven to level the playing field for women and men in the world of work, home, and sports. But it's crucial to acknowledge that women are different in one arena: health.

Until recently, most doctors and medical researchers assumed that (reproductive organs aside) male and female bodies were pretty much alike. In blood and bone, heart and liver, women were thought to be like men, only smaller. The male body was accepted as the prototype for both sexes. Many of the studies conducted up until the mid-1980s were conducted only on men, and the results were assumed to apply to women. Fortunately, the tide has turned. Today more than half of participants in health studies are women. Moreover, researchers are scrutinizing illnesses that affect mostly women, such as multiple sclerosis and rheumatoid arthritis. Clinical trials for new drugs, vaccines, and medical devices nearly always include female subjects.

It turns out that in matters of health, gender really matters. It matters from head to toe, from mind to midriff. It matters throughout our life span. Our gender affects everything from the makeup of our bones and the architecture of our joints, to our skin's response to sunlight and aging, to how we experience pain, react to drugs, and cope with stress.

Consider your heart. It's only about two-thirds the size of a man's, with smaller coronary arteries that supply it with blood and oxygen. And it beats differently, with a higher rate even during sleep. Many women think of cardiovascular disease as a "man's condition." But although men may have more heart attacks, more women die as a result of them. Every year, half a million women die from heart disease—50,000 more women than men. More women than men have a second heart attack within a year of the first one. And although both sexes share the same risk for stroke, women more often die from the event. Later in this book, you'll learn in detail about the unique nature of your heart and the important differences in your cardiovascular system.

When it comes to immunity, being female has some advantages. We're lucky in having enhanced immune responses compared with men, which increases our resistance to many types of infection. We tend to make more antibodies, perhaps due to the effects of estrogen. But there's a dark side to this boosted immunity. It means that our immune defenses more often turn against us, attacking our own organs and tissues. As you'll read in Part VI, "In Our Defense," women are almost three times as likely as men to develop autoimmune diseases, most often during childbearing age. Of the 1.5 million people with systemic lupus erythematosus—a chronic autoimmune disease that inflames the blood, skin, joints, kidneys, and other organs and body systems—90 percent are women.

We women are different in every system of the body, and the brain is no exception. Brains can be a prickly topic, of course. If you want to create a ruckus, just broach the subject of gender differences in mental skills. But the differences are there.

On tests of intelligence and problem solving, women perform as well as men, though they often use different areas of the brain and distinct mental strategies to execute the same tasks. It's not news that men and women think differently. What's new is our understanding of the underlying anatomical and biological sex differences in the brain and their effect on everything from how we process driving directions, to how we experience pain and stress, to the kinds of mental deterioration we may experience with aging. Researchers have learned lately that women tend to have more persistent and severe pain, though we manage it better and have more coping strategies than men do. We make more stress hormones and have a harder time turning them off. Estrogen "prolongs the secretion of the stress hormone, cortisol," explains my colleague Marianne J. Legato, MD, in her book on gender-specific medicine, *Eve's Rib*. "So a woman feels more stressed in the moment than a man in the same situation." Moreover, because estrogen activates more extensive networks of neurons in the female brain, we often have more detailed memories of stressful events. We also react to stress in different ways.

As you'll learn in Chapter 23, "Mental Health," women also show different patterns of mental illness and disease. Whereas men are more likely to have schizophrenia and alcohol or drug addiction, women have more depression, anxiety, and eating disorders. In brain aging, our gender is better off in one sense: Our stores of estrogen make us less susceptible than men to age-related loss of tissue and increase in fluid in the brain, which can cause a decline in mental abilities such as memory or the learning of new concepts. On the other hand, because we live longer, we're more vulnerable to degenerative brain disorders such as dementia, which hit the brain later in life.

Our gender also bestows both gifts and betrayals where medications are concerned. Painkillers such as ibuprofen don't work as well in women. Even as common a medication as aspirin provides different benefits. It offers men some protection against heart attack but not stroke; in women, it has precisely the opposite effect. Some medications are downright dangerous for us because of our gender. In the late 1990s, eight out of the ten medicines removed from market shelves were pulled because they presented real dangers to women. Many of these drugs were common antibiotics and antihistamines, such as Seldane. The primary focus of this book is prevention, so apart from offering some general advice on medications, we don't explore them in depth. To ensure safety, discuss any drugs you take with your health care provider and pharmacist. If you find that something you've taken is causing unexpected effects, contact your health care provider immediately.

WHAT MAKES US DIFFERENT?

So what biological wizardry makes our bodies and our brains so different, so female?

It begins, of course, with the X chromosome, which is truly gargantuan by comparison with the much punier Y. It carries a rich store of 1,098 genes to the Y's 78. Possessing a double dose of the X chromosome protects us from many diseases. When one of the genes in a pair is defective, having two copies comes in handy. Men, having only one X, possess no such backup and so more often have color blindness, hemophilia, and muscular dystrophy. Our extra X genes also mean that women may have as many as 130 more active genes per cell than men do, which may help explain some of our differences.

Our marvelous XX chromosome package finds its way into every cell in our body. It has always seemed incredible to me, but it's true: The 3 billion bits of information in your DNA, neatly packaged in 23 pairs of chromosomes, are present in all body cells. Among those 23 are your sex chromosomes, which determine the direction of your sexual development, from single fertilized cell to sentient human being.

Genes may set up our sex, but that's only the beginning. Our gonads release sex hormones that bathe the fetus early in gestation, creating sex-specific changes in every cell, tissue, and organ in the body, including the brain. These sex hormones "wire" the brain, organizing its systems of neurons that mediate behavior later in life—and they continue to do so after birth, influencing the mature neural systems in our adult brains.

Through this mix of genetics and hormone production, the brain is "hardwired" to be male or female from the moment it begins developing in the womb, until we die. As

Legato writes in *Eve's Rib,* "It isn't an exaggeration to say that the brain is as sexual an organ (if not truly more so) than the ovaries or testes."

This doesn't mean that our brains are "set." Our genes and sex hormones may direct the wiring of our brains and continue to shape our biology throughout life. But environmental factors and the way we live our lives matter equally in shaping the brain. Virtually every thought we have, every action we take, can shape, modify, and strengthen neurons and their connections. The real wonder of the brain is this remarkable plasticity; the brain is never a "finished" work but creates and re-creates itself from cradle to grave.

Clearly, though, hormones are powerful players, with effects that reach far beyond our reproductive systems and continue throughout life, surging and waning at various stages from puberty through our reproductive years and into menopause and beyond. One way they exert their potent effects is by regulating genes, turning them on and off in different cells and tissues. This may help explain a striking new scientific discovery: Thousands of genes that are the same in both sexes actually behave differently in the organs of men and women—another possible reason we may respond in our own way to the same drug or disease.

In the past decade or so, we've learned that estrogen not only dictates when and how we menstruate, it also directs how our feet grow, how well we repair our tissues and organs, how we respond to stress (too much or too little estrogen can trigger depression in response to stressful events), and the way we think, learn, and remember. A high level of the hormone appears to stimulate nerve cells. It also boosts bloodflow to some regions of the brain and can enhance the brain's use of glucose, its main source of energy. Moreover, abundant estrogen can help create more elaborate connections between neurons, which may improve learning and memory. On the flip side, estrogen may bear partial responsibility for our greater vulnerability to lung cancer by boosting the effects of carcinogens such as tobacco smoke, radon, and cooking fumes.

BACK TO BASICS

We know that who we are as individuals is rooted in our genes. When I look in the mirror, I see my mother's eyes and nose. If I could look deeper, I might see my higher risk of macular degeneration and cataracts, a legacy from my grandmother. Genes are the body's blueprint, determining not just our gender, eye color, and hair texture but also the likelihood of developing specific diseases. Physicians may soon have at their fingertips new ways of individualizing treatment based on this new understanding of our genetic makeup.

I have very mixed feelings about putting too much emphasis on the promise of genetically tailored or "personalized" treatment, though. There's very little you can do about the genes you possess, except to know your own family history and be vigilant about getting appropriate screenings and regular checkups. And the truth is, the really serious health issues facing most women today have less to do with our genes and more to do with our environment, lifestyle, and behavior. Our surroundings (family, work, neighborhood, community, and society) and our experiences in life (what we eat, how much we sleep, where we live, how we exercise, what we think about) all play a huge role in determining how good we feel on a given day and how healthy we are over the course of our life span.

Take cardiovascular disease. Our behavior determines 65 percent of our risk for this disease. Cardiovascular disease is preventable if we know what to do and take action now. Or consider obesity. Genes may give us the propensity to get fat, but our lifestyle and behavior determine whether we actually put on weight.

Our country spends a huge amount of research money on specialized health studies that come back around to the same message. The most important things you can do to stay healthy are also the simplest. Here are the five key actions:

1. Create a healthy food environment. (See Chapter 26.)
2. Configure your week to build in physical activity. (See Chapter 27.)
3. Have the self-confidence to make needed changes in your lifestyle. (See Chapter 24.)
4. Make taking care of yourself a joyful routine.
5. Find a health care provider you trust (see Chapter 28) and be informed about your own health: That's what this book is about! You can start today by taking the Smart Woman's Health Assessment on the following pages.

The Smart Woman's Health Assessment

Knowledge is power. This is especially true when it comes to your own health; that's why we begin this book with a targeted self-assessment. Being familiar with your own body and the numbers and measurements that reveal your basic health status is both empowering and essential to good self-care. The health assessment you'll find here is not the standard assessment that you might get from a doctor. It focuses primarily on your behaviors in relation to nutrition, physical activity, and mental health. I'm a big believer in knowing your health numbers—but not just the typical ones that your health care provider will obtain during visits, such as your blood pressure, lipoprotein profile (including cholesterol levels and triglycerides), and fasting blood glucose. These are important, of course, and I include them in other chapters. However, this assessment is aimed at helping you know where you stand on more atypical measures of overall health. I urge you to take the time to complete this health evaluation before you read this book. It consists of eight assessments:

1. Body mass index
2. Waist circumference
3. Vitamin D level
4. Nutrition and food-related behaviors
5. Physical fitness and movement-related behaviors
6. Self-efficacy level
7. Joy quotient
8. Family history

Most of these assessments can be completed right now, with just a pen or pencil; some will take time to complete; one will require a visit to your health care provider. Try to finish all of them—within a couple of weeks, if possible. Knowing the results will help you better understand where your health concerns lie and where to best focus your efforts at prevention. Throughout this book, I will refer back to these assessments and discuss ways to help you address the risk areas you identify here.

To complete this health assessment you will need:

- A visit to your health care provider to obtain measurement of your serum vitamin D level. If you've had it measured already, call for the results. However, chances are good that your health care provider will not have assessed your vitamin D level. When you get this assessment, ask to have your blood pressure taken and your blood lipid and fasting blood glucose levels measured at the same time. You'll need these later in the book to fully assess your risk for heart disease and diabetes.
- A body weight scale
- A tape measure to determine your waist circumference and your height
- A nearby track or treadmill where you can do a walking test
- An exercise mat or towel
- A stopwatch or a watch with an easy-to-use second hand
- A yardstick
- A pen and a calculator
- Some time to talk with relatives

1. BODY MASS INDEX

Body mass index (BMI) is a calculation of your weight in relation to your height. BMI is related to several important health conditions, including heart disease, type 2 diabetes, cancer (especially breast and colon), and osteoarthritis. To calculate your BMI, weigh yourself in the morning with minimal or no clothes to get as close as possible to your true body weight. You should also measure your height in the morning, when you are tallest (as a result of your spine elongating during sleep). Stand with your back against a flat surface and have someone place a ruler on top of your head, parallel with the floor. Mark your height on the wall and then measure with a tape measure. Once you have these measurements, use the chart at right to calculate your BMI.

Body weight = _____ pounds

Height = _____ feet _____ inches

BMI = _____

HEIGHT	WEIGHT (LB)																						
5'0"	92	97	102	107	112	118	123	128	133	138	143	148	153	158	163	168	174	179	184	189	194	199	204
5'1"	95	100	106	111	116	122	127	132	137	143	148	153	158	164	169	174	180	185	190	195	201	206	211
5'2"	98	104	109	115	120	126	131	136	142	147	153	158	164	169	175	180	186	191	196	202	207	213	218
5'3"	101	107	113	118	124	130	135	141	146	152	158	163	169	175	180	186	191	197	203	208	214	220	225
5'4"	104	110	116	122	128	134	140	145	151	157	163	169	174	180	186	192	197	204	209	215	221	227	232
5'5"	108	114	120	126	132	138	144	150	156	162	168	174	180	186	192	198	204	210	216	222	228	234	240
5'6"	111	118	124	130	136	142	148	155	161	167	173	179	186	192	198	204	210	216	223	229	235	241	247
5'7"	114	121	127	134	140	146	153	159	166	172	178	185	191	198	204	211	217	223	230	236	242	249	255
5'8"	118	125	131	138	144	151	158	164	171	177	184	190	197	203	210	216	223	230	236	243	249	256	262
5'9"	121	128	135	142	149	155	162	169	176	182	189	196	203	209	216	223	230	236	243	250	257	263	270
5'10"	125	132	139	146	153	160	167	174	181	188	195	202	209	216	222	229	236	243	250	257	264	271	278
5'11"	129	136	143	150	157	165	172	179	186	193	200	208	215	222	229	236	243	250	257	265	272	279	286
6'0"	132	140	147	154	162	169	177	184	191	199	206	213	221	228	235	242	250	258	265	272	279	287	294
6'1"	136	144	151	159	166	174	182	189	197	204	212	219	227	235	242	250	257	265	272	280	288	295	302
6'2"	140	148	155	163	171	179	186	194	202	210	218	225	233	241	249	256	264	272	280	287	295	303	311
BMI	18	19	20	21	22	23	24	25	26	27	28	29	30	31	32	33	34	35	36	37	38	39	40

BMI scores are organized into the following categories:

< 18.5	underweight
18.5 to 24.9	healthy weight
25 to 29.9	overweight
30 to 39.9	obese
> 40	extreme obesity

In general, the higher your BMI category, the greater your risk for chronic disease. This is especially true for obese and extremely obese individuals. The overweight category is less clear. Research demonstrates that if you are overweight but fit (see fitness assessments below), you do not have a greater than normal risk. The unfortunate reality, however, is that most overweight women are not fit, and so they are at greater risk for chronic disease. It's important to note that being below weight is also not healthy. Having a BMI below 18.5 puts you at risk for a number of chronic diseases, especially mental health disorders and cancer. (See Chapter 10 for more detail on body weight and energy balance.)

2. WAIST CIRCUMFERENCE

Abdominal obesity (a large waist) is a risk factor for heart disease and type 2 diabetes. For women, the risk of these two diseases goes up with a waist size that is greater than 35 inches. To measure your waist circumference, stand and place a tape measure next to your skin around your waist, just above your hip bones. Exhale completely and then take the measurement.

Waist circumference = _____ inches

Generally, if your waist circumference is greater than 35 inches, the only way to decrease it is to lose weight by eating a little less and exercising more.

3. VITAMIN D LEVEL

Vitamin D is an important nutrient obtained by the body primarily through exposure to direct sunlight and food sources such as milk and sardines with bones; low levels are linked to a number of serious health conditions, such as osteoporosis, cancer, cardiovascular disease, diabetes, and poor immune function. At least a third of adults in the United States have deficient or marginal vitamin D status. People who live in the northern part of the country (where your skin can't make vitamin D in the wintertime) have the lowest levels, on average; those who live in the south tend to have the highest levels. Your blood levels will be given to you in either ng/mL or nmol/mL.

Vitamin D blood (25-hydroxyvitamin D) level = _____ ng/mL
or nmol/mL

VITAMIN D STATUS	ng/mL	nmol/mL
Deficient	≤ 20	≤ 50
Marginal	21 to 29	52.5 to 72.5
Optimal	≥ 30	≥ 73

These are the newest criteria recommended by experts in the field. They are more stringent than those currently listed in US government guidelines. I expect that within the next several years, these new guidelines will be adopted by the government. If you have a vitamin D level lower than optimal, you should talk with your health care provider about vitamin D supplementation. (See the box Vitamin D and Calcium on pages 164–165.)

4. NUTRITION AND FOOD-RELATED BEHAVIORS

For this assessment, you will need to look at your nutritional intake and behaviors related to food. I encourage you to take the time to do this assessment. Although it provides only a snapshot of what and how you eat, it will give you a general idea of your pattern of eating.

STEP 1. ASSESSING YOUR FOOD INTAKE

On a piece of paper, list ALL food and drink you consumed yesterday (don't include measurements, such as ounces, weight, or number of glasses, etc.).

Now score what you've consumed by referring to the list below and placing a plus sign, a negative sign, or a zero next to each food or drink. Of course, there are thousands of different foods, and I can't possibly list them all here, but this overview provides scoring for the general categories into which most foods fall. Use your judgment in scoring foods that do not appear below.

Pluses

Put a + (plus sign) next to any fruit or vegetable without added sugar, low- or fat-free dairy without added sugar (yogurt and milk), fish (not fried), raw or dry-roasted nuts (unsalted), seeds, legumes, beans, non-meat vegetable proteins (e.g., eggs and soy), and 100 percent whole-grain foods, including whole-grain cereals.

Negatives

Next, place a − (minus sign) next to most processed foods, fried foods of any kind, chips, cookies, cakes, candies of all types (though I would love to put chocolate in the plus category, I really can't), sugar-sweetened beverages, highly sweetened energy and granola bars, ice cream and other frozen dairy desserts, sugar-sweetened yogurts, cuts of meat (beef, pork, lamb, and chicken) that are not lean, refined-grain foods (pancakes, waffles, muffins, etc.), salty, ready-made foods such as pizzas and frozen dinners, high-fat sauces, dips, gravies, dressings, and more than one alcoholic beverage.

Neutrals

Finally, place a 0 (zero) next to all other foods. Most likely these will consist of 100 percent fruit juices, lean meats (beef, pork, lamb, and chicken), most canned soups, pasta, white bread, white rice, low-salt crackers and pretzels, and potatoes and other foods that don't easily fit into other categories.

Tally the total number of +, −, and 0 signs.
Total + = _____ Total − = _____ Total 0 = _____

STEP 2. ASSESSING YOUR FOOD-RELATED BEHAVIORS

Do you regularly:

Eat while watching television?	Yes	No
Eat while driving?	Yes	No
Eat sugar-sweetened beverages?	Yes	No
Eat out?	Yes	No
Skip breakfast?	Yes	No
Eat at your desk?	Yes	No
Eat late at night?	Yes	No
Eat mindlessly?	Yes	No

For the food intake section, you should have twice as many healthy "plus" food choices as "negatives" and "zeros." If you don't, consider shifting your food pattern to include more positives (such as fruits, vegetables, whole grains, low- or nonfat dairy, and fish); even more important, try to include fewer negatives. (See Chapter 26.) It's fine to have "negatives" in your usual pattern of eating—in fact, it's important to enjoy these foods occasionally—but you don't want them to outnumber the positives. I love my ice cream and chocolate, but I try to make sure that these treats are just that—treats—and that the majority of my eating consists of wholesome food. For the food behavior section, it is healthiest to have as many "no's" as possible. These behaviors are linked to excessive calorie intake. If you've answered "yes" to several of these questions, use the suggestions in Chapter 24 to learn new strategies to change your behaviors.

5. PHYSICAL FITNESS AND MOVEMENT-RELATED BEHAVIORS

For this assessment, you will test your fitness and examine your behaviors related to physical activity. It will take some time to complete, but it's very important.

STEP 1. AEROBIC FITNESS, MUSCLE STRENGTH, AND FLEXIBILITY

This assessment will measure your fitness level compared with that of other Americans your age. The test was developed by the President's Council on Physical Fitness and Sports. For full instructions and to submit your results, go to Adultfitnesstest.org.

- **Aerobic fitness.** The first part of the test is the 1-mile walk. To do this test you should be healthy and capable of walking a mile. You will need to find a standard ¼-mile track (often located at schools or parks) where you can complete four laps. Or you can walk on a treadmill (with the incline at zero) for a distance of 1 mile. You will need a stopwatch to time your walk. You also need to be able to take your pulse (by holding the fingers of one hand against the wrist of the other, just at the base of your thumb) to measure your heart rate.
- It's best if you do this test with a partner, who can assist you in timing your results.

- Start the stopwatch at the beginning of the walk and stop it at the finish line. Just after you cross the finish line, have your partner count off 10 seconds while you measure your pulse rate.
- If you are a runner, you can run for this test, but time yourself for a 1.5-mile run and then capture your heart rate.
- **Muscular strength and endurance.** Women tend not to think about the importance of their own strength. But muscular strength and endurance are vital, not only for good health and the ability to complete basic household or work tasks, but also for enjoying recreational physical activities, such as tennis, rock climbing, and sailing. Although there are many ways to measure strength and endurance, two fitness tests—the half situp and the modified pushup—are offered at the adult fitness Web site Adultfitnesstest.org. You can find complete instructions for these assessments there.
- **Flexibility.** Maintaining flexibility as we age is critical for many daily activities and for minimizing our risk of injury. A good assessment for flexibility is a sit and reach test using a yardstick for measurement. You can find complete instructions on the adult fitness Web site.

Scoring. For all of the above tests (1-mile walk, half situp, modified pushup, and sit and reach), log in your results at Adultfitnesstest.org to obtain your score. If you rank in the 90th percentile in each of the categories, you're maintaining an excellent level of fitness. If you fall below this, there is room for improvement. Ideally, you want to be in the 75th percentile or above. If you fall below the 50th percentile, you need to work on your fitness.

I can't emphasize enough how important it is to know your level of physical fitness. In recent research at Tufts, we have found that women across the country are seriously out of shape. One study published in 2009 demonstrated that midlife women living in the Midwest had such poor cardiovascular fitness that they would actually qualify for a heart transplant. This is why I have included this assessment—it may be the most important one of all.

STEP 2: ASSESSING YOUR MOVEMENT-RELATED BEHAVIORS

Do you regularly:

Limit television viewing to no more than 2 hours a day?	Yes	No
Limit sitting to less than 2 hours at a time without getting up?	Yes	No

Walk regularly more than a mile at a time?	Yes	No
Break a sweat from physical activity at least once a week?	Yes	No
Perform any physical activity for *at least* 30 minutes at a time three or more days per week?	Yes	No
Strength train or lift weights two or more days per week?	Yes	No
Choose to be active when you have some extra time?	Yes	No
Do occasional errands or commute by walking or biking?	Yes	No
Take the stairs instead of the elevator?	Yes	No

The behaviors above are related to healthy physical activity habits. The more you answered "yes," the better! Also, the more sedentary your work is, the more important it is for you to be active, answering "yes" to as many of the above questions as possible. These are smart behavior choices that can help lower your risk for serious health conditions and diseases, including heart disease. (See Chapter 27 for a full physical activity program.)

6. SELF-EFFICACY LEVEL

Self-efficacy—the belief in your own abilities, especially to bring about change—strongly influences every aspect of your health and well-being. It's especially important when you are trying to change behaviors to improve your health. Below are three sets of questions to help you understand your level of self-efficacy in general, and in the areas of nutrition and physical activity in particular.

Use the following scale to answer the questions:

1 = Not at all confident

2 = Slightly confident

3 = Moderately confident

4 = Very confident

5 = Extremely confident

GENERAL SELF-EFFICACY

1. I can always manage to solve difficult problems if I try hard enough.   1 2 3 4 5

2. I am certain I can accomplish my goals.   1 2 3 4 5

3. I am confident that I can deal effectively with unexpected situations.   1 2 3 4 5

4. If I am in trouble, I can think of a good solution.   1 2 3 4 5

5. I can handle whatever comes my way.   1 2 3 4 5

NUTRITION

In the following situations, how confident are you that you can eat plenty of healthy foods such as fruits, vegetables, and whole grains and avoid sugary, processed, salty, and otherwise unwholesome foods?

1. When I am tired   1 2 3 4 5

2. When I am in a bad mood   1 2 3 4 5

3. When I feel I don't have time   1 2 3 4 5

4. When I am traveling   1 2 3 4 5

5. When I am working a lot   1 2 3 4 5

6. When I am with family on vacations   1 2 3 4 5

7. During my normal everyday life   1 2 3 4 5

PHYSICAL ACTIVITY

In the following situations, how confident are you in your ability to be physically active?

1. When I am tired   1 2 3 4 5

2. When I am in a bad mood   1 2 3 4 5

3. When I feel I don't have time   1 2 3 4 5

4. When I am traveling   1 2 3 4 5

5. When I am working a lot   1 2 3 4 5

6. When it is raining or snowing   1 2 3 4 5

7. When I am with family on vacations   1 2 3 4 5

8. During my normal everyday life   1 2 3 4 5

Scoring. A score of 3 or higher in any of the situations described above indicates that you have good self-efficacy (in general or in the particular health behaviors—nutrition and physical activity). If you scored below 3, don't despair; the information presented in this book will help you boost your self-efficacy. (See Chapter 24, "Making Change.") Self-efficacy is very behavior-specific. You may have excellent self-efficacy in one kind of health behavior, but not in another. If you're working to change a specific health behavior such as quitting smoking, you can amend the above questions to better suit that behavior.

7. JOY QUOTIENT

Our mental health is as important, if not more important, than our physical health. Ideally, we want to be sound in both body *and* mind. Chapter 23 of this book discusses at length the elements of good mental and emotional health, including joy or contentment. The following questions are designed to help you understand this aspect of your mental health: How joyful are you?

Read the following 10 statements and score them on the scale.

1. I am usually in a very good mood.

Not at all		Mostly No		Somewhat		Mostly Yes		Always	
1	2	3	4	5	6	7	8	9	10

2. Each day I find time for something I enjoy.

Not at all		Mostly No		Somewhat		Mostly Yes		Always	
1	2	3	4	5	6	7	8	9	10

3. I feel successful in my life.

Not at all		Mostly No		Somewhat		Mostly Yes		Always	
1	2	3	4	5	6	7	8	9	10

4. I feel very connected to people.

Not at all		Mostly No		Somewhat		Mostly Yes		Always	
1	2	3	4	5	6	7	8	9	10

5. Each day when I go to bed, I feel fulfilled.

Not at all		Mostly No		Somewhat		Mostly Yes		Always	
1	2	3	4	5	6	7	8	9	10

6. When I wake up in the morning, I look forward to the day.

Not at all		Mostly No		Somewhat		Mostly Yes		Always	
1	2	3	4	5	6	7	8	9	10

7. When I think about the future, I am optimistic.

Not at all		Mostly No		Somewhat		Mostly Yes		Always	
1	2	3	4	5	6	7	8	9	10

8. My life is filled with meaning and purpose.

Not at all		Mostly No		Somewhat		Mostly Yes		Always	
1	2	3	4	5	6	7	8	9	10

9. I am very engaged in what I do.

Not at all		Mostly No		Somewhat		Mostly Yes		Always	
1	2	3	4	5	6	7	8	9	10

10. Others enjoy spending time with me.

Not at all		Mostly No		Somewhat		Mostly Yes		Always	
1	2	3	4	5	6	7	8	9	10

If you averaged 7 or above on these statements, your life is most likely very joyful. If you averaged 5 or below, I urge you to find ways to bring more joy into your life. (See Chapter 23, "Mental Health.")

8. FAMILY HISTORY

Learn as much as you can about your family's medical history. Knowing the illnesses experienced by your parents, grandparents, and other blood relatives can help you take action to keep yourself and your family healthy. If you know that close relatives have had cancer or heart disease, for example, then it's important to be vigilant about getting regular screenings for these diseases and to pay close attention to warning signs.

Not long ago, my close friend Zoe told me a revealing story about her family history. Zoe's dad, a university professor, died at age 42 while he was running. Both his father and his grandfather had died at an early age from heart disease. But because both of these relatives had smoked and not taken very good care of themselves, Zoe's dad had believed that they died early because of poor lifestyle habits. He had taken very good care of himself, so he assumed he would be safe. But it turns out that a rare genetic disorder runs in his family, causing very high blood cholesterol levels in family members. If he had known this at an early age, he could have taken medications that may have prevented his premature death.

This is an unusual case, but it does illustrate how important it is to know the details of your family history. You should be aware of any family members who may have been diagnosed with a disease or passed away at an early age. This information will help you and your health care provider decide whether you need genetic testing or counseling or whether you should take precautionary measures, such as getting more frequent health screenings, making lifestyle changes that will help ward off the full development of the condition, or taking medications to help you lead as healthy and long a life as possible.

(If you were adopted or your parents died before you could obtain this information, you most likely won't have access to it. In that case, you should do what you can with regular assessments.)

To begin chronicling your family's medical history, record on a separate sheet of paper the following questions about each of your family members, including your parents, grandparents, and siblings. Fill in the answers and give the information to your health care provider during your next physical or checkup.

Family member _____

Current age or age at death ____

Alive: ☐ Yes ☐ No

If deceased, cause of death _____

If alive, list chronic conditions and age at onset, if any _____

_____

Any substance abuse? _____

If you have completed this health assessment, congratulations! You have accomplished an important step toward taking charge of your own health. You have a much better understanding of the nature of your individual health needs and concerns. Review the results now, and on a separate sheet of paper, jot down a few notes about your specific areas of concern that you'd like to keep in mind as you read this book.

productive Choices Fertility and Preg
nopause Sexual Abuse and Sexual A
n Teeth Hair and Nails Body Weigl
etabolism Blood Sugar Eating and Exc
scles Bones JointsHeart and Blood L
d Respiration Common Infectious Dis
toimmune Disease Cancer Vision He
ell, Taste, and Touch Mental Health
nce Abuse Making Change Managing
d Sleeping Well Shifting Your Food Env
nt Getting Active Screenings and H
intenance Reproduction Sexuality and
l Health Reproductive Choices Fertilit
egnancy Menopause Sexual Abuse and
l Assault Skin Teeth Hair and Nails
eight and Metabolism Blood Sugar E
d Excreting Muscles Bones Joints Hear
od Lungs and Respiration Common I
us Diseases Autoimmune Disease Ca

PART I

Sex for Life:
Reproductive and Sexual Well-Being

My interest in women's health grew out of my fascination during graduate school with how beautifully orchestrated our bodies are. I'm very glad I'm a woman—I think we're truly amazing creatures. But our reproductive systems and our sexuality are complicated, and it takes some effort to understand how things work. How can I best care for my reproductive organs? How can I prevent disease? How can I fully enjoy being female? Part I is designed to help you understand your female self, how your reproductive system changes as you age, and how to keep it as healthy as possible throughout your lifetime.

As women, we're much luckier today than we were even just a couple of decades ago. In nearly every aspect of reproductive health, from birth control to health care providers, we have more choices than ever before. There is much more open dialogue about reproduction and about the real risks of unsafe sex. We have more reliable guidance on maintaining a healthy pregnancy. And we've come a long way in understanding what many women consider the big hurdle or "change of life" in reproductive health: menopause. Although there are definite drawbacks to menopause, such as unpleasant physical symptoms and loss of estrogen (the hormone that keeps our bones strong), I speak from experience in saying that there are some advantages. There are also excellent new options available to help mini-mize menopause-related symptoms and reduce the risk of health problems as we age and our hormones change.

Whatever your stage in life, I urge you to take your reproductive health seriously. Know your choices. And perhaps most important, find an excellent reproductive health expert to guide you.

Part I also explores the nature of a healthy sex life and describes how it can be a potent and positive force to enhance your relationships and your sense of yourself. Views of what makes for satisfying and pleasurable sexual activity differ from woman to woman and often change as you go through the stages of life. It's a good idea to become an authority on your own body in this realm as in others, to learn what excites you and gives you the most pleasure.

These **S.M.A.R.T.** behaviors will help you keep your sexual health and reproduc-tive system in top shape:

1. Be comfortable with your sexual and gender identity.
2. Find a health care provider you're comfortable talking with about your sexual and reproductive health.
3. Be aware of your full range of choices for birth control, fertility issues, menopause symptoms, and other aspects of reproductive health.
4. Avoid extremes of body weight and exercise.
5. Know your partner's sexual history.
6. Always use condoms to ensure safer sex.
7. Strive for good communication and frank discussion with your sexual partner.
8. Enjoy your sexuality.
9. Understand what is normal for your body so that you know when to seek medical care.

1

Reproduction

The female reproductive system is an intricate and complex set of organs that carry out an amazing variety of tasks, from producing sex hormones to nurturing the miracle of new life. They include internal organs—ovaries, fallopian tubes, uterus, vagina, and accessory glands—and also the vulva, which covers the opening to the vagina. A woman's main reproductive organs are two ovaries—each about the size and shape of an almond—located on either side of the uterus. Ovaries produce eggs (ova) and sex hormones. Over the course of a lifetime, they produce, store, and release about 450 eggs in a process known as ovulation.

Two slender 4-inch fallopian tubes, or oviducts, connect the ovaries with the uterus. The end of each tube near the ovary is funnel shaped and fringed with fingerlike extensions called fimbriae that draw the egg into the tube. When an egg is released from your ovary, the fimbriae catch it and help push it along the fallopian tube in its 7-day journey to the uterus. Because the egg is only fertile for about a day, fertilization occurs in the fallopian tubes before the egg moves to the uterus.

Your uterus, or womb, provides the fertilized egg with a nurturing, hospitable environment in which to grow. The uterus is a powerful, muscular organ, normally about the size and shape of an upside-down pear. Its 1-inch-thick muscular walls can expand to accommodate a full-term fetus and help push the baby out during labor. The lining of the uterus, known as the endometrium, is where a fertilized egg arriving from the fallopian tube embeds and develops. If the egg is not fertilized, it dries up and, roughly 2 weeks later, exits the body along with menstrual flow consisting of sloughed tissue from the endometrium.

Your uterus opens to your vagina at the cervix, a strong, thick-walled opening normally no wider than a straw but capable of expanding to allow the passage of a baby. Within the cervix are glands that secrete mucus. This mucus varies in consistency from tacky and sticky to thin and clear and either assists or impedes sperm, depending on the time of your cycle.

From the cervix, the vagina runs about 4 inches to the vaginal opening. A hollow, accordion-like muscular tube lined with mucous membranes that keep it moist, the vagina is where the erect penis is inserted during sexual intercourse. It also serves as the birth canal and as a passageway for menstrual flow from the uterus. The vagina expands during sexual arousal and, especially, during childbirth. The lower third of the vagina is laced with many nerve endings and includes the Gräfenberg spot, or G-spot, a sensitive spot roughly the size of a dime, 2 to 3 inches up just past the pubic bone; for some women, it is an area of erotic sensitivity. During sexual arousal, small glands on either side of the vagina known as Bartholin's glands may also swell and lubricate the passage. The opening to the vagina is known as the introitus; at birth it may be partially covered with a membrane of tissue called the hymen. It was once thought that a torn hymen was evidence of sexual intercourse, but that's simply not true. A hymen can be easily stretched, abraded, or torn by physical activity, use of tampons, masturbation, and other activities.

Your external genitalia, also known as your vulva or pudendum, include the mons pubis, the fleshy area just above your vaginal opening; the labia majora and labia minora, the two skin flaps surrounding the vaginal opening, which help keep bacteria out of the vestibule of the vagina; and the clitoris, a highly sensitive structure rich in blood supply and nerves, which swells during sexual arousal. Your clitoris is the only part of your body that is designed solely for pleasure.

While your breasts are not strictly necessary for procreation, they are part of your reproductive system and are sensitive to female hormones. Each breast has a raised nipple surrounded by a circular pigmented area called the areola, which contains muscles that make your nipple stand erect in response to touch and, sometimes, to cold. Your nipples contain openings for milk ducts within the breast. Inside, your breasts have lobes of glandular tissue (known as mammary glands) that include the sacs and tubes that make milk. The lobes are separated by protective fat and supported by connective tissue. The shape of your breast is determined by the amount and distribution of fat. The function of your mammary glands is regulated by estrogen and progesterone from your ovaries and, from your brain, prolactin and oxytocin—two hormones involved in breast development and milk production, among other things.

Female Reproductive System

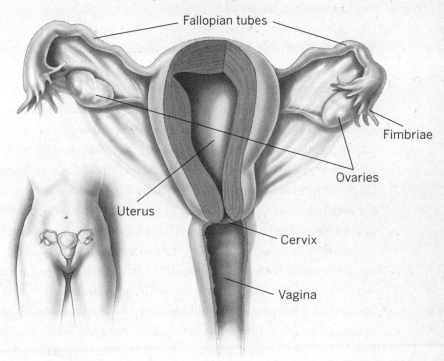

The main organs of the female reproductive system include two ovaries, a pair of fallopian tubes (capped by fimbriae), and the uterus. An ovary releases the egg, which is swept by the fimbriae into the opening of the fallopian tubes, and from there, travels into the uterus.

Although we tend not to think of it this way, the brain is a powerful sexual organ, integral to both reproductive and sexual life. The pituitary gland, for instance, a structure about the size of a pea located just beneath the hypothalamus at the base of the brain, sends signals to the ovaries to prepare your eggs for ovulation. Both the hypothalamus and the pituitary gland play an important role in regulating female hormones.

YOUR REPRODUCTIVE CYCLES

A finely tuned array of interacting sex hormones orchestrates your reproductive cycles. At puberty, the pituitary gland in the brain begins to secrete two key hormones: follicle-stimulating hormone (FSH) and luteinizing hormone (LH). These hormones stimulate your ovaries to make other hormones, including estrogen. Toward the end of puberty, your ovaries begin to release eggs—one per month—as part of your monthly menstrual cycle. The cycle has four phases:

1. **Follicular.** This phase begins just after menstruation ends and lasts for 6 to 13 days. The pituitary releases FSH and LH, stimulating the growth of a group of egg follicles, only one of which will eventually make a mature egg. Estrogen promotes the thickening of the endometrium in preparation for a fertilized egg.
2. **Ovulatory.** On around day 14 of your cycle, a mature egg is released into the fallopian tube—the process called ovulation. At this time of the cycle, your cervical mucus may become clear, copious, and stretchy, a state hospitable to sperm. The cervix opens a little.
3. **Luteal.** In this stage, progesterone and estrogen further stimulate the development of the endometrium. If there's no fertilization, however, the hormone levels drop. At this phase, the endometrium may produce prostaglandins—hormonelike substances that can trigger the cramps, breast tenderness, and mood swings of premenstrual syndrome.
4. **Menstrual.** The endometrial buildup, about 2 to 6 tablespoonfuls of blood and tissue, is expelled out of the uterus by uterine contractions. Normal menstrual flow can be light or heavy, regular or irregular, and can last from 3 to 7 days. After this, the endometrium rebuilds itself, and the cycle begins anew.

A girl's first period, called menarche, may occur anytime between the ages of 9 and 16. Although there are few statistics, it's widely believed that the age of menarche decreased by 2 to 3 years between 1900 and 1970, most likely due to better nutrition and health care. Today, some 10 percent of American girls reach menarche by age 11 and 90 percent by age 13.75. The average age of menarche in healthy American girls is 12.5, but it's perfectly normal to start menstruating at either end of the age spectrum. I didn't get my period until I was 16. At the time, I thought I was abnormal because all of my friends had already begun menstruating. But now I realize I was just at the older end of the age range. Once menarche takes place, most young women will have reached a height within an inch or two of their adult height. Some girls develop body image issues at menarche and during puberty. (This mental health issue is discussed in Chapter 23.)

After menarche, it can take up to 2 years or even more for a young woman to establish regular menstrual cycles. The typical menstrual cycle ranges from 20 to 40 days, with an average of about 28 days. However, there is great variation here, too. Some women experience irregular cycles for much of their premenopausal lives. I had very irregular periods until I got pregnant at the age of 27. Sometimes men-

Women's Menstrual Cycle

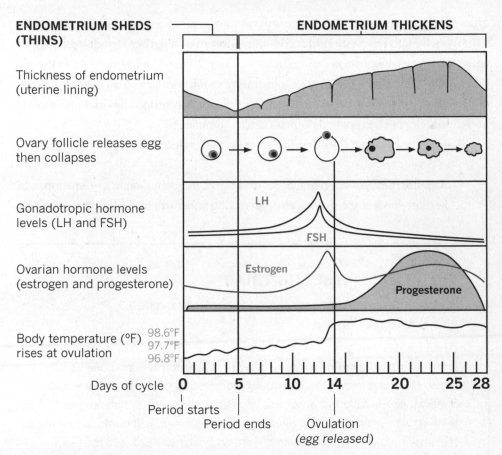

ENDOMETRIUM SHEDS (THINS)

ENDOMETRIUM THICKENS

Thickness of endometrium (uterine lining)

Ovary follicle releases egg then collapses

Gonadotropic hormone levels (LH and FSH)

LH

FSH

Ovarian hormone levels (estrogen and progesterone)

Estrogen

Progesterone

Body temperature (°F) rises at ovulation

98.6°F
97.7°F
96.8°F

Days of cycle 0 5 10 14 20 25 28

Period starts

Period ends

Ovulation
(egg released)

A woman's menstrual cycle includes a range of interacting events that prepare her body for pregnancy each month. The endometrium thickens; the ovary releases an egg in response to messages sent by the gonadrotropic hormones LH and FSH and the ovarian hormone estrogen. Rising progesterone levels stimulate the building up of the endometrium to provide a healthy environment for a fertilized egg to implant. If fertilization and implantation do not occur, progesterone levels drop, and the endometrium Is sloughed off during menstruation. Body temperature rises just after ovulation and stays higher by about 0.4°F for 5 to 10 days, until menstruation.

strual irregularities are due to hormone imbalances; consulting a physician can help clarify this.

A woman's reproductive cycles continue from menarche to menopause, when hormone levels change and reproductive cycles halt—usually in the late forties or early fifties. Cycles often get shorter first and then are erratic. But the pattern varies: Each woman's body follows its own script.

DISORDERS OF THE MENSTRUAL CYCLE

Menstrual patterns normally change and vary over the course of a lifetime. Flow may shift from light to heavy; monthly cycles may shorten or lengthen. In adolescence and again during perimenopause, women may experience irregular bleeding. After the age of 35, cycles often shorten. However, some menstrual irregularities such as the absence of periods or infrequent, prolonged, or heavy periods may reflect underlying disorders and should be checked out by a women's health clinician.

Among the common disorders of the menstrual cycle are:

- **Amenorrhea.** Amenorrhea, or the absence of menstruation in a premenopausal woman who is not pregnant, can occur during puberty or later in life. It can be a seri-

THE FEMALE ATHLETIC TRIAD
The link between disordered eating, amenorrhea, and low bone density

When I was a new graduate student in nutrition at Tufts University in 1984, my first research study explored the link between amenorrhea and bone density. Two previous studies had shown that young women who were amenorrheic had lower bone density—probably because of low estrogen levels. To find out more about the link, we recruited a group of young athletic women, half of whom had regular menstrual cycles and half of whom were amenorrheic. Because the laboratory I worked in was part of a nutrition research center, we were interested in finding out whether there were any nutrition issues involved in the association.

The results were surprising. As in the earlier studies, we found that the women who were amenorrheic had lower bone density despite being similar to the other women in weight and activity levels. But our nutrition studies also uncovered something new: The amenorrheic women had disordered eating habits. These women reported eating considerably fewer calories than the women with normal menstrual cycles, despite being similar in weight. In addition, about two-thirds of them were not getting enough protein in their diets. They were also engaging in some atypical eating patterns, skipping meals or eating very tiny meals 20 or 30 times a day. It appeared that this disordered eating and/or calorie restriction, not body weight or abundant exercise, was causing their amenorrhea.

ous condition that may affect fertility and bone health. (See the box The Female Athletic Triad below.) Primary amenorrhea is not beginning menstruation by age 16. It may be caused by chromosomal abnormalities, problems with the hypothalamus or pituitary gland, structural abnormalities in the reproductive system, or anorexia. Secondary amenorrhea is missing several periods in a row once you have gone through menarche. Amenorrhea can be a normal result of breastfeeding or an intended effect of some kinds of birth control pills or the progesterone-containing IUD. (In these cases, it has none of the implications for fertility and bone health characterized by true secondary amenorrhea.) Or, it can be caused by stress, certain medications such as antidepressants and antipsychotics, polycystic ovary syndrome (PCOS), eating disorders such as anorexia or bulimia, low body weight, thyroid malfunction, premature menopause, and other disorders.

When we published the study in the *American Journal of Clinical Nutrition* in 1987, it made national headlines and spurred a flurry of follow-up studies. The concept was later labeled the Female Athletic Triad.

Since then, much has been learned about the triad. We now know that amenorrhea among athletes is not normal—and not healthy. It increases their risk of infertility and also of stress fractures when they're young and osteoporosis in their later years. In the past, many female athletes thought it was convenient to be amenorrheic. But we now know that amenorrhea results in lower levels of estrogen and other hormones, and this is not good for bones. We also know that the cessation of menstrual periods among many (though not all) athletic women is most often caused not by high volume of exercise but by calorie restriction or disordered eating. Women who engage in rigorous exercise will most likely maintain regular menstrual cycles as long as they hold a stable body weight and eat well.

If you or someone you care about has irregular or absent menstrual periods, seek out a health care provider who can help you determine the root cause of the problem. You may want to start by consulting an endocrinologist. If an eating disorder is present, seek psychological help. Eating disorders are a mental health issue and should be addressed by a mental health expert. If there are serious nutritional deficiencies, you may also need to consult a nutritionist.

You should consult your health care provider if:

○ You're age 16 or older and you've never had a menstrual period

○ You've begun menstruating but have missed three or more consecutive periods

• **Premenstrual syndrome (PMS).** Roughly three-quarters of menstruating women experience some kind of premenstrual symptoms, ranging from mood changes to bloating and breast tenderness, especially from their late twenties to early forties. For some women, these symptoms may be so severe that they interfere with daily life. This condition is called premenstrual syndrome. Among the symptoms are severe irritability, tension, anxiety, mood swings, or difficulty concentrating, as well as pronounced physical symptoms such as breast tenderness, abdominal bloating, fatigue, acne, food cravings, and increased appetite. Symptoms most often occur in the second half of the menstrual cycle and resolve within a few days of the onset of menses.

For relief or control of mild PMS symptoms, you can try making lifestyle changes:

○ Get aerobic exercise—at least 30 minutes three times a week.

○ Reduce stress through relaxation techniques such as yoga and/or deep breathing.

○ Get adequate sleep.

○ Take a nonsteroidal anti-inflammatory drug (NSAID) such as ibuprofen.

If making these lifestyle changes doesn't ease your symptoms and they continue to seriously affect your health and well-being, you may wish to consult with your health care provider about taking other medications, such as diuretics or antidepressants. Research suggests that new lines of oral contraceptives show promise in helping with both physical and emotional symptoms.

• **Dysmenorrhea.** Dysmenorrhea, or menstrual pain, affects roughly half of all premenopausal women. There is an increased risk among women who smoke, drink, are overweight, or began menstruating before the age of 11. Other risk factors include stress, excessive caffeine use, and a family history of menstrual pain.

Dysmenorrhea can occur without pelvic disease but can also be a symptom of underlying pelvic disorders, such as endometriosis, uterine fibroids, pelvic inflammatory disease, or ectopic pregnancy.

The more common form is marked by recurrent cramps and lower abdominal pain that may extend to your back and down the back of your legs, and sometimes by headache, nausea, vomiting, and diarrhea. It is thought to be caused by an excess of prostaglandins, which trigger uterine contractions. The pain most often starts within hours of menstrual flow and peaks in the first day or two. It is usually treated with nonsteroidal anti-inflammatory drugs.

The treatment of cramps caused by pelvic disorders may vary, depending on the type of underlying disease.

- **Menorrhagia.** Menorrhagia refers to excessive or prolonged menstrual bleeding. Relatively heavy menstrual bleeding is a common concern, especially for young women in the first year or two after menarche and for older women nearing menopause. Menorrhagia is defined as menstrual flow so heavy it soaks through one or more sanitary pads or tampons every hour for several hours in a row, or flow that lasts longer than 7 days. If you experience these symptoms, you should seek medical help. The cause of menorrhagia can be anatomic (polyps or fibroids, for instance) or hormonal, in which case oral contraceptives can sometimes be used to control bleeding.

- **Polycystic ovary syndrome (PCOS).** PCOS is relatively common, affecting about 1 in 10 women. It is a condition of excess androgens (male hormones—all women have some) and insensitivity to insulin. This causes lack of ovulation and sometimes excess hair growth, especially on the face (hirsutism), and small ovarian cysts. It is also associated with an increased risk for type 2 diabetes. Treatment usually focuses on symptoms. Lifestyle interventions such as exercise and weight loss can be effective, but medications are often used to regulate the cycle, reduce hirsutism, and induce ovulation in those who wish to get pregnant.

VAGINAL HEALTH

It's important to understand that a healthy vagina is a complex ecosystem, home to many different types of microbial species, including bacteria and fungi. Among these is lactobacillus, a species that produces hydrogen peroxide and helps keep the vagina slightly acidic. Infection results when there's a shift in the populations of these normal vaginal bacteria, and one type overwhelms the others.

Also normal and healthy is the mucus, or "discharge," from your vagina and cervix. Mucus may vary in color, consistency, and scent depending on the phase of your menstrual cycle, use of contraception, sexual activity, and medications. It's unwise to try to get rid of mucus with douching or other methods, because this can upset the bacterial population and acid balance vital to your health. However, if your mucus is greenish in hue, irritating, or odiferous, or if you experience spotting with blood between periods, you should see your health care provider because this could be a sign of an infection or other problem.

Here are some self-care steps to keep your vaginal environment healthy:

- Avoid public hot tubs and baths, which are breeding grounds for bacteria.
- Avoid douching, which may change the balance of normal vaginal bacteria in harmful ways and may force bacteria up the vagina into the upper reproductive organs.
- Avoid scented or harsh soaps, and scented tampons or sanitary pads, which may irritate the vulva.
- Rinse well after soaping your genital area during showering.
- Wear fast-drying and breathable underwear during the day; if you need to wear hose, wear brands that have a breathable crotch and aren't too tight. (See the box Über Undies—Cotton Out, High-Tech In on the next page.)
- Do not wear underwear while sleeping.
- Always wipe from front to back after urinating or defecating.

VAGINAL INFECTION

Vaginitis, or vaginal inflammation, is a condition of the vagina that can result in abnormal vaginal discharge, odor, itching, irritation, or pain. The cause is usually a change in the normal balance of vaginal bacteria or an infection. The three most common types are:

- **Bacterial vaginosis (BV).** A common vaginal condition in women of childbearing age, BV results from overgrowth of one group of bacteria normally present in the vagina. In the United States, it affects some 17 percent of pregnant women. Symptoms include a thin, grayish vaginal discharge and a fishlike vaginal odor, particularly during menstruation or after unprotected intercourse; vaginal itching or burning; and pain during intercourse and, occasionally, during urination. BV can be treated with antibiotics such as metronidazole or clindamycin, although it often recurs.

- **Candidiasis, or yeast infection.** Candidiasis is most often caused by a naturally occurring fungus called *Candida albicans*. Some 75 percent of women experience at least one yeast infection in their lifetime. Symptoms include itching (especially on the vulva), redness of the vulva, vaginal irritation, thick, clotted white discharge, burning on urination, and pain during intercourse. I really encourage women to see their doctor if they get a yeast infection. Treatment consists of vaginal antifungals, vaginal boric acid, or oral fluconazole. Uncontrolled diabetes, and the use of antibiotics or the contraceptive sponge, diaphragm, or spermicides, is associated with more frequent yeast infections. If you are taking a course of antibiotics for an illness, it's a good idea to consume yogurt with active lactobacillus cultures to reduce your risk of yeast infection.

ÜBER UNDIES—COTTON OUT, HIGH-TECH IN

For years, we have been told by our doctors and by the media to wear cotton underwear to avoid infection. Considered a "breathable" fabric, cotton was thought best for areas of the body where moisture might be an issue. I no longer subscribe to this cotton recommendation for skivvies. Although cotton is breathable, if it gets wet it's slow to dry. With the advent of new clothing technology, there are now numerous sports-type fabrics on the market that are more breathable and quicker drying than cotton, and also more antimicrobial (which may help decrease yeast infections). Gynecologists are now recommending that women use underwear made from these fabrics.

Most athletic brands, such as Patagonia, Under Armour, REI, Adidas, and Nike, have excellent high-tech underwear in many different styles. There is a catch to these über undies, however: They're expensive. You can get a pair of cotton underwear for less than $5, but you may have to pay upwards of $18 for a pair of high-tech panties. Because they're quick drying and very durable, though, you can get away with buying just a few pairs and keeping them for longer. I try to take advantage of seasonal sales to get these undies at a more affordable price.

- **Trichomoniasis.** This disease is caused by a parasite that is commonly transmitted by sexual intercourse. It may also be contracted from moist objects, such as towels, clothing, or toilet seats that have been in contact with the genitals of infected individuals. Some two million to three million women in the United States are infected with trichomoniasis each year. Symptoms include vaginal discharge that smells foul and is sometimes yellow-green and frothy; itching, burning, or redness of the vulva; and pain on urination. Treatment is usually oral metronidazole for both a woman and her sexual partner.

Other conditions of the vaginal area, such as skin conditions or allergic reactions, can be confused with vaginitis. Sometimes a biopsy of the area is required to diagnose these. If you have recurrent vaginal symptoms, be sure to visit your health care provider.

UTERINE HEALTH

I tend not to think much about my uterus now that I am past having babies. But like my skeletal muscles or heart or skin, it requires care and attention, including regular checkups, to remain healthy. If your periods become irregular or marked by excessive bleeding, or if you develop pelvic pain or another symptom that could signal a uterine disorder, you should see a health care provider. Among the more common conditions and diseases affecting the uterus are:

- **Uterine fibroids.** These are benign fibrous tumors inside the uterus that may range in size from "seedlings" barely less than an inch in diameter to some the size of a grapefruit. They are common, affecting as many as 7 in 10 women, but they rarely cause symptoms severe enough to require treatment. Symptoms most often appear in women in their late reproductive years (35 and beyond) and may include pelvic pain and cramping, heavy vaginal bleeding, frequent urination, constipation, hemorrhoids, pain during sexual intercourse, miscarriage, and infertility. In the past, uterine fibroids were a common reason for hysterectomy, but more and more choices are now available. If troublesome symptoms persist, medical treatment and surgical procedures can shrink or remove fibroids. In severe cases, partial or total hysterectomy is an option.
- **Endometriosis.** With endometriosis, the uterine lining, or endometrial tissue, implants and grows outside of the uterus, often affecting the ovaries, uterus, and

VAGINAL "REJUVENATION" AND COSMETIC VAGINAL PROCEDURES

When I was on a train last fall with two colleagues in women's health, one of them brought me up to speed on this disturbing new industry—procedures to surgically alter women's vaginas for cosmetic reasons. These procedures are marketed by some physicians as a way of enhancing appearance or sexual enjoyment. Among the types are so-called vaginal rejuvenation, revirgination, and G-spot amplification. Vaginal rejuvenation (also known as designer vaginoplasty) is promoted as a tightening and toning of a woman's vaginal muscles, especially after childbirth. Revirgination involves repairing the hymen in an attempt to reproduce a virginal state. G-spot amplification entails injecting collagen into the front inner wall of the vagina.

Although some types of genital surgeries are performed for valid medical reasons, such as pain or disfigurement, there is no proven benefit whatsoever for cosmetic vaginal procedures, and the surgery carries serious risks. The American College of Obstetricians and Gynecologists has issued a warning against these procedures, stating that they are neither safe nor effective. Their potential risks include scarring, chronic pain, infection, nerve damage, and difficulty having sexual intercourse.

"I've had patients coming into the office to ask for this, having seen it promoted in women's magazines," says Dr. Hope Ricciotti, an OB-GYN at Harvard Medical School. "It's viewed by some women as the new thing—you get a breast enhancement when you're young and vaginal rejuvenation when you're older. But there is no evidence that these procedures make any difference to sexual pleasure," she emphasizes, "and the risks far, *far* outweigh any possible benefits."

fallopian tubes. These implants follow the same hormonal cycles as normal uterine tissue, growing each month. But because the tissue can't leave the body through the uterus and vagina, it builds up, which can lead to inflammation and bumps, nodules, and scarring in the pelvis, involving nearby organs. Women typically develop the disease not long after they begin to menstruate. The cause is unknown, but the condition can run in families. Treatment includes pain medication, hormone therapy, and surgery ranging from laparoscopy to hysterectomy.

- **Adenomyosis.** In this condition, the endometrial lining of the uterus grows into its muscular outer walls. It typically occurs late in childbearing years and disappears after menopause. Its cause is unknown. It occurs more often in women who have given birth or who have had Cesarean sections, fibroid removal, or other uterine surgery. For many women, adenomyosis causes no symptoms; others may experience heavy or prolonged menstrual bleeding, sometimes with blood clots, severe dysmenorrhea, bleeding between periods, swelling or tenderness in the lower abdomen, and pain during intercourse. Treatments such as anti-inflammatory medications and hormone therapy can ease discomfort, but the only cure is hysterectomy.

2

Sexuality and Sexual Health

There are few things more complex than a woman's sexuality. Our sexual selves are fundamental to our sense of self and well-being, bound up with our reproductive capability; our emotions and self-esteem; our physical transformations as we mature and age; our experiences, attractions, expectations, and thoughts about our sexual relationships; our family of origin; our religion; and a host of other components. Given its importance, you would think we would have plenty of open dialogue about sexuality. But the sad truth is that few of us talk about our sexuality with anyone, even our partners. And most doctors are not well equipped to discuss the subject with their patients. When I think back, I realize that in my younger years, I never once had a conversation with my parents or any doctor about sexuality or sexual health. I got lucky and married a good man who was very willing to talk openly.

In this section, we emphasize the importance of frank discussion—whether it's with your doctor about your sexual health, with your partner regarding your relationship and mutual sexual needs, or with your children about the importance of reproductive health and safety. Sexual topics are notoriously difficult for people to talk about openly, but good reproductive and sexual health depend on it

GENDER IDENTITY AND SEXUAL ORIENTATION

Gender identity is our sense of ourselves as female, male, or something else, e.g., people who are transsexual (biologically one sex but feel themselves to be the other, and sometimes take hormones or have operations to change their sex), transgender (who challenge traditional boundaries of male and female), or intersex (who have a combination of chromosomes such as XXY rather than an XX or XY and may have genitals that are not completely male or female).

Sexual orientation is defined as our attraction—emotional, romantic, or sexual—to another person. Following are common terms used to describe different sexual orientations:

- **Straight or heterosexual.** Women or men sexually attracted to members of the opposite sex.
- **Lesbian.** Women who are attracted to women.
- **Gay or homosexual.** Women or men who are attracted to members of their own sex.
- **Bisexual.** People who are sexually attracted to both men and women.
- **Questioning.** People who are exploring their sexual orientation.
- **Asexual.** People who are not experiencing or acting on sexual attraction.

Scientists and medical professionals agree that people do not choose to be gay, straight, transsexual, or bisexual and cannot voluntarily change their sexual orientation. Rather, sexual orientation emerges for most people at an early age, before sexual experience, and is determined by a complex mix of biological, psychological, and environmental factors that differ from person to person.

All forms of sexual orientation are perfectly normal. Our society has come a long way in accepting this and in respecting differences. But we still have a long way to go toward full acceptance and guarantees of equality. For instance, there are still people in our society who are under the misconception that homosexuality is a mental illness or an emotional or social problem and that homosexual couples cannot effectively parent. Research clearly shows that this is not the case. Homosexuality is not an illness of any sort. Moreover, like heterosexual couples, lesbian, gay, transsexual, and bisexual couples can be excellent parents: Studies of groups of children raised by homosexual parents and by heterosexual parents suggest that there is no developmental difference in the two groups in terms of intelligence, psychological adjustment, social adjustment, and popularity with friends, and that the sexual orientation of a parent does not dictate the sexual orientation of a child. Homosexual men can raise physically and emotionally healthy girls; lesbians can raise healthy boys. As long as the family unit is stable and nurturing, children thrive.

The most important thing is to be comfortable with your own sexual identity and to help those you love—siblings, children, parents, friends—be comfortable with theirs.

SEX AND SEXUALITY

For most women, a healthy sex life is an important part of overall physical, emotional, and mental health. As Pepper Schwartz says, sexual desires and needs are part of a magnificent body that has evolved over thousands of years and shouldn't be dismissed or ignored.

"Sexual activity is something positive to share with other people, to nurture bonds, trust, and intimacy," says Pepper. A sociology professor at the University of Washington and a relationship expert, Pepper believes that we should view the capacity to experience sexual joy and ecstasy as a splendid gift we've been given to use and enjoy as we wish rather than as something shameful or irrelevant—which it is only too often in our society. Although this is a field with many authorities, I particularly admire the views of Pepper, who is a friend and colleague. "Our culture often makes us feel bad about what the body does naturally," she says, "whether it's menstruating, going to the bathroom, or enjoying sex. But we were designed to do these things; they're vital to our mental and physical well-being."

Not only is sexual activity an important part of maintaining a strong relationship with a partner, but it is also good for individual emotional and physical well-being. Sexual activity can improve cardiovascular health. It boosts heart rate and causes the release of a cascade of hormones, including adrenaline, noradrenaline, prolactin, DHEA, and testosterone—many of which work to protect the heart. With orgasm comes the release of oxytocin, a hormone that lowers blood pressure and calms and relaxes the body. Sex can also provide pain relief—from menstrual cramps, back pain, migraines, and arthritis—perhaps because sexual stimulation and orgasm may trigger the release of corticosteroids and endorphins, which raise our pain threshold. It can even boost mood and relieve stress, thanks in part to the effects of endorphins and oxytocin.

Pepper points out that our need and desire for sex doesn't end when our childbearing years are over, nor does it cease if a relationship or marriage ends. If a woman doesn't have a partner—if she's a widow or has left a bad marriage or has made a choice not to be in a relationship, "that doesn't mean that she should cease to have sexual joy," Pepper says. "The gift of enjoying her own body is still available to her through masturbation. This is the biggest taboo we've created, that masturbation is somehow a 'waste' of sexual time and energy. It simply isn't so."

A healthy sex life depends on being comfortable with your gender identity and your sexual orientation, whatever it may be. It helps to have good self-esteem and self-image, so it's important to take care of your body so that you feel strong and self-confident. Good lovemaking with a partner requires feeling relaxed, trusting, and attractive.

Pepper identifies two important additional ingredients of good sexual relations. The first is communication. "Women often have the mistaken idea that their partners should know exactly what to do and where to do it," she says. "But our partners are not mind readers. You have to be willing to say what you like, what you enjoy, and then communicate this to your partner. If you don't say anything, and your partner misses, you may think, 'Boy, he just doesn't get it!' This happens between lesbians as well. You need to be able to say, 'That felt good, now do a little more of this.' Or, 'That's not quite it, there, to the right a little. Ah, that's it.'" Some people feel embarrassed about talking this way. But you have to get over that, and say to yourself, "If I truly want an intimate relationship, I need to be able to tell my partner what I want." Sometimes this is hard, especially if you're having difficulty with intimacy in your relationship outside the bedroom. Then you have to work on your relationship out of bed to have good relations in bed.

You have to be free of anger, says Pepper. "You can't be ticked off about the fact that your partner didn't take out the garbage or got home late for dinner. That's noise in the system. Healthy sex depends on letting go of anger, on having openness and positive energy."

TYPES OF SEXUAL ACTIVITY

Sex doesn't necessarily equal intercourse. Healthy lovemaking includes intimacy of all kinds. I define good sex as any kind of sexual activity that you want and enjoy, that is fully consensual, mutual, and equal, and that does not cause you or anyone else physical or mental harm. It can encompass a whole range of experiences, including but not limited to:

- **Caressing and kissing**—often a part of foreplay
- **Masturbation**—stimulating yourself, which is a good, risk-free way of learning what you like and what you don't like
- **Mutual masturbation**—masturbating a partner as part of foreplay or for sexual satisfaction
- **Oral sex**—stimulating the clitoris and vulva or the penis with the mouth
- **Vaginal sex**—inserting the penis into the vagina in various positions and movements. This is what's most commonly considered sex, but for many women, it does not result in orgasm because it does not directly stimulate the clitoris.

In my view, the full range of fantasies and behaviors is healthy, as long as they don't lead to emotional or physical discomfort, conflict, or other problems. What each woman finds pleasurable is a very individual thing. And within a couple, it is also normal to experience differing preferences and desires for certain behaviors. It's important to find compromise and common ground, a pattern of behavior acceptable to both members. The key is to relax, take your time, and feel comfortable and confident. Experimenting or broadening your bedroom repertoire can be a good idea, especially if you're intent on keeping your sex life fresh and interesting. (See the box Sexual Aids on pages 24–25.)

How much sex is "normal"? One study found that 18- to 29-year-olds said they had sex an average of about twice a week; 30- to 39-year-olds, an average of 1.5 times a week; and 40- to 49-year-olds an average of just over once a week. About half of women 50 to 59 say that they have sex a few times or more each month. So what does this mean for you? Not much, really. What's considered a normal amount of sex varies tremendously depending on a wide range of variables—your health, your job and family situation, whether you have children at home (which can complicate intimacy), the status of your relationship, and your level of desire. The important thing is finding the pattern and frequency of sexual activity that's most satisfying and comforting for you at any phase of life.

Sometimes there's a disparity between your level of sexual desire and your partner's. Maybe your partner is not particularly interested, but you are—or vice versa. Balancing the needs and desires of a couple is an art form. If you're the one with a stronger libido, it's fine to say, "I have this need, can you help me out?" But the burden really is on the person with the lesser appetite to be gracious, helpful, and understanding, says Pepper. If you or your partner wants sex every day, that may be too much to ask, but you can negotiate. What's a fair compromise? Maybe a couple of times a week. "The point is that it's not a zero-sum game, all on my terms or all on yours," Pepper explains. "And it's fine to have a 'quickie' or to provide sexual satisfaction for a partner by means other than sexual intercourse. This is not an insult," she emphasizes. "It's good to mix it up." The essential thing is to communicate openly and honestly with your partner to come to an understanding about how to fulfill your mutual needs.

Many women find that they're too tired in the evenings to fully enjoy sex. If that's the case for you, try having sex at another time of day, in the morning, or on weekends. Try putting the kids to bed early. Most of all, take care of yourself and get a good night's sleep so that you are able to fully enjoy sexual activity.

LIBIDO

As with most aspects of sex and sexuality, libido among women ranges from very low to very high, and for any individual woman at any particular moment, it's influenced by a host of physiological and psychological factors. Not everyone has the same sex drive. "It's like anything—running, cooking, socializing, etc.," says Pepper. "Energy levels and desires differ. If a strong sex drive has always been central to your character, it's likely to stay that way. If you would just as soon play a round of golf, your sex drive is going to be less resilient over the years."

Low libido is a common complaint during the postpartum period and just after menopause. However, it's not always physiological in nature. Among women young and old, the problem may arise in a marriage plagued by the "hum of anger," as Pepper describes it. A lot of women confuse a partnership problem with low libido. "If you're experiencing low libido," she explains, "you have to ask yourself whether it's a sex problem or a 'Dave' problem—that is, is it a relationship issue? If Brad Pitt or George Clooney (or for that matter, Kate Winslet or Penelope Cruz) walked in the door and said, 'Babe, you're the one,' would you be uninterested?"

However, if you love your partner and want to have sex but have no capacity for arousal, then you may be dealing with depression, a side effect of a medication, or a physiological issue, perhaps involving problems with nerve endings, bloodflow, or hormones, and should seek help from a health care provider.

ORGASM

Technically speaking, orgasm is the rhythmic, involuntary contractions of the uterus and vagina. It begins with an excitement phase that includes increased bloodflow in the erectile tissue of the clitoris and in the labia minora, ovaries, and breasts. Muscle tension increases, the vagina enlarges, and the uterus elevates. Breathing and heart rate quicken. The end result is an intense wave of pleasure, followed by resolution—feelings of peace and sexual satisfaction.

A majority of women don't orgasm during coitus. This is because the "in-out" motion of coitus doesn't offer the steady, circular pressure and stimulation many women require for orgasm. Direct clitoral stimulation and breast play are often the keys to intensifying a woman's arousal and orgasm. Research shows that heightening sexual tension by stopping and restarting stimulation before climax can also lead to a more intense orgasm. Many women enjoy continued gentle stimulation afterward.

"We don't know why some women are easily orgasmic during intercourse, while others need direct stimulation of the clitoris," says Pepper. "What we do know is that the mind has to be very focused, accepting, and concentrated. If the mind wanders and worries intervene, if the mind is 'spectatoring,' watching itself and you, then orgasm is very unlikely. The mind has to be tightly focused on pleasure." Sometimes women find it handy to concentrate on a fantasy as a kind of helping mechanism to focus the brain.

It's also important for the clitoris and vagina to stay highly lubricated. Artificial lubricants such as K-Y jelly, Wet, or Astroglide, or simple vegetable oil, can help with lubrication so that touching is pleasurable and doesn't result in irritation. This is especially important as we get older.

SEX AND EMOTIONAL ISSUES

Sexual desire and sexual satisfaction are rooted in the mind. To become sexually aroused, you need to feel self-confident, be free of anxiety, and be able to focus. So it's not surprising that your mental and emotional concerns have a profound impact on your sexual health. Untreated anxiety or depression, stress, relationship conflicts, anger, self-esteem issues, body-image concerns, a past history of sexual abuse, teachings in childhood, and other issues can contribute to sexual problems. If your mental or emotional well-being is interfering with your sex life, you may want to see a mental health professional or a sex or marriage therapist.

SEX AND AGING

Women are living longer than ever, and many expect to be sexually active throughout their lives. It was once thought that menopause inevitably diminished a woman's desire for sex. This is simply not true. A woman's interest in sex and sexual intimacy can continue during and after menopause and, often, well into old age. Moreover, studies suggest that a woman's capacity for orgasm and sexual fulfillment continues indefinitely. (I am banking on this.) Her sexual satisfaction often grows rather than diminishes in later years, in part because worries about unwanted pregnancy are no longer a concern and because she may have more time and fewer parenting responsibilities.

(continued on page 26)

SEXUAL AIDS

(or my trip to the sex toy boutique)

I never thought that someday I would be offering advice on sexual aids. But use of sex toys, as they're sometimes called, has become more commonplace, and many women enjoy using them not only to address issues such as difficulty reaching orgasm but also simply to spice up their sex life. For instance, recent national surveys suggest that 53 percent of all women report having used a vibrator, most often for shared pleasure. Sexual aids may also be useful for people who are physically impaired.

Generally the best selection is found at a specialty store. After interviewing Pepper Schwartz, I decided that I needed to take a trip to such a store. I have to admit that it took me close to 6 months to get my nerve up. I just couldn't imagine walking into a sex toy shop and asking for help. As it turned out, I discovered a shop on Newbury Street in Boston, right next to the salon where I get my hair cut. Newbury Street is one of the nicest upscale shopping streets in Boston. I figured that I would be as comfortable as I could be walking into that store. I scheduled my hair appointment and left work early to walk to the salon.

When I reached the store, I froze; my heart rate went up and my palms grew sweaty. But I finally mustered my courage and walked in. To my surprise, the place was bright, clean, and welcoming. Although there were some wild items on the shelves, nothing made me uncomfortable. I went up to the desk and introduced myself to Chad, a very courteous, clean-cut young man. I mentioned that I was doing some research on sex toys for a women's health book. He explained to me how the industry is working hard to change the public's perception of sex toys and the boutiques that sell them. He pointed out that his store was well lit and sold no pornographic books or magazines. There were no black lights or strange music. Chad showed me around the store and explained the various toys and how they work. I had no idea there was such a range of sexual toys for sale. I spent about a half hour with Chad and felt very comfortable and at ease. I even left with a purchase and am happier for it.

Sex toys range from vibrators and dildos (the two most popular items) to lubricants, restraints, and flavored body paints. "These toys can do their job very efficiently," says Pepper. "They're not a substitute for a partner, of course, but they can help produce stronger feelings in yourself and your partner. If the two of you are intimate and trusting enough to play with them, you can have a lot of fun and even produce ecstasy."

Vibrators were first patented in the 19th century to assist physicians in treating women said to be suffering from "hysteria." (Physicians actually treated women by bringing them to orgasm with the help of these tools. You have to wonder about some of these "doctors"!) These days, vibrators come in all shapes and sizes. Some women use them during masturbation. Others use them during foreplay with a partner or to achieve orgasm during intercourse.

Dildos, said to be used since classical times, are available in a range of sizes (from 4 inches to a staggering 16 inches) as well as various colors and materials, from skinlike to textured. Some couples find them helpful in dealing with issues of premature ejaculation and erectile dysfunction.

Sex toys can be found online, at pharmacies and convenience stores, through mail-order catalogues, and at sex boutiques such as the one I visited, as well as larger shops, some of which are like big department stores with three floors and walls packed with more models than you can imagine. I encourage you to take a trip to one of these stores—you'll be amazed at the variety of offerings. They are often staffed by young women and men like Chad who are professional and candid and can help you find what you're looking for.

"Go ahead and experiment," advises Pepper. "See what you can add to life. What are you afraid of? Too much pleasure?"

However, most women do experience changes with menopause that affect their sexual activity. Even before menopause, as early as the late thirties, many women notice a reduction in the secretion of fluids that act as natural lubricants during arousal. This is easily remedied with use of vaginal lubricants and moisturizers such as such as K-Y jelly, Astroglide, Albolene, or Silk-E. As a woman approaches menopause and the amount of estrogen in her body declines, the problem may be compounded by a thinning and loss of elasticity in the vaginal tissues. Some 20 to 45 percent of peri- and postmenopausal women report vaginal dryness. As the labia covering the genitals shrink and become thinner during menopause, they sometimes expose more of the clitoris, which can reduce its sensitivity or even produce an unpleasant sensation. These changes, known as postmenopausal vagina (PMV), may contribute to discomfort during intercourse, diminishing the pleasure of sex. If a woman halts sexual activity for a few months, and then resumes it, sex can be quite painful despite the use of lubrication. Fortunately, the condition is usually easily treated with low-dose local estrogen tablets, gels, and creams, and the Estring, a Silastic ring that is inserted into the vagina every 3 months, which all work to restore vaginal moisture and suppleness. In addition, regular (weekly) sexual intercourse can actually help prevent PMV by stretching the vagina and boosting its supply of blood and lubrication.

If you're experiencing discomfort or pain during intercourse, it's important not to try to "tolerate" it but to get treatment right away. Even just a few sessions of painful intercourse can disrupt the ability to feel arousal, because the anticipation of pain may block the neurological pathways involved in the sensation of arousal.

With the onset of menopause, some women report a loss of interest in sex. If you feel this loss of libido may be related to a relationship problem, it's important to address the underlying issue. The problem may also arise because of menopausal symptoms such as vaginal dryness, hot flashes, night sweats, and insomnia. Some loss of libido may be related to hormones, especially in women who have had their ovaries surgically removed. If you have problems with diminished libido that you feel are physiological in nature, you may want to talk with your health care provider.

As we age, talking with our partners is more important than ever. Be candid about how you're feeling physically and emotionally and be flexible about catering to your changing needs. You may want to explore such strategies as sensual massage, creative foreplay, and sexual variety (as well as toys) to help you sustain a healthy sex life. Don't forget to make dates with your partner, opportunities to relax and get reacquainted.

SEXUAL DYSFUNCTION

Many women have sexual difficulties at some point in their lives. The key here is to determine whether the problem is yours or your partner's (male erectile dysfunction, perhaps) or an issue between the two of you.

A common concern for women is low or absent libido. Or it may be pain during intercourse or waning sexual responsiveness or sensation—the reduced ability to become aroused, stay aroused, or achieve orgasm during sexual activity.

In medical circles, any sexual concern that persists or recurs and causes a woman personal distress or negatively affects her relationship with her partner is known as female sexual dysfunction (FSD). A 2005 study by researchers at Yale School of Medicine and the Albert Einstein College of Medicine found that FSD affects almost half of all women. The causes are varied and complex. Experts agree that the female sexual response involves not only physiology but also emotions, experiences, relationships, and beliefs. Changes in any one of these components can affect your sexual drive, arousal, and satisfaction.

FSD may occur at any age, but it's more common during times of hormonal transition, such as postpartum or at menopause. During pregnancy, after childbirth, or while breastfeeding, women often experience diminished libido.

Dyspareunia, persistent or recurring pain during intercourse, is the most commonly reported sexual complaint. Surveys indicate that one in five women experiences physical pain with sex at some point in her life. The pain may be a burning or aching pain. It may be constant or intermittent, localized or diffuse. It may occur with each penetration or only with certain partners or in certain situations. Dyspareunia is common with first-time intercourse because the vaginal channel is tight. Over time, the vagina becomes more elastic and adapts to penetration. Experts suggest using plenty of water-based lubricant and penetrating very gradually. The location of pain in dyspareunia may vary and can occur:

- As superficial pain with penetration. This can result from:
  - Inadequate lubrication because of insufficient foreplay, or menopausal changes, or after childbirth or during breastfeeding
  - Inflammation or infection of the skin in the genital area
  - Allergic reaction to birth control products, such as foams or jellies
  - Vaginismus, or involuntary muscle spasms in the vaginal wall
  - Anatomic position of the cervix, which may expose it to "bumping" during intercourse

- Vestibulitis, a condition that causes stinging or burning at the vaginal opening
- Vulvodynia, a serious condition marked by chronic discomfort or pain of the vulva, with burning, stinging, or irritation in the genital area without the presence of infection or skin disease. The type and severity of symptoms vary and may occur with tampon use, exercise, and other daily activities.
- As deep pain with thrusting, which may arise from:
  - Some conditions such as endometriosis, uterine fibroids, cystitis (inflammation of the bladder), and other diseases
  - Infections of the cervix, uterus, or fallopian tubes
  - Scarring from surgeries or medical conditions

If you are experiencing pain during intercourse or other persistent sexual problems, see your health care provider. The problems are often treatable through a combination of therapies that may include treating an underlying medical condition, hormone therapy, medication, desensitization therapy (which involves learning vaginal relaxation exercises that can decrease pain), and addressing emotional or mental health issues that may develop as a result of the dysfunction.

In addition, making the following lifestyle changes may alleviate pain and improve your sexual health:

- Avoid douching and using scented bath products, such as body washes and shower gels, which can irritate your genital area and dry up your natural lubrication.
- If contraceptive creams or jellies cause discomfort, try switching to another brand or a different form of birth control.
- Avoid tobacco use and excessive alcohol consumption.
- Strengthen your pelvic muscles, which are involved in pleasurable sexual sensation, by doing Kegel exercises. (See the box Kegeling on page 145.)
- Talk to your partner about what feels good and what doesn't.
- Experiment with positions. Sharp pain during thrusting can result from the penis striking your cervix or stressing your pelvic floor muscles, triggering cramping pain or aching. Try being on top of your partner during sex, which will help you control the depth of penetration.
- Use lubricants such as K-Y jelly or Astroglide or plain vegetable oil to make penetration more comfortable.
- Take your time with sex. Enjoy longer foreplay to help stimulate your natural lubrication.

WHEN SHOULD I SEEK HELP?

If you and your partner are experiencing persistent or serious problems with sexual practices or performance (such as lack of sexual desire or satisfaction, difficulty reaching orgasm, premature ejaculation, etc.), it's important to seek help from a knowledgeable family physician and/or counselor or therapist. Many women turn to close friends or a family doctor to get a referral to a reputable counselor or therapist. The American Association of Sex Education Counselors and Therapists (AASECT) lists specialists across the country.

SEX AND ILLNESS

Any illness or disability that affects your mental or physical health or well-being may also affect your sex life. Hormonal problems, high blood pressure, or chronic illnesses, such as cardiovascular disease, arthritis, cancer, diabetes, or depression, may affect sexual function and sexual interest. These conditions may decrease libido, alter genital sensation, or decrease frequency or intensity of orgasm. They can cause vaginal dryness, muscle tightness or spasms, bladder or bowel dysfunction, or pain during sex.

Moreover, certain medications used to treat illnesses, including antidepressants, blood pressure medications, antihistamines, and chemotherapy drugs, can have sexual side effects, reducing sex drive and the ability to achieve orgasm.

If you think a health condition—or the medication used to treat it—is affecting your sexual health, it's important to talk openly with your partner and your health care provider. Where medications are concerned, your doctor may be able to prescribe a different medicine or a dosage that reduces sexual side effects. It may also help to adapt the type of sexual activity you engage in and how you approach it:

- Talk to you partner about how you feel and how to deal with sexual activity in a way that will satisfy both of you.
- Plan sexual activity for the time of day when you are most rested and relaxed and when your health concerns are least troubling.
- After eating, wait for at least a couple of hours before having sex.
- Take any necessary pain medications a half hour before sex.
- Take your time with foreplay and caressing. Any kind of loving touch can be both healing and comforting.
- Experiment with different positions to find the ones that are most comfortable for you and allow for gentle movements.
- Try using lubricants to ease vaginal discomfort with intercourse.

SEXUALLY TRANSMITTED DISEASES (STDs)

Sexually transmitted diseases are infections spread from person to person through vaginal, anal, or oral sex with an infected individual. More than 15 million new cases of STDs are reported each year in this country; women are twice as likely as men to contract one of these diseases. They may be transmitted even by someone who has no symptoms, and they are sometimes difficult to treat. It is far better to prevent infection in the first place. If left untreated, some STDs can lead to liver disease, pelvic inflammatory disease, cervical cancer, an increased risk of HIV/AIDS, infertility, and complications with pregnancy, such as early onset of labor and uterine infection after delivery. They can also have harmful effects on a baby before, during, and after birth. These include low birth weight, eye infections, pneumonia, hepatitis, meningitis, liver disease, and stillbirth. At annual physical exams, be sure to discuss STDs with your health care provider to determine whether you need to be tested.

All women need to be vigilant about practicing safer sex. As my colleague Pepper says, sex involves trading fluids and germs. We can't pretend there aren't deadly diseases out there, as well as diseases that can affect our fertility and cause serious health problems. We have to think of sex as something we prepare for.

The bottom line is this:

- *Don't have sex without asking your partner whether he or she has an STD.* "This can be a real problem for people who are embarrassed about talking openly," says Pepper. "But this embarrassment can be deadly. You have to say, 'Look, I would like to be as free as possible with you. What do we need to worry about?' It's not very sexy, so it's unlikely to come up unless you purposely address it—and you absolutely have to."
- *Don't have sex without a condom; and for sex between women, use a dental dam.* Make sure you have condoms and *use* them. Apart from abstinence, condoms are by far the most effective preventive measure against STDs. As Pepper puts it, "You have to be willing to say to your partner, 'No condom, no deal. It's nothing personal—just my health behavior.'"

If you're in a relationship that you are certain is monogamous, and you and your partner have been tested to ensure that you are free of sexually transmitted disease, then your sexual activity is probably safe. However, many women believe that their partners are faithful, and it turns out that they aren't; the opposite is true as well. It's important to be cautious. Unless you have a trusting, longstanding, mutually faithful relationship with someone who has been tested for STDs and has had no or few other sex partners, you should ask about your partner's health status with regard to STDs and *use condoms*. If you or your partner is having sex with more than one person, you should discuss the risks with your health care provider and take immediate action to protect yourself.

Sexually transmitted diseases include:

- **Human papillomavirus (HPV).** HPV is the most common sexually transmitted disease. More than six million cases are diagnosed every year in this country. HPV describes a group of viruses that may cause abnormal growths on the body, from warts to cervical cancer. There are more than 30 sexually transmitted strains of HPV, which can infect the genital areas of both men and women, including the skin of the penis, vulva, and anus, and the linings of the vagina, cervix, and rectum.

  Some HPV infections cause genital warts—single or multiple growths or bumps that are soft, moist, pink, or flesh-colored that appear in the genital area, including the thigh—which may appear within weeks or months of sexual contact with an infected person.

  HPV infections may also trigger cellular changes in the cervix. These abnormalities are most often detected by a Pap test. Infections with "low-risk" types of the virus (such as types 6 and 11) cause mild changes that usually resolve without treatment. Infections with high-risk types (such as types 16 and 18) don't resolve as easily; some advance to cervical cancer. Each year, about 11,000 women in this country are diagnosed with invasive cervical cancer and close to 4,000 women die from the disease.

  At least half of all sexually active men and women acquire genital HPV infection at some point in their lives. By age 50, 8 out of 10 women have been infected. Most people with HPV infection do not experience any symptoms, yet they can transmit the virus to a sex partner.

  There is no cure for HPV infection. Getting regular Pap tests to detect precancerous and cancerous cells on the cervix, along with thorough medical follow-up, can prevent HPV-triggered changes in the cervix from developing into life-threatening cervical cancer.

  The only certain way to prevent HPV is to refrain from all sexual activity. The fewer partners a woman has, the less likely she is to get HPV. However, even women with only one sex partner can be infected if her partner has been infected by previous partners.

Condoms, when used properly, may lower the risk of getting HPV. However, they do not fully protect against HPV because the virus can infect areas not covered by a condom.

The good news is that a powerful new preventive tool against HPV infection and cervical cancer is now available. The vaccine Gardasil protects women

THE HUMAN PAPILLOMA VIRUS (HPV) VACCINE

In 2006, the US Food and Drug Administration (FDA) approved the use of the Gardasil vaccine in girls and women ages 9 to 26 for protection against certain strains of HPV. Ideally, girls should receive the HPV vaccine before they become sexually active. But even women who are already sexually active will derive some benefit from HPV vaccination, because it can protect them from contracting HPV infections by viral types to which they have not yet been exposed. The vaccine is routinely recommended for 11- and 12-year-old girls and for girls and women age 13 through 26 who have not yet been vaccinated even if they are already sexually active.

Some parents have concerns about the vaccine because it is so new. I admit that I had some reservations of my own about whether or not to have my teenage daughters vaccinated. So not too long ago, I asked two of my colleagues who are experts in obstetrics and gynecology for their opinions. One colleague said to wait a while if I was feeling uneasy. The other asked, "How old are your girls?" I told her they were 15 and 17. Both colleagues said in unison, "Get the vaccine now." The evidence on the efficacy and safety of this vaccine is very strong, and the potential benefits of girls getting it before they are sexually active are significant.

When my girls went to the doctor together for the series of three shots, they had a great experience. They were offered counseling by our pediatrician on the benefits and limitations of the vaccine, as is required by law, and wore their adhesive bandages to school as a symbol of a rite of passage.

Research is currently under way to determine whether vaccinated women will require booster shots in the future and to determine the safety and efficacy of a single-shot vaccine for women older than age 26. Because the vaccine doesn't protect against every type of HPV, it's important for women to continue getting regular Pap tests and practice safe sex to reduce exposure to HPV and other sexually transmitted diseases.

against infection by the four HPV types mentioned above (6, 11, 16, and 18), which together cause 70 percent of cervical cancers and 90 percent of genital warts. Ideally, women should receive the HPV vaccine before they become sexually active. (See the box The Human Papilloma Virus (HPV) Vaccine at left.)

- **Chlamydia.** One of the most common STDs in the United States, chlamydia is caused by the bacterium *Chlamydia trachomatis.* It is often a silent, symptomless disease. However, it can trigger cervicitis, or inflammation of the cervix, and urethritis, inflammation of the lining of the urethra, which causes pain with urination. If left untreated, it can lead to pelvic inflammatory disease (PID). This can be a cause of infertility. When symptoms do occur, they include abnormal vaginal discharge, burning during urination, and bleeding between menstrual periods. Treatment is oral antibiotics for a woman and her partner.

- **Genital herpes.** Most cases of genital herpes are caused by one of two kinds of herpes simplex viruses (HSVs), type 1 or type 2. These viruses can be easily transmitted by skin-to-skin contact, even when there is no evidence of infection. Symptoms range from nonexistent to severe (during an "outbreak") and may include painful bumps, blisters, or open sores on or near the genitals (which usually heal after 2 to 4 weeks); vaginal discharge; fever; headache and muscle aches; painful, itching, or burning urination; swollen glands in the genital area; and pain in the legs, buttocks, or genital area. Treatment includes oral antiviral therapy, but there is as yet no cure. Using condoms reduces but does not eliminate the risk of infection with genital herpes.

- **Gonorrhea.** Gonorrhea is caused by the bacterium *Neisseria gonorrhoeae,* which grows easily in warm, moist areas of the reproductive tract, including the cervix (the most common site for women), uterus, and fallopian tubes, and the urethra. It can also grow in the mouth, throat, eyes, and anus. Symptoms occur in women in only about 50 percent of cases and are sometimes mistaken for bladder or vaginal infections. They include pain or burning during urination, vaginal discharge that is yellowish and sometimes bloody, and bleeding between menstrual periods. If left untreated, gonorrhea can lead to pelvic inflammatory disease. Treatment is antibiotics.

- **Pelvic inflammatory disease (PID).** An infection of the uterus, fallopian tubes, or other reproductive organs, PID occurs when bacteria migrate upward from the vagina or cervix into the reproductive organs. It is a common complication of chlamydia and gonorrhea. Some 10 to 30 percent of women with these infections develop PID. The condition can cause chronic

TEEN SEX AND STDs

There's some good news in recent reports about teen sexual activity in the United States. In the past 10 years or so, there has been a decrease in the percentage of 15- to 19-year-old girls who report having had sexual intercourse—from 50 percent in the early 1990s to 45 percent more recently. The proportion of teen girls who reported having sex before the age of 15 declined from 19 percent in the 1990s to 13 percent during this decade. There has also been a 36 percent decline in the rate of teen pregnancy during the same time span, due primarily to higher contraceptive use and, to a lesser degree, to more teens choosing to postpone sexual activity. Some 83 percent of female teens reported using contraceptives during their most recent sexual encounter.

Still, many young women are at risk for unplanned pregnancy and for sexually transmitted diseases. Roughly one in three young women becomes pregnant at least once before the age of 20—an alarming fact. Half of the almost 19 million new cases of STDs each year occur among 15- to 24-year-olds, even though they comprise only a quarter of the sexually active population.

These are distressing statistics. The reality is that sexually active teenage girls are at greater risk for STDs—in part because they may have more than one sexual partner (some 10 percent of teen girls report having had four or more

pelvic pain, infertility, and ectopic pregnancy (when a fertilized egg implants inside the fallopian tube or elsewhere outside the uterus), which is a leading cause of pregnancy-related deaths for women in the first trimester. Women under the age of 25 are most at risk for the disease because their cervix is not fully matured (making them more vulnerable to sexually transmitted infections linked with PID), as well as women with multiple sex partners and women who douche. Symptoms vary, but often include lower abdominal pain, fever, pain during intercourse or urination, vaginal discharge with a foul odor, and irregular menstrual bleeding. When chlamydia causes PID, women may have few symptoms even though the disease is causing serious damage to reproductive organs. Prompt treatment with antibiotics can cure the disease and prevent damage.

sexual partners) and because they may not use condoms or may use them incorrectly. In addition, a teen girl's risk of chlamydia is higher because during adolescence the cervix is not yet matured and the lining of the uterus is more exposed to bacteria.

This is yet another argument for postponing sexual intercourse. But if a teen girl decides to have sex, at the very least she should provide herself with the best possible protection against unwanted pregnancy and STDs. As a mother, I believe that you have a responsibility to educate your teenage daughter(s) about birth control and health protection. In so doing, you are not encouraging her to have sex. You can tell her that you want her to postpone having sex until she's emotionally ready and has fulfilled her goals, whatever they may be. But you should also tell her that if she decides to have sex (against your best advice), this part is not optional: To protect herself from STDs, she must use a condom and use it correctly, for the sake of her health and her future.

What about boys? Parents should also have frank discussions about sex with their sons, emphasizing the same key points and encouraging them to take responsibility in their sexual relations.

- **Hepatitis B.** This form of hepatitis is a serious liver disease caused by the hepatitis B virus (HBV). One out of 20 people in the United States has been infected with HBV at some point in their life. Infection with HBV occurs through contact with blood, semen, and other body fluids. You can contract the illness by having sex with an infected person or sharing contaminated needles. The disease can also be spread from an infected mother to her infant during birth. Although some people with the disease have no symptoms, others have symptoms such as yellow skin or yellowing of the whites of the eyes (jaundice), fatigue, mild fever, headache and muscle aches, loss of appetite, nausea or vomiting, abdominal discomfort, dark-colored urine and pale gray bowel movements, or joint pain. For some, hepatitis B can become a chronic infection, which may lead to cirrhosis, liver cancer, or liver failure. There are currently no medications available to treat acute HBV infection, but chronic infections can be treated with antiviral drugs. The best prevention against the disease is the hepatitis B vaccine.

- **Human immunodeficiency virus (HIV).** HIV is a virus that attacks and progressively weakens the body's immune system. The virus can cause acquired immune deficiency syndrome, or AIDS. You can contract HIV through sexual contact or exposure to infected blood or tissue, from infected mother to infant during delivery and breastfeeding, and from blood transfusion and organ transplantation. Some women experience no symptoms for 10 years or more. Symptoms include extreme fatigue; rapid weight loss; low-grade fever and night sweats; frequent oral yeast infections, vaginal yeast infections, and other STDs; pelvic inflammatory disease; changes in menstrual cycles; and red, purple, or brownish blotches on or beneath the skin or inside the mouth, nose, or eyelids. Women are more susceptible than men to infection with HIV. Especially vulnerable are women with other STDs, which may cause lesions in the vulva, vaginal lining, or cervix, or changes in the immune system. You can prevent HIV/AIDS by using safe sex practices and avoiding injectable illegal drugs. (For more information on HIV/AIDS, see Chapter 17.)

- **Syphilis.** Syphilis is caused by the bacterium *Treponema pallidum* and is passed between individuals during vaginal, anal, or oral sex through direct contact with a syphilis sore. These sores occur mainly on the external genitals or in the vagina, anus, or rectum, but they may also appear on the lips and in the mouth. In the United States, there were an estimated 36,000 cases of syphilis in 2006. Those who are infected with syphilis often experience no symptoms for years, yet they remain at risk for later complications if they are not treated. The disease is hard to diagnose because its symptoms resemble those of other diseases. In the early stage of the disease, a single, small, round, and painless sore, or chancre, appears, usually in the genital area but sometimes in the mouth. If the infection is not treated, it moves to the next stage, causing skin rashes on the hands and feet and lesions in mucous membranes, as well as fever, swollen lymph glands, sore throat, patchy hair loss, headaches, weight loss, muscle aches, and fatigue. If the infection remains in the body, it can damage the brain, nerves, eyes, heart, blood vessels, liver, bones, and joints. In its early phases, syphilis is curable with penicillin.

WHAT ARE THE RISKS OF STDs
WITH DIFFERENT TYPES OF SEXUAL ACTIVITY?

- **Caressing and kissing.** Generally a low-risk activity, except if you or your partner has cuts or sores on your body or in your mouth, which can increase the risk of infection.
- **Masturbation.** Risk free.
- **Mutual masturbation.** Low risk, unless fluids such as vaginal secretions or semen come into contact with cuts or sores.
- **Oral sex.** Low risk, unless you have sores or ulcers in your mouth. Condoms or oral shields such as dental dams can protect you (see below). (It's best not to brush your teeth before oral sex because you can nick your gums.)
- **Vaginal sex.** High risk of sexual infection, including HIV. Use of a condom can offer protection. Spermicides can actually increase risk.
- **Anal sex.** High risk of sexual infection, including HIV, due to cuts, sores, and abrasions. Use of a condom can offer protection.

HOW TO AVOID GETTING AN STD

- **Abstain from sex** or **be faithful** to one partner free of infection. The best protection from contracting an STD is abstaining from sexual intercourse except in a long-term mutually monogamous relationship with a partner known to be free of infection.
- **Use latex condoms** consistently and correctly every time you have intercourse.
- **For oral sex, use a dental dam.** These are thin pieces of latex that help reduce the transmission of STDs by acting as a barrier to body fluids during oral-vaginal or oral-anal sex. Dental dams are placed over the anus or vagina before sexual contact and are made in a variety of sizes and flavors.
- **Never share sexual aids or drug paraphernalia** such as needles, syringes, water, or "works."
- **Be aware that most methods of birth control will not protect you from STDs.** These include birth control pills and shots, spermicides, implants, and diaphragms.
- **Get regular pelvic exams.** Talk with your health care provider about how often you need them and speak openly and honestly about any STDs you or

your partner has had or may have presently. Many tests for STDs can be done during an exam. If you are pregnant, or age 25 or under and sexually active, or if you have new sex partners or multiple sex partners, the Centers for Disease Control and Prevention (CDC) recommend yearly chlamydia testing.

- **Be informed.** For more information, call the Centers for Disease Control and Prevention at (800) 232-4636 or visit the CDC Web site for STDs at www.cdc.gov/std.

- **Most important, talk to your partner before you have sex,** about whether he or she may have a sexually transmitted disease.

WHAT TO DO IF YOU HAVE AN STD OR THINK YOU OR YOUR PARTNER MIGHT HAVE ONE

If you experience genital symptoms that may be signs of STD infection, such as unusual sores, odorous vaginal discharge, burning while you urinate, or bleeding between periods, you should stop having sex and see your health care provider.

If you or your sexual partner is diagnosed with an STD, you should:

- Get treatment.
- Get tested for other STDs, including HIV.
- Get vaccinated for hepatitis B, if you have not already done so.
- Notify your recent sex partners so they can be screened for STDs and, if necessary, treated. Informing a partner about STD status can be very difficult, but it must be done before initiating sexual activity.
- Do not resume sexual activity until all sex partners have been examined and treated.
- When you resume sexual activity, use condoms or other forms of effective barrier contraception.

3

Reproductive Choices

Some people in my family might raise their eyebrows at my offering expertise in the area of reproductive choices, given that my first pregnancy was unexpected (though happily concluded with the birth of my son, now 21). After this, I managed to have two planned pregnancies and then successfully stopped reproducing through the effective use of birth control.

I speak from experience when I say that whether you're trying to prevent pregnancy or achieve it, the timing of ovulation is one of the most important things to understand about your own body.

In women of childbearing age, ovulation occurs roughly once a month, when a mature egg is released from one of your two ovaries. The egg then enters the adjacent fallopian tube leading to the uterus. If you have unprotected sexual intercourse at around this time, sperm ejaculated from the man's penis may travel up the vagina and through the uterus to reach the egg in the fallopian tube. If a sperm cell penetrates and fertilizes the egg (known as conception or fertilization), the egg begins developing as it travels down the fallopian tube. Eventually it implants in the lining of the uterus and develops over the course of 9 months into a baby. Even without intercourse, it's possible for sperm ejaculated in or near the labia to move up the vagina and fertilize an egg.

You can roughly calculate the time of ovulation by noting the starting day of your last menstrual period (LMP). Most women ovulate between day 11 and day 21 of their cycle, counting from that first day of your LMP. Sexual intercourse during this time increases the chance of pregnancy.

BIRTH CONTROL

Most American women are fertile for about 35 years, from about age 13 to 48. If you wish to avoid having children at any stage during this time, it's important to select a birth control method that's right for you and best fits your reproductive health needs at each life stage.

There are more than a dozen kinds of contraception available today that vary in their efficacy, ease of use, safety, risks, cost, and other factors. Some forms work by preventing the ovaries from releasing an ovum (e.g., birth control pills); others, by blocking the release of sperm or preventing sperm from entering the vagina or cervix (condoms, etc.). Choosing among the options to find what is most comfortable and appealing is a highly personal health care decision. Here are some questions to consider in making your choice:

- How effective is the method at preventing unplanned pregnancies? If you would consider an unplanned pregnancy unacceptable for you and your partner, then you should pick a highly effective method. Efficacy is measured by the number of failures or unplanned pregnancies in 100 women using that method for 1 year (sometimes noted as a percentage, e.g., a 21 percent failure rate, which means that there are 21 unplanned pregnancies out of each 100 women using this method over a period of 1 year).

- How effective is the method at preventing STDs, including HIV? If you have more than one sex partner, or have any concerns at all about STDs, condoms should be used in addition to other methods.

- How safe is it? Some methods carry health risks: For example, for women over 35 who smoke, birth control pills present risks.

- Are you interested in temporary protection or long-term (or even permanent) protection? If you are certain that you do not want to have children, permanent methods may be a reasonable choice.

- Is your partner willing to participate in ensuring protection?

- How comfortable are you with planning ahead for sex?

- How careful are you about following directions?

- Can you afford this method and easily obtain it? Does it require a prescription, or, for minors, parental consent?

Among the available birth control methods are:

Abstinence. Completely refraining from sexual intercourse is, of course, a cheap, failsafe way of avoiding pregnancy and preventing STDs. However, for most women this is not a realistic option.

Contraceptive barriers. These methods prevent sperm from meeting egg by physical or chemical blocking. They range from condoms and cervical caps to sponges and spermicides and vary in their effectiveness, which depends on consistent and correct use. *Only a condom is an effective method for reducing risk of sexually transmitted infections.*

- **Male condom,** also called a rubber. Among the most popular birth control barriers, a condom is a thin sheath placed over an erect penis before intercourse, preventing the passage of semen into the vagina. It can be used only once. Condoms have been proven to protect against STDs, including HIV. Those made from latex are best at preventing pregnancy and protecting against STDs. (For women with latex allergies, there are latex-free alternatives such as polyurethane.) They are available at most drugstores and grocery stores at relatively low cost. They should not be used with oil-based lubricants such as Vaseline or petroleum jelly, lotions, or oils, which may damage them and reduce their effectiveness at both preventing pregnancy and reducing the risk of STDs. Lubricants that are not oil-based, such as K-Y jelly or Astroglide, are safe to use. If condoms are used consistently and correctly, their failure rate is only about 3 percent.

- **Diaphragm.** A diaphragm is a shallow latex cup with a professionally fitted springlike rim that holds it in place in the vagina, so that it acts as a barrier to the passage of semen into the cervix. It requires fitting and training for use. A health care provider can measure your vaginal canal to fit you with the correct size and demonstrate proper usage. Before sex, the inside of the dome of the diaphragm (the side covering your cervix) is filled with spermicide and the diaphragm is put into place over the cervix. After intercourse, the diaphragm must be left in place for 6 to 8 hours. Then it should either be removed or more spermicide should be added with an applicator. The device should not be left in place for more than 24 hours after sex. If properly used, the diaphragm can provide effective birth control; however, because of improper use in the first year, the typical failure rate is estimated at 20 percent.

- **Cervical cap.** The cervical cap is a fitted, soft, cup-shaped latex device, smaller than the diaphragm, which fits over the base of the cervix to act as a mechanical barrier to sperm migration. The cap is filled one-third full with spermicide before insertion. It can be inserted as long as 8 hours before intercourse and left in place for as long as 48 hours and provides continuous contraceptive protection for multiple sessions of intercourse. The cervical cap is more effective for women who have not yet had children (childbirth affects the shape of the cervix), with a failure rate of 10 to 20 percent for childless women, compared to 20 to 40 percent for women who have delivered children.

- **Vaginal sponge.** The sponge is a soft, circular polyurethane device that fits over a woman's cervix and contains spermicide that blocks and absorbs semen for 24 hours. It is inserted just before intercourse or several hours in advance, then left in place for at least 6 hours. It is available over-the-counter and is for one-time use only. Its failure rate is 14 to 16 percent, though that rate may be as high as 28 percent in women who have had children.

- **Female condom.** A female condom is a polyurethane sheath designed to prevent pregnancy by acting as a barrier to the passage of semen into the vagina. It measures about 3 inches in diameter and 6.5 inches in length, is open at one end and closed at the other, and contains two flexible rings. It can be placed inside a woman's vagina as many as 8 hours before intercourse. The ring at the closed end serves as an insertion mechanism and internal anchor. The other ring forms the external edge of the device and remains outside of the canal after insertion. Like the male condom, it is intended for one time use only, and should not be used together with a male condom. However, it is not considered an effective form of birth control, with a failure rate of 21 percent.

- **Spermicides.** These chemical barriers contain substances that kill or inactivate sperm. Vaginal spermicides come in the form of foams, creams, jellies, films, suppositories, and tablets. They are not highly effective when used alone (with a 29 percent failure rate) but are more so when combined with physical barrier devices such as condoms, diaphragms, or cervical caps. Some spermicides require a waiting period before they become effective, and all must be reapplied before each session of intercourse. *They do not provide protection again STDs* and may in fact increase susceptibility by irritating the vaginal lining.

Hormonal contraceptives. A highly effective method of preventing pregnancy, hormonal contraception works by preventing ovulation, changing cervical mucus to reduce sperm mobility, and/or preventing the implantation of the embryo. These contraceptives may take the form of birth control pills, mini-pills, 3-month pills, injections, implants, skin patches, and vaginal rings. Most use a combination of estrogen and progestin. For women who want to steer clear of estrogen, progestin-only methods are available. *Hormonal contraceptives do not protect against HIV/AIDS or other STDs.* Among the choices are:

- **Birth control pills.** Also called oral contraceptives, or just "the Pill," birth control pills use a combination of the hormones estrogen and progestin to prevent ovulation from occurring. They are obtained by prescription only and if used consistently (taken every day) are considered highly effective, with a failure rate of 2 to 8 percent. If you are taking other medications, you should speak with your doctor about whether they may interfere with the Pill's efficacy. Side effects include dizziness, headaches, breast tenderness, irregular menstrual cycles, mood disturbances, nausea, bloating, and decreased libido. Oral contraceptives may increase risk for blood clots, heart attack, and stroke. You should not smoke while taking the Pill because it increases these risks. (If you are over age 35 and a smoker, most health care providers will not prescribe oral contraceptives.) You should not use the Pill if you have a history of cardiovascular disease, blood clots in the legs or lungs, or breast, uterine, or liver cancer. There are several new forms of oral contraceptives:
  - A spearmint-flavored, **chewable birth control pill**—designed to encourage compliance with a daily regimen of pill taking—is now available by prescription.
  - A **3-month combination pill** became available in 2003. The current version, known as Seasonique, is taken daily for 3 straight months, or 84 days, followed by 1 week of inactive pills, when you have a period (often lighter than normal), then another 3 months of active pills, and so on. The 3-month pill provides year-round protection and is equal to the regular pill in effectiveness, though it does have some side effects, such as spotting and breakthrough bleeding.
  - The **mini-pill.** For women who cannot take estrogen, an alternative is the "mini-pill," which contains only progestin. Its effectiveness is slightly lower than the combination pill.
  - **"No more period" pill.** In spring of 2007, the FDA approved the first continuous-use drug product for prevention of pregnancy. Known as Lybrel, the 28-day-pill pack contraceptive stops the body's monthly preparation for pregnancy by lowering its production of the hormones necessary for pregnancy. Women who use Lybrel do not have a regular menstrual period but

sometimes have unscheduled bleeding or spotting and some bloating. It was once thought that women needed to menstruate to keep the reproductive system healthy, but the latest research indicates that most women suffer no ill effects from halting menstruation for a period of time.

My colleague Hope Ricciotti, an OB-GYN at Harvard Medical School, tells me that as long as women are confident they will have no trouble remembering to take birth control pills every day, then these are a good option for them. For women who may find this difficult, there are other hormonal options, including:

- **Skin patch.** The skin patch (Ortho Evra) is a small adhesive square embedded with the hormones estrogen and progestin, which release slowly through the skin and into the bloodstream. You can stick it on your shoulder, lower abdomen, or buttocks. It works for 1 week and then must be replaced with a new one. You use the patches for 3 weeks in a row (three patches), separated by 1 week off, when you menstruate. If used consistently and correctly, the skin patch is considered as reliable as other hormonal contraceptives, with a failure rate of 1 to 8 percent, though it may be less effective for women who weigh more than 200 pounds or are obese. The patch delivers a higher dose of estrogen than the Pill, which may increase the risk of blood clots. Side effects include skin irritation, breast tenderness, mood changes, decreased libido, and nausea or vomiting.
- **Vaginal ring.** The vaginal ring (NuvaRing) is a flexible ring about 2 inches in diameter that is inserted into the vagina and releases progestin and estrogen for a period of 3 weeks. After this, it is removed for a week, and you get your period. Then you put in a new ring. If used correctly, it has a 1 to 8 percent failure rate. Risks include vaginitis, and in women who smoke, blood clots and stroke.
- **Hormone injections.** Progestin may be delivered by injection. Depo-Provera, the only version of injectable contraception available in this country, prevents pregnancy for as long as 90 days. It has a 3 percent failure rate and is a good choice for women who may have trouble sticking with a regimen of daily pill taking. Side effects include irregular periods, breast tenderness, mood changes, and weight gain. Long-term use of the injections may cause bone loss, but once use ceases, bone density returns to normal.
- **Progestin implants.** Implants are small rods about the size of a matchstick, surgically implanted beneath the skin of the upper arm. The implant known as Implanon, approved in 2006, releases a steady dose of progestin to prevent pregnancy for up to 3 years and has a 1 to 8 percent failure rate. Side effects include

headache, depression, and bleeding. It is not recommended for women with a history of breast cancer.

- **Intrauterine devices (IUDs).** Among the safest, most comfortable, and most effective of contraceptive devices, IUDs are small plastic devices inserted in a woman's uterus by a medical professional. They are more than 99 percent effective and may be left in place for 5 to 10 years. The Paragard IUD is hormone free and prevents fertilization for up to 10 years. Though it's often called a copper IUD, it's actually a flexible plastic "T" sheathed with copper. Its main side effect is heavier (and sometimes longer) menstrual bleeding and cramping. The Mirena IUD, a similar plastic T that releases a tiny amount of levonorgestrel (a progestin), is effective for 5 years. The progestin has a direct effect on the uterus, thinning the lining and making the uterine walls less prone to cramping. Women typically experience irregular spotting during the first 3 to 6 months on the Mirena, with little to no cramping. By 6 months, bleeding is usually very light or nonexistent. Hormonal side effects are rare.

  The majority of women do very well with IUDs, and it's unfortunate that more OB-GYNs don't recommend them. For most women, especially women seeking birth control following a pregnancy, IUDs may be the most effective method with the fewest side effects. The main side effect is irregular bleeding, and there is only a very slight risk of infection, infertility, and perforation of the uterus during insertion. IUDs are used more often in Europe than in the United States. The devices have gotten a bad rap in the United States because one model that was on the market in the 1960s, the Dalkon Shield, caused pelvic infections. Experts assert that today's models are safe, though they may be more difficult to insert in women who have not given birth and they should not be used by women at risk for chlamydia or in a nonmonogamous relationship, because pelvic infection from an STD can be more dangerous with an IUD in place.

NATURAL METHODS

- **Fertility-awareness method (FAM).** A form of natural family planning, FAM, also referred to as the rhythm method, involves observing signs of ovulation and avoiding unprotected intercourse during a woman's fertile period. Most commonly used is the "symptothermal" method to determine the beginning and the end of the fertile period. FAM is often used by those who have religious or cultural beliefs that prohibit use of birth control drugs and devices. However, it is not an effective form of birth control. The typical failure rate is about 20 percent.

This method requires charting changes in basal body temperature (temperature on waking) and cervical mucus and recording them on a calendar. The couple refrains from unprotected sex for several days before and after the suspected dates of ovulation. Women with irregular periods or irregular body temperature patterns or frequent infections of the reproductive tract should avoid this method.

- **Breastfeeding, or lactational amenorrhea method.** This method is based on the idea that breastfeeding can inhibit the production of hormones necessary for ovulation. It is effective only for the first 6 months after delivery, only if the woman's period has not yet returned, and only if breastfeeding is used as the exclusive method of feeding, with nursing at least every 4 hours during the day and every 6 hours at night. If these criteria are met, the method can have a failure rate as low as 2 percent.

- **Withdrawal, or coitus interruptus,** is the practice in which a man withdraws his penis from a woman's vagina and away from her genitalia before ejaculating in order to prevent fertilization. However, because sperm are often released before ejaculation, the method has a high failure rate of about 27 percent and obviously does not protect against STDs.

PERMANENT BIRTH CONTROL

Ending fertility is the most common form of birth control for women over the age of 35 who are absolutely sure they do not want to have children (or more children). Each of the three options currently available is more than 99 percent effective. They include tubal ligation and Essure for women and vasectomy for men. It is important to be certain of your decision, because these methods are usually irreversible.

- **Tubal ligation** is a surgical procedure in which the fallopian tubes are permanently cut or blocked to interrupt passage and prevent fertilization. About a million American women a year choose to have their tubes "tied." The procedure is commonly done during a Cesarean section if a woman does not want to have more children. Temporary postoperative side effects include fatigue, abdominal and shoulder pain, dizziness, and intestinal gas. The procedure involves all of the risks of surgery, as well as rare complications, such as injury to the bowel, bladder, or abdominal blood vessels, and pelvic infection.

- **Essure** is a permanent, incision-less sterilization procedure in which small springlike metal coils are inserted through the vagina and cervix to the top of the uterine cavity and into both fallopian tubes. Within 3 months, scar tissue grows around the coils, forming a barrier that prevents sperm from reaching eggs. During the first 3 months after the device is inserted, other forms of birth control are required. After this period, a special x-ray is taken to confirm that the tubes are blocked. Risks include pain immediately after the insertion procedure and a small risk for ectopic pregnancy.

- **Vasectomy** is a technique for sterilizing men that involves cutting the vas deferens (the tubes that carry sperm from testes to penis), which prevents sperm from passing into the seminal fluid. It's a relatively simple procedure, performed in a doctor's office or clinic, with local anesthesia. It does not affect a man's sexual function, and serious side effects are rare. Failure rates are less than 1 percent, but effectiveness varies with the experience of the surgeon and surgical technique.

Emergency contraception (birth control after sexual intercourse) is a drug or device that prevents pregnancy after a contraceptive fails or after unprotected sex. It is not intended for routine use and does not work in women who are already pregnant (i.e., it does not cause abortion). The two types of emergency contraception available in the United States include emergency contraceptive pills (ECPs), also known as "morning-after" pills, and the copper IUD (Paragard).

- The only ECP currently in use in this country is Plan B (now available over-the-counter for women age 17 and older and by prescription for younger women). The first tablet must be taken as soon as possible after sexual intercourse, ideally within 3 days (though some studies show that it may be effective for up to 5 days). The second tablet is taken 12 hours later. Plan B is 89 percent effective. Side effects are rare but include fatigue, headache, nausea, abdominal pain, and menstrual changes.
- The copper IUD must be inserted within 7 days of sexual intercourse. It is considered more effective than ECPs, reducing the risk of pregnancy by more than 99 percent. It can be removed after a woman's next period, or left in place as a birth control method.

UNWANTED PREGNANCY

Finding out that you are pregnant can be the most thrilling moment in your life—or among the most devastating. Either way, early detection is extremely important.

If you suspect that you are pregnant, don't delay getting confirmation from a health professional or a home pregnancy test. These inexpensive tests, available in drugstores and grocery stores, can detect pregnancy starting about 2 weeks after ovulation. It's best to take them a week after your missed period. The tests measure human chorionic gonado-tropin (HCG), a hormone produced by your body just after a fertilized egg implants in your uterine lining. Most home tests work by detecting HCG in your urine with a special dipstick; it's important to follow the directions carefully. If you're confused about the test or the results, call the manufacturer (usually there's a toll-free number listed in the instructions). Your doctor can offer a more sensitive blood test to detect HCG.

For women who face an unwanted pregnancy, there are a number of options to consider. It's important to seek help from an unbiased counselor—a social worker or other individual trained in pregnancy counseling—to discuss your full array of choices. A well-qualified counselor can assist you with the difficult decisions that lie ahead and help you sort through your options. (It's important to note that some places that promote themselves as providing "counseling services" for problem pregnancies are in fact promoting an antiabortion agenda.)

Among your choices is to keep the pregnancy and the baby and figure out how to work the child into your life. Another option is keeping the pregnancy, and surrendering the baby to adoption. There are many families who wish to adopt, including some with couples who are not able to have a biological child of their own. Adoptions may be open or closed. In an open adoption, you meet the family and get to know them so that you are more comfortable with your choice. Open adoptions can also result in a continued role for you with the child after birth. A closed adoption is one that is confidential and means that after you give birth, you have no contact with the child or adoptive family. Occasionally closed adoptions include concessions that allow the child to seek you out when he or she reaches adulthood.

Abortion is another option. Since the passage of the historic *Roe versus Wade* Supreme Court decision in 1973, women have had the choice of legal abortion. Based on the right to privacy, the *Roe v. Wade* decision held that a woman, with her doctor, could choose abortion in the earlier months of pregnancy without restriction, and with restrictions in later months. Abortion is a difficult choice and one that must be made with an understanding of all of the options and consequences. Laws vary by state, so you will need to find out what regulations may apply in your state. In some places, you may need to wait 24 hours after consulting with a counselor at an abortion clinic. Some states require a parent's involvement if you are under 18.

There are several types of abortion. The prescription drug mifepristone (also known as RU486) can be used to end pregnancy within the first 2 months. This is called a medical abortion. The drug blocks the progesterone needed for pregnancy to continue and can be used for up to 49 days after the start of your last menstrual period. It's important to consult with your reproductive health specialist or health care provider before using this drug and to schedule follow-up visits. It's also essential to have ready access to a medical care facility in case of an emergency. You should not use the drug if you have an ectopic pregnancy, an IUD in place, or problems with your adrenal glands. You should also avoid it if you've had long-term treatment with certain steroids, or if you have bleeding problems, are taking blood thinners, or have had an allergic reaction to mifepristone, misoprostol, or similar drugs.

A medical abortion is administered during the 49 days since the start of a woman's last menstrual period. It involves taking three pills at a clinic, hospital, or medical office under a doctor's supervision. The pills stop the embryo from growing and cause the uterus to contract and expel the pregnancy-related tissue. The result is a very heavy period usually accompanied by cramping. Two days later, a return to the medical facility is required for an examination to make sure that no tissue remains in your uterus to cause infection. Risks include infection and heavy bleeding. In rare cases, the treatment may fail or be incomplete, requiring a surgical procedure to complete the abortion.

A surgical abortion is performed from about 6 weeks after the last menstrual period until 20 weeks and after in some states. During this procedure the woman is given a local anesthesia or sometimes some sedation, and a small suction or vacuum is used on the uterus to remove the pregnancy tissue. This procedure must be done at a medical facility, and the woman usually needs to stay in the facility for a short time to make sure there is no adverse reaction or heavy bleeding. Risks include infection, heavy bleeding, and perforation of the uterus.

Overall risks of a legal abortion to a woman's health, especially when it is performed under 12 weeks, are very low, and far fewer than the risks of delivering a pregnancy at term.

The most important thing to remember if you're facing an unwanted pregnancy is to get the support you need, understand your options, and work with someone you trust—an unbiased social worker or health care provider—to make a decision that's right for you.

4

Fertility and Pregnancy

Fertility is the ability to become pregnant. The average woman in peak childbearing years, ages 20 to 35, with no fertility problems has about a 20 to 30 percent chance of getting pregnant in any given menstrual cycle. However, this can vary a great deal from woman to woman. For some women, trying to get pregnant is as simple as having a few sessions of unprotected intercourse; for others, it can be a long and difficult process.

I feel very lucky that I was able to get pregnant easily. Many of my friends have had problems with fertility, and I've seen their struggles. In truth, I thought I would have trouble because of my irregular periods. I think it helped that I had my children when I was in my twenties and early thirties.

There's no perfect time to have a baby. Though some women may argue with me, I believe that if you are certain that you want children, it's better to have babies earlier in your career, provided that you have a good support system and are in good health and relatively secure financially. Some of my colleagues in women's health go as far as to suggest that it's unwise to wait too many years. The problem, of course, is that a woman's fertility diminishes significantly with age. "The biological clock is nothing to sneeze at," says OB-GYN Hope Ricciotti. "People think of 35 as a kind of cutoff, but fertility really lies on a continuum." A woman's fertility peaks in the late teens and early twenties and declines gradually in the early thirties and then more rapidly in the late thirties, as the ovaries produce fewer viable eggs of good quality. For this reason, women who choose to delay pregnancy into their late thirties and early forties are more likely to encounter problems with infertility. For some women, menopause and the end of fertility may arrive prematurely, before the age of 40. A few women can still conceive in their fifties, although this is rare. Most women who bear children at this age do so with donor eggs. Preserving fertility by freezing eggs is also becoming more common, especially in Italy, but it has been slow to catch on in this country.

WHEN AM I FERTILE?

Each month, your pituitary gland produces a hormone called luteinizing hormone (LH) that stimulates your ovary to release an egg in the process known as ovulation. This tends to occur near day 14 of your menstrual cycle (if you have a consistent 28-day cycle), but this varies from woman to woman and from cycle to cycle. Ovulation occurs 14 days before your next period—and you know just when that is only after the fact. Once the egg has been released, it begins its 24- to 36-hour journey through the fallopian tube. This is the best time to conceive. Sperm cells can live in your reproductive tract for 48 to 72 hours, so if you're trying to get pregnant, it's good to have sex about every other day during the 3 or 4 days surrounding ovulation.

HOW CAN I TELL WHETHER I'M FERTILE?

It's helpful to keep track of your cycles on a menstrual calendar or fertility awareness chart, marking the day your period begins each month and noting the number of days you menstruate. As I mentioned, the time from the first day of your period until ovulation may vary, but it is typically about 2 weeks. Here are some other ways to watch for the major signs of fertility:

- **Basal body temperature (BBT).** Track your waking, or basal body, temperature with a special oral BBT thermometer that shows temperatures in increments of tenths of degrees rather than fifths. Take your temperature every morning before you get out of bed and track the results on a chart, noting the pattern of lows and highs. Before ovulation, your waking temperature will likely range from 97.0°F to 97.5°F. Ovulation typically causes temperature to rise 0.5°F to 1.6°F—either gradually or suddenly—to a range of 97.5°F to 98.6°F, where it remains for about 14 days and then drops just before menstruation. You are most fertile during the 2 to 3 days before this temperature rise. If you don't see this two-phase temperature pattern—low before ovulation and high after—you should consult a medical practitioner to make sure that you're ovulating. Your

BBT is a great indicator of pregnancy, too. When I was in my twenties, because I kept such close track of my BBT, I knew within 2 weeks that I was pregnant—even before I took a pregnancy test—because my temperature had risen and stayed high. (In fact, I suspected after only several days.)

- **Cervical mucus.** Keep an eye on your vaginal secretions and note when they become more copious and wet, clear, and slippery, like raw egg whites. This is a sign that ovulation will soon occur. The most fertile time in your cycle is the last day you have this slippery cervical mucus, so it's best to have intercourse on all days that you experience this kind of secretion.

- **Ovulation predictor kit.** Available without a prescription at most pharmacies, ovulation predictor kits are about 99 percent accurate in identifying the surge of luteinizing hormone (LH) that triggers ovulation. LH is present in your urine and surges 24 to 48 hours before ovulation. "These predictor kits let you know exactly when to have sex—on the day you experience your ovulation surge and again on the next day," says Hope Ricciotti. "Women get so stressed about the timing; this kit takes the pressure off." But be careful not to over-target sex: By waiting too long, couples may miss the window. The kits range in price from $20 to $50. According to Hope, one of the most cost-effective types of kit is a reusable electronic test kit such as Clear Plan Easy Fertility Monitor. Ovulation predictor kits are not recommended as a method of tracking ovulation in order to avoid pregnancy.

Other ways to improve your chances of conceiving:

- Have sex regularly, two or three times a week.
- Avoid alcohol, smoking, and drug use, all of which may impair your ability to get pregnant.
- Maintain a healthy body weight: Being either overweight or underweight can affect your body's production of the hormones necessary for conception and pregnancy. Negative energy balance (taking in less energy than you expend), any type of energy intake restriction, or disordered eating will increase risk of infertility.
- Avoid vaginal lubricants.
- Avoid use of medications that may make it difficult to conceive, including some prescription drugs and over-the-counter medications such as nonsteroidal anti-inflammatory agents (NSAIDs, e.g., ibuprofen and naproxen).

INFERTILITY

Infertility is classically defined as the inability to conceive after 12 months of having well-timed, frequent, unprotected sexual intercourse. (This rule of thumb applies only to women under the age of 35.)

The biological clock ticks for every woman, regardless of how fit she is or how well she takes care of herself. Although some women give birth to healthy children into their forties, many face issues of infertility as early as their thirties. They also face higher miscarriage rates and greater risks of birth defects. If you're set on having children, I would recommend planning for pregnancy in your late twenties and early thirties. If you choose to delay, be aware of the possible consequences.

Infertility can be a stressful, heartbreaking problem, and it's far more common than people realize, affecting more than six million couples in the United States—some 10 percent of those of reproductive age. In her OB-GYN practice, Hope urges women to be proactive about their fertility. "Time is of the essence," she says. "Don't wait." You should consult a fertility specialist if you're under age 35 and you haven't gotten pregnant after a year of unprotected intercourse, after 6 months if you're age 35 to 40, or after 3 months if you are over age 40.

Infertility may be caused by a single problem or a combination of problems in one or both partners. Roughly a third of infertility cases are due to factors affecting women; a third, to factors affecting men; and a third, to a combination of factors in both partners. Many cases are unexplained, and the source of the problem remains a mystery.

Among the causes of infertility in women are:

- Age. Because of aging eggs, a significant decline in fertility occurs in women during their mid- to late thirties. By your mid- to late forties, you may have just a few good eggs left.
- Anovulation (failure to ovulate) or other ovulation disorders
- Fallopian tube damage or obstruction, most often caused by chlamydia
- Endometriosis
- Polycystic ovary syndrome (PCOS)
- Elevated prolactin, the hormone that normally stimulates milk production
- Early menopause
- Uterine fibroids
- Pelvic adhesions

- Hormonal imbalance, which may result from thyroid dysfunction or hypothalamic-pituitary disorders caused by tumors, injury, excessive exercise, or malnutrition
- Being overweight
- Being underweight, especially as a result of eating disorders such as anorexia nervosa or bulimia
- Some prescription drugs, including steroids, blood pressure medications, and antidepressants, which can impair fertility
- Diseases such as cancer (and its treatment), sickle cell disease, diabetes, kidney disease, and other medical conditions
- Smoking
- Alcohol use. It's okay to have a glass of wine or one beer a day. However, if you are trying to conceive, drink only in the first half of your menstrual cycle, prior to ovulation, if at all.

For men, fertility problems can result from:

- Problems with the production or function of sperm, which may arise from varicose veins in the scrotum, undescended testicles, deficiency of testosterone, genetic defects such as Klinefelter's syndrome, repeated infections with STDs such as chlamydia and gonorrhea, and other factors
- Impaired delivery of sperm due to erectile dysfunction, premature ejaculation, oil-based lubricants, blockage of the ejaculatory ducts, and other problems
- Health and lifestyle factors such as malnutrition, obesity, emotional stress, alcohol or drug use, cancer treatments, and other medical conditions
- Age—men over age 40 may be less fertile than younger men
- Exposure to environmental factors such as tobacco, toxins, pesticides and other chemicals, and heat

Diagnosing the underlying problem involves testing all of the steps along the path from ovulation to pregnancy and may take up to a year to complete. The workup can include the following:

- Taking a general medical history of you and your partner
- Monitoring ovulation
- Gynecologic examination
- Hormonal profile

- Evaluation of ovarian reserve, or the capacity to grow normal eggs
- Semen analysis
- Uterotubogram or hysterosalpingogram, an x-ray that determines whether there are blockages in the fallopian tubes
- Endometrial biopsy to determine whether you're ovulating normally and to evaluate your uterine lining
- Laparoscopy, a technique that allows a physician to view your ovaries, fallopian tubes, and other reproductive organs
- Pelvic ultrasound
- Genetic testing

INFERTILITY TREATMENT

Infertility treatment is a complex field beyond the scope of this book. However, what follows is some general guidance. Resources for further information are listed at the end of this book. (See Resources section.)

How infertility is treated depends on its cause and the age of the partners involved. About half of couples who are treated for infertility become pregnant. The vast majority of cases that are successfully treated (about 90 percent) are addressed with medication or surgery or both.

Treatment for female infertility relating to hormonal imbalance or ovulation disorders often involves the use of fertility drugs such as clomiphene citrate (Clomid, Serophene), human menopausal gonadotropin (Repronex), and other medications. These drugs, which include natural hormones and synthetic substances, increase the chance of multiple births and their use requires careful monitoring.

Surgical techniques such as microsurgery, balloon-catheter techniques, and laser surgery can be used to correct blockages or other problems in the fallopian tubes, to remove endometrial adhesions and scar tissue, and to correct structural problems in the cervix and uterus. These procedures are less common now that in vitro fertilization (IVF) is available.

About 5 to 10 percent of cases of infertility are treated through assisted reproductive technologies. The most common form is IVF. Since 1978, more than three million children worldwide have been conceived through IVF, which involves taking drugs that trigger the development of multiple eggs. Then the eggs are removed from the woman's ovaries and, in a laboratory dish, fertilized with a man's sperm. Three to 5 days later, the resulting embryos are implanted in the uterus. IVF is often used when a woman has blocked fallopian tubes, endometriosis, ovulation disorder, or unexplained infertility. The procedure requires frequent blood tests and daily hormone injections. It also involves some risk of multiple pregnancy, bleeding or infection, low birth weight, and birth defects.

Whatever form it takes, treatment for infertility is often an emotional roller-coaster ride. The drugs and surgical procedures can be unpleasant, and there is always the issue of uncertain outcome. It may help to set a limit on the number and kind of procedures acceptable from an emotional and financial point of view. You may also wish to explore other options early in the process, such as adoption. It's important for you and your partner to talk about your feelings and to seek support from friends, family, and support groups or counseling services. Stress-reduction techniques such as relaxation training may also be useful in easing anxiety and tension. (See Chapter 25.)

ON THE HORIZON

In the next decade or so, we may see common use of several new potential treatments for infertility:

- **In vitro maturation (IVM).** This process eliminates the need for expensive fertility drugs to trigger egg development. Immature eggs are extracted from the ovaries and matured in a Petri dish until they are ready for fertilization; after 3 to 5 days, the embryos are transferred to the womb.
- **Stem cell therapy.** Scientists are attempting to turn stem cells into sex cells (both sperm and eggs). If the considerable technical and practical obstacles involved can be overcome, this therapy would give couples who cannot produce eggs or sperm of their own the opportunity to have a biological child.
- **Ovarian tissue transplant.** This process involves surgically removing a section of ovarian tissue and freezing it for future use, when it may be thawed and reimplanted—either in the donor herself or in another recipient. Ovarian tissue transplant has the potential to restore fertility to women who have become infertile due to cancer therapy and to women beyond childbearing age.

PREGNANCY

For women who welcome it, pregnancy is an exciting time of major physical and emotional change. Not every woman loves being pregnant, but I did—seeing my body change, feeling this little being growing inside of me. The amazing experience of the baby's first kicks inside can be magical.

Taking good care of yourself before and during pregnancy is critical for your health and for the baby's. If you're planning to get pregnant, be sure to get a preconception checkup to evaluate your health and identify any risks that might affect your pregnancy. You'll want to discuss with your health care provider which birth control method you have been using; any lifestyle issues that may affect your pregnancy; and your complete medical history, including childhood diseases such as chicken pox and rubella. Make sure that your vaccinations are up-to-date (including TdaP—tetanus, diphtheria, and pertussis) so that you are properly protected against diseases that might harm your baby. See your dentist for a checkup and teeth cleaning.

If you have any chronic medical condition such as asthma, diabetes, high blood pressure, obesity, epilepsy, or any sexually transmitted disease, you should talk with your health care provider about ensuring that these conditions are under control.

Also, you'll want to discuss any medications you may be taking, including herbal medications. Depending on your family health history and your partner's, your health care provider may advise you to see a genetic counselor to assess your risk of having a child with a birth defect. If you're planning to get pregnant, in addition to visiting your health care provider, you should:

1. **Take folic acid to reduce the risk of birth defects**—800 to 1,000 micrograms of folic acid a day beginning at least 3 months before you get pregnant and during the early phase of your pregnancy. Folic acid has been found to reduce by 50 to 70 percent a woman's risk of having a baby with a serious birth defect of the brain and spinal cord.

2. **Stop smoking and avoid secondhand smoke.** Tobacco smoke can cause serious health problems for your developing baby.

3. **Avoid exposure at home and at work to toxic chemicals** such as pesticides, solvents, paints, lead from water pipes, and other dangerous substances that can cause birth defects or increase your risk of miscarriage. Always wear protective gloves and/or a mask when working with cleaning products and other hazardous chemicals and work in a well-ventilated area.

4. **Eat a healthy diet.** Go for a range of nutritious foods, including high-quality proteins, legumes, fruits, and vegetables, especially leafy green vegetables like spinach and romaine lettuce, which are packed with vitamins. (See Chapter 26.)

5. **Maintain a healthy weight.** If you're carrying extra pounds, lose weight before you start trying to get pregnant. Do not wait until you're trying to get pregnant, because losing weight then may harm your chances of getting pregnant or your baby. If you are underweight, try to gain a few pounds prior to conception. (See Chapter 9.)

6. **Get regular exercise** to help maintain a healthy weight and reduce stress. Pick a fitness activity that works for you, such as swimming, walking, or yoga, and try to exercise for at least 30 minutes most days of the week. (See Chapter 27.)

7. **Don't drink alcohol.** Alcohol puts you at risk for miscarriage and can seriously affect the physical and mental health of your baby. If you do drink prior to conception, consume no more than one drink a day and only during the first 2 weeks of your cycle, prior to conception.

8. **Don't use illegal drugs,** which can increase the risk of miscarriage and preterm labor.

9. **Avoid infections and toxins of all types.** Wash your hands often with soap and water. As much as possible, stay away from children with colds or other illnesses. Avoid any food that may be unsafe, such as undercooked meats and eggs, unwashed fruits and vegetables, unpasteurized milk products, and fish with high levels of mercury. Stay away from cat feces, because they may be a source of toxoplasmosis, an infection that can cause birth defects. (Have someone else in the family change the cat litter!) Avoid contact with rodents, including pet mice, guinea pigs, and hamsters, which can carry harmful diseases.

10. **Reduce your stress.** Avoid stressful situations when you can. Rest when you need it. Use relaxation techniques such as meditation, yoga, tai chi, or deep breathing to lower stress levels. (See Chapter 25.)

HOW DO I KNOW WHETHER I'M PREGNANT?

Early signs of pregnancy vary from woman to woman and from pregnancy to pregnancy. Here are some common symptoms of early pregnancy:

- Missing your period
- Tenderness, tingling, or enlargement of breasts
- Feeling nauseous or throwing up
- Increase or decrease in appetite; food cravings or aversions
- Feeling unusually tired, emotional, or weepy

- Experiencing irregular spotting, sometimes caused by implantation bleeding, which occurs when a fertilized egg implants in the uterus

An easy, convenient way to find out whether you're pregnant is to take a home pregnancy test. As mentioned above, these tests detect pregnancy within about 2 weeks of conception. If your test is positive, make an appointment with your health care provider as soon as possible. The earlier you know that you're pregnant, the earlier you can begin good prenatal care.

CHOOSING YOUR PRENATAL HEALTH CARE PROVIDER

Prenatal care to monitor your pregnancy can be provided by a doctor, (e.g., an obstetrician-gynecologist, or OB-GYN; a perinatologist, or high-risk obstetrician; or a family doctor) or a midwife or other health care professional. Who you pick can have a big impact on your experience, so it's important to find a practitioner who best matches your personal preferences and the needs of your pregnancy. You should pick someone you trust, someone who listens carefully to your concerns and offers helpful advice, someone who is comfortable with your positions on pregnancy and childbirth and who can deliver your baby at the place you choose. You may also wish to consider whether your insurance covers the provider.

Women giving birth in hospitals may also choose to employ a doula, a woman skilled at attending to a mother before, during, and after labor, to coach her through the birthing process. Research suggests that women who are attended by a doula require less medication during labor and have a lower rate of Cesarean section.

TAKING CARE OF YOURSELF WHILE YOU'RE PREGNANT

During the 266 or so days of a full-term pregnancy, your body undergoes a host of major changes. Your immune system adjusts to the presence of a foreign body, your baby growing inside your own tissues. Your blood volume is greatly expanded to supply nutrients and oxygen to the baby. You breathe more deeply. Your kidneys filter more harmful substances from your body, and your digestive system slows to better absorb nutrients. Your hormones prepare your breasts to make milk. All of these changes require adaptation and may stress your body. For this reason—and because the health of your baby is intimately linked with your own health—it's essential to take good care of yourself. This involves going faithfully to your prenatal appointments, eating well, getting exercise and plenty of rest, and avoiding harmful substances.

- **Get regular prenatal care.** During pregnancy, it's essential to get regular prenatal checkups to monitor your health and the health of your baby.

- **Eat right.** Your diet should include the usual components of a well-balanced diet: plenty of whole grains, vegetables, fruits, low-fat dairy foods, and lean proteins, especially fish rich in omega-3 fatty acids. There is solid research indicating that eating plenty of low-mercury fish with omega-3s during pregnancy enhances fetal brain and nervous system development. As far as we know, fish oil supplements—an alternative source of omega-3s—do not contain mercury. In Europe, doctors recommend that pregnant women take a 200 milligram supplement of DHA, a type of omega-3 fatty acid. Although this is not recommended in the United States, I believe that it should be now that we have abundant data on the benefits of omega-3s to fetal brain development. In addition, during pregnancy you have specific nutritional needs, including folic acid and iron. Your doctor may recommend that you take a prenatal supplement, but there is little data on the benefits of supplements apart from folic acid and iron.

  Some foods may contain substances or infectious agents harmful to your baby. You should avoid:
  - Raw fish, especially raw shellfish; fish with high levels of mercury, including swordfish, shark, king mackerel, tilefish, and blue-fin tuna; refrigerated smoked seafood
  - Luncheon meats, hot dogs, refrigerated pâtés, and meat spreads
  - Raw or lightly cooked eggs
  - Soft cheeses and other foods made with unpasteurized milk
  - Unpasteurized juices
  - Raw vegetable sprouts, such as alfalfa, mung bean, and radish
  - Herbal supplements

- **Gain the appropriate amount of weight.** There is more and more evidence that overeating and gaining too much weight during pregnancy may raise your baby's risk of developing chronic diseases in adulthood, such as type 2 diabetes and heart disease. The Institute of Medicine guidelines recommend the following:
  - **If you are underweight,** gain up to 40 pounds.
  - **If you are ideal weight,** gain 25 to 30 pounds.
  - **If you are overweight or obese,** gain no more than 15 pounds.

  Pregnancy is not a time to attempt weight loss.

- **Get regular exercise.** When you're pregnant, it's important to continue exercising, for your health and the health of your baby. If you have been inactive, pregnancy is a perfect time to start becoming more active. Research suggests that regular exercise during pregnancy can help prevent gestational diabetes (diabetes that develops for the first time during pregnancy)—and for those women who already have it, bring the condition under control.

Most women can and should exercise during pregnancy. Check with your health care provider first to make sure there are no medical reasons for you to avoid physical activity, such as heart or lung disease, incompetent cervix, placenta previa, multiple pregnancy, preterm labor, or hypertension. If you get the green light, you should try to get at least 150 minutes of moderate exercise per week. Walking and swimming are great activities. You want to avoid activities that put you at risk for falling (e.g., horseback riding) or for excessively high body temperature (such as exercising in the extreme heat). If you experience symptoms such as dizziness, labored breathing, headache, chest pains, muscle weakness, vaginal bleeding or leakage of fluid, or preterm labor, stop exercising immediately and call your health care provider.

If you have been very active prior to becoming pregnant, you should be able to continue being active for the first two trimesters unless your doctor tells you otherwise. Generally, very active women need to reduce the intensity and volume of exercise as their pregnancy progresses.

- **Enjoy having sex** as long as it's comfortable for you. Unless you have a high-risk pregnancy, sex during pregnancy is safe for both you and your baby. Ask for guidance from your health care provider. It's vital to avoid STDs while you're pregnant, so be sure to practice safe sex: Have sex with only one partner who has no other sexual partners and/or use a condom.
- **Avoid excessive stress and get plenty of rest.**
- **Avoid harmful substances** that can damage your baby, including:
  - Alcohol
  - Tobacco
  - Illegal drugs
- **Avoid medications and herbal preparations** that may cause birth defects, low birth weight, or other damage to your baby. These include prescription drugs such as isotretinoin (Accutane), a treatment for severe acne; drugs for psoriasis such as etretinate (Tegison) and acitretin (Soriatane); thalidomide; and ACE inhibitors used to treat high blood pressure (such as captopril and enalapril). Nonprescription medications such as ibuprofen (Advil) and aspirin and herbal supplements may also be harmful.
- **Avoid exposure to unnecessary radiation such as x-rays.**

PREGNANCY AFTER AGE 35

Some 20 percent of women in this country have their first child after the age of 35. Most deliver healthy babies. But women who get pregnant in their mid- to late thirties and forties do face some special risks:

- **Miscarriage.** For women in their twenties, the rate of miscarriage is about one in ten. The risk rises to one in five during the late thirties, and one in two in the early forties.
- **Pregnancy-related complications.** Older women also run a higher risk of pregnancy-related complications, such as high blood pressure, gestational diabetes, and placenta previa, which can lead to Cesarean delivery. (About 47 percent of first-time mothers over age 40 have a Cesarean delivery, compared with about 21 percent of first-time mothers under age 30.)
- **Multiple births.** Older mothers have a higher risk of multiple births in part because of greater use of fertility treatment or assisted reproduction technologies.

RISK OF DOWN SYNDROME

It is important for women to know that their risk of having a baby with Down syndrome increases significantly with age. Down syndrome (also known as trisomy 21) is a condition in which an extra copy of chromosome 21 causes delays in development, resulting in intellectual disabilities from mild to severe.

Chance of having a baby with Down syndrome

AGE	RISK
25	1 in 1,250
30	1 in 1,000
35	1 in 400
40	1 in 100
45	1 in 30
49	1 in 10

- **Birth defects.** Older mothers have a greater likelihood of having babies with chromosomal birth defects, such as Down syndrome. (See the box Risk of Down Syndrome at left.) Experts used to recommend that pregnant women age 35 and older get prenatal testing such as amniocentesis or chorionic villus sampling to diagnose or rule out chromosomal problems. But both procedures carry a small risk of miscarriage. We now have less invasive blood and ultrasound tests that can predict the risk of Down syndrome. Consult with your health care provider to weigh the risk against the value of knowing the test results.
- **Premature delivery.** Women over age 40 are 40 percent more likely than younger mothers to deliver prematurely, before 37 weeks.

Because of these special risks, it's especially important for women over 35 to get good prenatal care. Keep in mind that most problems that arise can be successfully treated, and most women in this age group have healthy pregnancies and healthy babies.

POSTPARTUM ISSUES

The postpartum period after your baby arrives is technically defined as the 6 weeks following delivery. For many women, this is a time of physical and emotional upheaval as severe as the changes experienced during pregnancy. About 8 out of 10 new moms feel sore, sad, anxious, and irritable in the days and weeks after delivery. It's important to recognize that giving birth to a baby is exhausting, and that it will take time for your body and mind to recover. It may take many weeks before you begin to feel like yourself again. Gradually increase your activity, but be sure to pay attention to your body's signals. If you feel tired, slow down. Get as much rest as you can, especially when your baby sleeps. Put off all unimportant tasks, limit visitors, and avoid any strenuous work. Ask for help from dependable friends and relatives with household necessities such as grocery shopping, cleaning, laundry, and making meals. Remember that the best way to care for your baby is to care for yourself.

Here are some things to expect in the 4 to 6 weeks after delivery:

- Postpartum blues and postpartum depression
- Vaginal soreness

- Vaginal discharge
- Afterpains
- Difficulties with urination
- Hemorrhoids
- Hot flashes and night sweats as your hormones readjust
- Sore breasts
- Temporary skin changes and/or hair loss
- Disinterest in sex
- Six-week postpartum checkup

After six weeks, you should see your health care provider for a checkup. This may include an examination of your vagina, cervix, and uterus to make sure you're healing well, a breast exam, and weight and blood pressure checks. If any postpartum issues noted above are still a concern for you, this is a good opportunity to discuss them and seek help.

BREASTFEEDING

Most of us are aware that breastfeeding is good for babies. Breast milk contains the proper balance of nutrients to help babies grow, as well as antibodies to protect them against infections, and infants find it easier to digest breast milk than commercial formula.

Less well known are the benefits to your own health. When your baby nurses, your body releases oxytocin, a hormone that makes your uterus contract and shrink. The pleasure of the close interaction and the satisfaction of feeding your baby can help alleviate postpartum blues. Breastfeeding can also help you lose weight. And finally, there is evidence to suggest that it may have a protective effect against the later development of some types of cancer and certain risk factors for heart disease.

But breastfeeding can be a challenging task, requiring persistence and practice, especially in the first few weeks after the baby is born. To learn proper technique, be sure to ask for guidance from a maternity nurse or lactation support specialist. To keep up your milk supply, it's a good idea to feed your baby frequently, because this stimulates your breasts to make more milk.

I had expected breastfeeding to be very easy, and it wasn't. I got mastitis several times—one of the most painful conditions I've ever experienced. Luckily, nursing, hot baths, and medication cleared up the infections quickly. With time, I became very comfortable nursing my babies at home and in public.

When you're nursing, make sure you're in a comfortable place with good back support; hold your baby close to you. Keep up your nutrition and try to limit your intake of caffeine and alcohol. Follow these tips for taking good care of your nipples:

- Let them air-dry after you breastfeed and keep them dry between feedings.
- Keep them free of cleansers when you bathe.
- Use olive oil or another natural oil if they're dry or cracked.

If you're having trouble, don't be discouraged. Get help from a lactation consultant or your pediatrician if you need it, especially if you're experiencing pain during breastfeeding or your baby is not gaining weight.

WEIGHT CONTROL AFTER PREGNANCY

If you're like most women, you'll be keen on getting your body back after pregnancy. You would love nothing better than to toss out those maternity shirts and elastic pants and squeeze into your beloved skinny jeans. But few women bounce right back to their normal weight after pregnancy and delivery. Typical weight gain during a normal pregnancy is 25 to 35 pounds. How a 7-pound baby can create so much additional body weight in its mother is a mystery to many of us. Most women lose about 10 to 15 pounds during birth and a little additional weight during the first week after delivery. However, reclaiming your old, pre-pregnancy body takes time, perhaps 6 months or longer. After all, it took you a year to get that way; it typically takes a year to get back. The best plan is slow, gradual weight loss (about a ½ pound a week), achieved by nursing, healthy eating, regular exercise, and sufficient sleep.

5

Menopause

I'm now fifty and just recently hit menopause. Last year I experienced my first hot flashes, and recently, my periods came to an end. After I got a hormone test from my OB-GYN, she sent me an e-mail saying, "Well, it looks like you've crossed to the other side. Watch your waist." I was surprised by how happy I was to be finished with my periods. For some women, I know, this is not necessarily a milestone to celebrate. But I was elated to have made it through one of life's major passages.

In simple terms, menopause is when a woman stops having menstrual periods, signaling the end of her fertility. It's not a single event but a gradual process that occurs in stages over several years' time. It's usually confirmed by the absence of a period for a full year (absent other obvious causes). It takes place, on average, between the ages of 40 and 58, but some women may go through it as early as their thirties and, in rare cases, as late as their sixties. Onset of menopause may occur earlier than normal as a result of genetics, autoimmune disorders, or medical intervention, such as surgical removal of the ovaries or chemotherapy or radiation that damages the ovaries.

Though there are definite drawbacks to menopause, such as the loss of estrogen (which raises our risk of osteoporosis) and creeping weight gain, there are also advantages: no more menstrual issues and no need for birth control. I'm ecstatic to be done with menstruation. I love knowing that I won't ever again have to struggle to change a tampon when I'm mountain climbing or worry about getting my period while running a race!

Menopause is often called the "change of life," an expression that resonates with many women, because it often coincides with other emotional, social, and physical changes. It's a time when women tend to be well established in their careers and free of the responsibility of caring for young children. Sometimes, menopause coincides with an empty nest or contemplation of retirement or cutting back to part-time work to explore personal interests. It's also a time of heightened risk of heart disease, osteoporosis, and breast cancer. Fortunately, there are many things you can do, from lifestyle changes to temporary hormone therapy, to minimize the unpleasant physical symptoms of menopause and reduce your risk of health problems.

We've come a long way in our understanding of menopause in the past few decades, and today there are plenty of good options for smoothly navigating its phases. Some women do not like using the term *symptoms* to describe the common changes (hot flashes, irregular periods, mood swings, etc.) that often accompany the transition period leading up to menopause because it suggests disease. It's important to recognize that menopause is not an illness or a disease but a natural, normal consequence of aging ovaries, which produce lower levels of estrogen and other hormones. Up to 20 percent of women sail through this period without experiencing any physical signs; about 70 percent endure some troublesome changes; and about 10 percent have severe symptoms.

The bottom line is that menopause is a perfectly natural process—not something that needs to be treated unless excessive hot flashes or other symptoms make you intolerably uncomfortable or deprive you of sleep.

The gradual transition of menopause occurs in three stages:

- **Perimenopause.** Perimenopause is the period leading up to menopause. Signs of this transition may begin some 2 to 8 years before a woman's menstrual periods end. The physical changes women experience during perimenopause are the result of shifting levels of ovarian hormones, including estrogen. These include irregular menstrual periods, hot flashes, sleep disturbances, mood swings, and, sometimes, vaginal dryness. Though fertility is low during this period, it's important to continue to use birth control if you do not wish to become pregnant: Pregnancy is still possible until a full year after your final menstrual period.

  If you begin to experience signs of perimenopause, it's a good idea to keep a careful record of your menstrual cycles and your symptoms. This will give you insight into the changes you're experiencing and will provide helpful information to discuss with your health care provider. Keep a notebook on your bedside table or in the bathroom and note when you have your periods, how long they are, and any other symptoms you may have. If your symptoms get so bad that you need help, this record can give your health care provider useful data.

- **Menopause.** Menopause itself occurs when your ovaries make so little estrogen and other ovarian hormones that your reproductive cycles stop altogether. The decreased levels of estrogen circulating in your body thin your uterine lining and halt your menstrual periods. Menopause is verified by the absence of a period for 12 consecutive months. Sometimes a blood test that measures levels of follicle-stimulating hormone (FSH) is used to confirm menopause. (FSH greater than 40 mIU/mL is a generally accepted indicator of menopause.) However, this test is not considered completely reliable, because FSH levels may vary during perimenopause. The lower levels of estrogen and other ovarian hormones and the higher levels of FSH and luteinizing hormone that mark menopause are responsible for the symptoms linked with it.

- **Postmenopause.** Postmenopause refers to all of the years following menopause (after your periods have ceased for a year or longer). This period is not the end of femininity or sexuality. Far from it. For many women, this is a golden age when they're liberated from worries about birth control, pregnancy, and periods; when their kids are grown and they have more freedom with their time; when they have more economic security, patience, and wisdom. Many postmenopausal women describe feeling happier overall, with renewed energy for work and greater libido. (Unfortunately, it is also a time when many women face later life without a partner because of divorce or death.)

SIGNS AND SYMPTOMS OF PERIMENOPAUSE

The changes experienced during perimenopause vary a great deal from one woman to the next: Some women have few or no signs or symptoms; others have one or more troublesome physical and emotional symptoms. The list below may seem daunting, but remember that there are several ways of managing these problems, and some women escape them altogether.

Among the most common signs are:

- **Irregular periods.** Changes in both menstrual flow and frequency of periods often characterize perimenopause. The cause is changes in the levels of estrogen and progesterone produced by the ovaries. Some 9 out of 10 women experience irregular periods for 4 to 8 years before menopause. Often, this irregularity takes the form of shortened cycles, longer or shorter periods of bleeding, lighter or heavier flow, or skipped periods.

- **Hot flashes.** Feeling beet red and overheated? Hot flashes are the most common cause of perimenopausal and menopausal discomfort, affecting some 75 to 85 percent of women. Though their cause is still a mystery, experts suspect they come about because of perimenopausal changes in the hypothalamus, the part of the brain that regulates our body temperature. It is thought that a hot flash occurs when your hypothalamus mistakenly responds as if your body were too warm. It triggers events to cool you off, spurring perspiration and dilating blood vessels near your skin surface to increase bloodflow there and release body heat (hence that flushed look). Hot flashes tend to last from a few seconds to several minutes and are sometimes accompanied by feelings of anxiety, irritability, and rapid heartbeat. Most women experience them for 3 to 5 years, though some are spared altogether and others have them well into their seventies and eighties. As I'm editing this chapter, I'm experiencing about 10 a day, but they're only a minor annoyance.

- **Sleep disruption.** When hot flashes occur at night, they can cause heavy perspiration, or night sweating, which may disrupt sleep. However, a new study suggests that some of the sleep troubles women typically blame on hot flashes may in fact be caused by true sleep disorders such as sleep apnea. If you are experiencing serious sleep disruption, you should consult with your doctor to see whether you're suffering from an underlying sleep disorder.

- **Mood swings.** Many women experience irritability, anxiety, and mild depression during perimenopause. The culprit may be fatigue from sleep loss. For most women, these emotional swings are temporary and manageable through healthy lifestyle adjustments.

- **Forgetfulness.** Some women experience memory lapses or forgetfulness during menopause. For me, this is the most distressing aspect of menopause. I find that I don't have the recall I once had. Memory issues were at one time chalked up to the effects of diminished estrogen on the brain. However, recent studies show that menopausal women show no sign of mental decline from estrogen loss. Instead, the memory issues may result from loss of sleep or from stress due to juggling work and family or caretaking adolescents or aging parents. Stress-reduction techniques can help. (See Chapter 25.) I also have a few tricks to help my memory: I always have a notepad on my desk or on the kitchen counter to jot down lists and notes to myself, and I try to put things I need to keep track of on a daily basis—keys or cell phone or glasses—in the same spot on a table next to the door or on my desk.

- **Vaginal and urinary problems.** Low levels of estrogen may cause vaginal tissues to become drier and less elastic. This can make sexual intercourse painful. Diminishing estrogen may also contribute to thinning of the lining of the urethra (the outlet for the bladder), causing leaking of urine and recurring urinary tract infections (UTIs).

- **Changes in sexual function.** Sexual arousal and desire may decrease during menopause for a variety of reasons, including lower levels of androgen, sleep disturbance, fatigue, mood swings, stressors, and vaginal dryness. It should be noted, however, that androgen levels do not fall off suddenly at menopause but rather taper over a woman's lifetime.

- **Loss of bone.** With diminishing estrogen, you start to lose bone more rapidly than you replace it, putting you at greater risk for osteoporosis.

- **Weight and waist gain.** The midlife weight gain that many women experience is not due to menopause or hormonal changes but to slowing metabolism brought on by aging and lifestyle. I believe that some weight gain and waist expansion is inevitable at this time of life. The key is to keep both of these areas of midlife expansion in check as much as you can. It may be necessary to reduce your consumption by a few hundred calories per day and increase your daily physical activity.

- **Shifting cholesterol.** Lower levels of estrogen may lead to shifts in blood cholesterol, increasing low-density lipoprotein (LDL), or "bad" cholesterol. This can boost your risk of heart disease.

STRATEGIES (AND TREATMENTS) FOR EASING MENOPAUSAL SYMPTOMS

The key to good health during perimenopause and beyond is healthy behavior, a positive attitude, and regular checkups, including Pap tests. (It also helps to have a supportive partner.) To minimize the changes associated with perimenopause, it's a good idea to exercise regularly—at *least* 30 minutes of moderate-intensity physical activity most days; eat a nutritious diet (including the usual balance of fruits, vegetables, and whole grains, and 1,300 to 1,500 milligrams of calcium and 1,000 IU of vitamin D each day); alleviate stress with relaxation techniques; and stay away from smoking.

In addition, here are some steps to ease the most common symptoms of perimenopause:

- **Regulate irregular periods.** Prescription hormones, such as low-dose oral contraceptives, can help regulate cycles. For more severe cases, involving heavy or otherwise abnormal bleeding or for anatomical issues such as fibroids that are contributing to the problem, surgical options are available, ranging from laparoscopy to hysterectomy.

- **Chill hot flashes.** Fortunately, a number of lifestyle changes can ease the discomfort of mild hot flashes:
  - Try one of the most useful and old-fashioned tools for cooling a hot flash: a handheld fan of any kind.
  - Dress in layers so that you can remove clothing when you feel too warm.
  - Sleep in a cool room.
  - Exercise regularly.
  - Identify your own hot flash "triggers" and avoid them. Triggers often include smoking, alcohol, caffeine, spicy foods, hot drinks, or a hot environment, indoors or out.
  - Try stress-reduction techniques such as deep breathing, yoga, and meditation. (See Chapter 25.)
  - If you get hot flashes at night, put an ice pack under your pillow and turn your pillow over when you wake up hot.
  - Wash your hands in cold water.

  Some women experience relief from hot flashes from over-the-counter and herbal therapies, such as topical progesterone creams, vitamin E (in supplement form, with less than 400 IU daily), foods with isoflavones (e.g., chickpeas, soybeans, and other legumes), which have weak estrogen-like effects, and black cohosh pills. However, there's little scientific evidence to prove the efficacy of these remedies: They may owe their impact to the power of the placebo effect. Studies show that women who took a placebo reported up to a 40 percent reduction in hot flashes.

If you've had breast cancer, be sure to talk with your health care provider before taking pills containing isoflavone, because they may increase cancer risk.

Hot flashes typically fade on their own, but if yours are severe and are causing you distress or interfering with daily life, discuss with your health care provider the option of taking estrogen for the short term, the most effective treatment.

- **Restoring restful sleep.** To increase your likelihood of getting a good night's sleep, be sure to avoid alcohol, caffeine, and nicotine later in the day, and especially in the evening. Get regular exercise during the day. In your bedroom, create an environment conducive to sleep—cool, dark, and quiet. Cultivate a nighttime routine that encourages sleep, such as reading, taking a warm bath, and/or drinking a cup of chamomile tea. Use relaxation techniques such as deep breathing or progressive muscle relaxation. If you still suffer from serious sleep disturbances, you should consult with your health care provider.

- **Stabilizing mood.** Make sure you take time for yourself. Emotional equilibrium depends on balancing your obligations of work and caring for others with your own need for self-nurture. It may also help to try stress-beating techniques such as deep breathing, yoga, massage, taking time to talk with friends, laughing, and setting time aside for activities you find pleasurable. If you don't get relief from these strategies, see your health care provider. (See also Chapter 23.)

- **Addressing vaginal problems.** Regular sexual activity helps minimize the effects of vaginal drying by boosting bloodflow to vaginal tissues. For many women, water-soluble lubricants such as Astroglide or K-Y jelly can help. If discomfort or pain persists, vaginal estrogens in the form of a cream, a tablet, or a ring may provide relief.

- **Addressing urinary problems.** To manage urinary incontinence, practice Kegel exercises (see the box Kegeling on page 145), drink plenty of water, and avoid foods and drinks that may irritate the bladder, including those high in caffeine and acid. If these measures do not help, you may wish to consult a continence educator or physician. To minimize the risk of UTIs, practice good hygiene, wiping from front to back. Avoid tight pants, drink cranberry juice, and stay away from irritants such as feminine hygiene products and scented bath products. Wear underwear made of one of the new quick-drying, antibacterial synthetic materials. (See the box Über Undies on page 13.) If you have become incontinent and the usual self-help remedies have not worked for you, see your health care provider. There are a number of options available to address the problem. (See Chapter 11.)

WHEN TO SEEK MEDICAL HELP

You should consult with your health care provider if you have any of the following symptoms, which may indicate an underlying gynecological health issue:

- Much heavier periods than usual (requiring a change of tampons or pads every couple of hours), with or without clots
- Periods lasting longer than 7 days (or 2 or 3 days longer than your usual period)
- Frequent periods (fewer than 21 days apart)
- Spotting or bleeding between periods
- Bleeding from the vagina after sexual intercourse
- Hot flashes that are interfering with your sleep or making your life miserable
- Any other symptom that is affecting your quality of life

HORMONE THERAPY

Hormone therapy (HT) is not recommended for use by every woman going through menopause. Women need to remember that menopausal symptoms are perfectly normal. Our bodies are designed to function with less circulating estrogen after menopause. However, HT is an option for women who seek relief from severe menopausal symptoms. It is still the most effective therapy to relieve hot flashes, night sweats, and vaginal dryness. Current recommendations are for short-term use at the lowest possible dose.

A little background: Until 2002, HT was the most common treatment for menopausal symptoms such as hot flashes and vaginal dryness and to protect against osteoporosis and cardiovascular disease. That year, the Women's Health Initiative (WHI), a comprehensive study of HT among postmenopausal women, reported its results. The WHI showed a small increased risk of breast cancer, blood clotting disease, stroke, and coronary artery disease among women taking combination estrogen-progestin therapy (Prempro) and a slightly increased risk of stroke for women taking estrogen-only therapy (Premarin). In addition, the study found that women taking either the combination or the estrogen-only therapy experienced an increase in mammography abnormalities. Most of these were false-positive results due to the increase in the density of breast tissue caused by exposure to estrogen. The studies also suggested that HT is *not* effective against memory loss, heart disease, heart attack, or stroke.

On the positive side, the WHI studies reported that women on HT (both combination and estrogen only) had a slightly lowered risk of osteoporosis and colon cancer.

Questions remain about the benefits and risks of HT, and follow-up studies are under way to resolve them. Participants in the original WHI study were older postmenopausal women; the new studies are aimed at determining whether the results can be applied to younger women who start HT early in menopause. However, because of the health concerns reported in the WHI study, many women have chosen to halt HT, and health care providers no longer routinely prescribe it.

These sorts of studies tell us what is right for a population but not necessarily for an individual. Before deciding on any form of treatment, talk with your health care provider about the risks and benefits in light of your personal and family medical history. In general, women with breast cancer or a history of blood clots should not take HT. If you decide to use HT to treat menopausal symptoms, the hormones should be taken in the smallest dose for the shortest time possible. Check regularly with your health care provider to see whether you still need treatment.

The new approach to HT involves tailoring treatment to your primary symptoms. Numerous forms are available, ranging from pills to patches to creams to gels, which offer different doses and different combinations of estrogen and progestin. To address specific symptoms, several forms of hormone therapy have been approved by the FDA:

FOR BOTH VAGINAL DRYNESS AND HOT FLASHES

- **Transdermal gel.** Estradiol gel is applied once a day to the arm to treat both vaginal discomfort and severe hot flashes.
- **Evamist (estradiol transdermal spray).** Evamist is a low-dose estrogen spray hormone therapy applied one to three times daily on the inner forearm.

FOR VAGINAL DRYNESS

- **Vaginal cream.** These include creams such as Estrace, Ortho-Dienestrol, Ogen, and Premarin, which release a small amount of estrogen that is absorbed by vaginal tissues.
- **Vaginal tablet.** An estradiol tablet, Vagifem, is inserted into the vagina with a disposable applicator.
- **Vaginal ring.** The estradiol ring (Estring) is a small silicone ring, inserted into the vagina like a diaphragm, that releases estrogen for 3 months. The estradiol-acetate ring (Femring) is used both for vaginal symptoms and to treat severe hot flashes and night sweats.

FOR HOT FLASHES AND NIGHT SWEATS

- **Oral.** Most HT used to treat hot flashes, night sweats, and vaginal dryness comes in pill form.
- **Lotion.** A white emulsion containing estrogen is applied to the thighs and calves on a daily basis to treat moderate to severe hot flashes and night sweats.
- **Patches.** Dime- to half-dollar-size estrogen patches of various doses, applied to the abdomen or upper buttock, are used for the treatment of hot flashes and vaginal discomfort.
- **Vaginal ring.** The estradiol-acetate ring (Femring) is used to treat severe hot flashes and night sweats, in addition to vaginal symptoms.

FOR MOOD SWINGS

HT is not effective in treating mood issues. However, your health care provider may recommend using low doses of an antidepressant medication. Before taking medications that may have side effects, consider other lifestyle options such as psychotherapy and increasing your physical activity levels.

There are several alternative drug treatments for hot flashes, such as Venflaxine and Fluoxetine, Gabapentin and Clonidine in pill or patch form.

productive Choices Fertility and Pregn
enopause Sexual Abuse and Sexual A
in Teeth Hair and Nails Body Weigh
etabolism Blood Sugar Eating and Excr
scles Bones Joints Heart and Blood L
d Respiration Common Infectious Dis
toimmune Disease Cancer Vision He
ell, Taste, and Touch Mental Health
ice Abuse Making Change Managing
d Sleeping Well Shifting Your Food Env
nt Getting Active Screenings and H
intenance Reproduction Sexuality and
Health Reproductive Choices Fertilit
egnancy Menopause Sexual Abuse and
Assault Skin Teeth Hair and Nails
ght and Metabolism Blood Sugar E
d Excreting Muscles Bones Joints Hear
od Lungs and Respiration Common I
us Diseases Autoimmune Disease Ca

PART II

Beauty Inside and Out

I'll make a confession here: I'm the kind of woman who takes pride in the fact that I didn't wear makeup for my own wedding—not even lipstick. When I look back at my wedding photos today, I'm really happy with the way I look. Though it may sound trite, I've always believed that beauty radiates from within; it comes from how you feel about yourself and how healthy and animated you are, not from the length of your eyelashes, the size of your breasts, or the texture of your skin.

When it comes to the façade we present to the world, good health is at least 80 percent of the game. Almost every year, I take a group of women on a weeklong mountain climbing expedition. We leave behind most of our normal toiletries and cosmetics, from basics such as soap and shampoo to luxuries such as lipstick and foundation. For some women, the Spartan conditions—no showering for a week, using only disposable wipes for hygiene—take some getting used to. But nearly all of them say afterward that this aspect of the experience was liberating. They're often surprised to realize that they're just fine with their dirty hair or crow's-feet. In fact, they say, it's wonderful to go for 7 or 8 days without looking in a mirror, to feel the glow from within. Our photos show these women on the peaks of mountains sporting their knit hats and cold red noses, radiant and beautiful!

There's no question that we need to take good care of our skin, teeth, hair, and nails, especially as we enter midlife and later years. While it's important to accept the natural effects of aging—and to a degree, let nature take its course—there are a few things we can do to minimize age-related changes. For me, this involves some simple strategies for helping my skin, hair, and nails maintain their health and strength, rather than resorting to surgery or complicated regimens involving multiple beauty products.

As far as cosmetics are concerned, I'm a minimalist. When I go into my teenage daughters' shared bathroom, I have to laugh. Both of my girls have always had lovely skin and hair. And yet the counters and cupboards are jammed with more cosmetics and hair and skin products than you can imagine. I have no idea what all of these potions do.

My own personal beauty routine is spare by comparison: It includes bathing on a daily basis, using moisturizing lotion (especially in winter), and applying sunscreen with a sun protection factor (SPF) of 30 or greater if I am going outside for any length of time. Beyond this, I do little. The one time in my life that I got a facial, I ended up with a bright red and inflamed face—which taught me that my skin is sensitive and that I likely have allergies to lanolins and certain animal products. When I give my public talks and make TV appearances, I do wear a little powder, lipstick, and mascara. No doubt these cosmetics improve my appearance. I know there are many women who don't feel their best unless they've put in time in front of the mirror. Every woman has her own beauty routine that's been shaped over the years by numerous influences, such as her family, her culture, her profession, and her comfort level with herself. As Gwyneth Paltrow once said, "Beauty, to me, is about being comfortable in your own skin. That, or a kick-ass red lipstick."

The most important thing is to be happy with who you are and what nature has given you. I find it deeply disturbing that some parents give their daughters the gift of a nose job or breast augmentation for their Sweet Sixteen. After all, beauty really does come in different packages. What we may view as imperfections—moles, crooked teeth, big nose, dense eyebrows, even wrinkles—are markers of our individuality.

To preserve your inner and outer beauty throughout life, I recommend that you follow these **S.M.A.R.T.** guidelines:

1. Protect yourself from the sun (with hat, sunglasses, and sunscreen).
2. Check yourself for skin and mole changes.
3. Cleanse your skin daily with soap and water and moisturize when necessary.
4. Avoid harsh beauty products for skin, hair, teeth, and nails.
5. Be gentle with hair care and minimize blow-dryer use and exposure to extreme heat from straightening and curling irons.
6. Keep nails clean and clipped.
7. Brush and floss your teeth daily.
8. See your dentist regularly.

6

Skin

If you had to give up a single organ, my guess is that your last choice would be your skin. The largest organ in your body (covering about 21 square feet and making up 16 percent of your body weight), it's also far and away the most beautiful—at its best, smooth and suffused with a healthy glow from within.

Skin is our shield, our guardian against excessive heat or cold, light, infection, and injury. It is our alchemist, transforming sunlight into a nutrient essential for health, vitamin D. It is a subtle communicator and a key sensor. Think of the pallor of fear, the flush of excitement, the blush of embarrassment. Think of the tingling pleasure of soft stroking on skin or the warning sear of a burn from a hot oven or steaming kettle. When we're happy and well, our skin glows; when we're ill, it reveals our poor health. And yet, as much as we value our skin, we tend to abuse it more than any other part of our bodies. We scour it with harsh soaps, detergents, and facials; we subject it to scrapes and cuts, to desiccating wind and extreme temperatures; we overexpose it to radiation and the damaging rays of the sun. And many women nip and tuck it as it ages.

You have only one skin; it's impossible to overemphasize the importance of keeping it in good shape. What are the best ways to protect, nourish, and improve this extraordinary organ?

THE SKINNY ON SKIN

Skin is the body's paramount protector thanks in large part to its outer layer, the epidermis. Though paper-thin, the epidermis is tough, elastic, waterproof, stain-resistant, self-replenishing, and breathable. The outermost layer of the epidermis consists of dead cells made of special fibrous proteins called keratins (from the Greek word *keratos*, meaning "horn"). These keratins, together with fatty lipids, form a hard shield that keeps in the body's natural moisture and keeps out excessive water, chemical irritants, allergens, and invading organisms. Dead epidermal cells are continually sloughed off and replaced every month or so by new ones. The epidermis also houses cells that make melanin, the dark pigment responsible for skin's color and its primary protection from the sun's damaging rays.

Just beneath the epidermis lies the dermis. This thick, soft layer is permeated with collagen and elastin, proteins that make skin not only strong and firm but also supple and elastic—at least until age and sun exposure break them down. The dermis is peppered with hair follicles, sweat glands, and oil-secreting (sebaceous) glands, and laced with blood vessels and exquisitely sensitive nerve endings—all guarded by roving white blood cells on the lookout for injured tissue or intruding microorganisms. The sebaceous glands, which abound in the face, scalp, chest, and genitals, exude waxy oil that lubricates

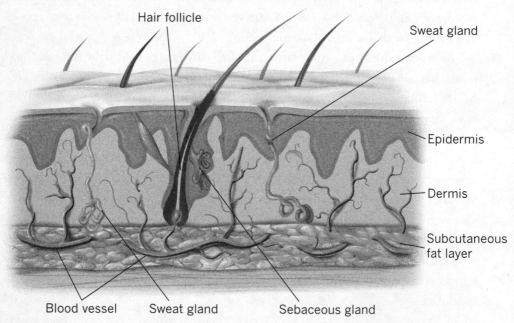

Hair follicle

Sweat gland

Epidermis

Dermis

Subcutaneous fat layer

Blood vessel   Sweat gland   Sebaceous gland

Skin has three layers: The outermost layer is the epidermis, a thick layer of living epidermal cells topped by a sheet of dead cells, which forms a waterproof shield at the surface. Within the epidermis are special cells called melanocytes, which make melanin, the substance that gives your skin color. The middle layer, the dermis, contains blood vessels, sweat glands and sebaceous oil glands, hair follicles, and nerve endings, which register hot and cold and pressure changes. The deepest layer is the subcutaneous fat layer, made mostly of fat, which insulates and cushions your body.

and shields the outer skin. The blood vessels and sweat glands help keep body temperature constant. All of this in an envelope of flesh only a couple of millimeters thick.

WHAT AFFECTS THE WAY YOUR SKIN LOOKS AND FEELS?

A host of factors may shape your skin's appearance and texture, from air pollution and climate to allergies and other health issues you may have, as well as medications you may be taking. Among the most important factors are:

Your skin condition. Some dermatologists divide skin into four basic groups:

Normal (no dry areas; no oily areas)
Oily (shiny skin, with no dry areas)
Dry (no oily areas; some flaking)
Combination (both oily and dry areas)

However, it's important to note that your skin, like the rest of your body, is in a constant state of flux, changing with age, hormonal and weight fluctuations, stress, seasons, and sun exposure.

Your age. As you grow older, your skin becomes drier and less elastic. Your glands produce less oil and sweat, and the collagen and elastin in the dermis break down—especially if they've been exposed to excess sunlight—resulting in wrinkles, loose skin, and a tendency to bruise more easily. After menopause, the outer layer of your epidermis renews itself more slowly. As skin thins and grows more transparent, blood vessels stand out more prominently. But many of the changes we associate with aging are in fact the result of sun damage.

Sun exposure. This is the biggest threat to your skin. Excessive exposure to sunlight causes damage to the skin known as photoaging—deep wrinkling, coarseness, a leathery texture—and an increased risk of skin cancer, including melanoma. Sun overexposure early in life increases the risk for melanoma. Chronic, excessive sun exposure throughout life boosts the incidence of the more common skin cancers, basal cell carcinoma and squamous cell carcinoma.

Whether you smoke. Smoking prematurely ages skin by decreasing bloodflow to it and by boosting levels of enzymes called matrix metalloproteinases (MMPs) that degrade collagen. In some people, it may create lines on the face, including crow's-feet, lip lines, and creasing known as marionette lines.

Your diet. Poor nutrition affects the skin's appearance and can accelerate skin aging.

Your hormonal cycles. The hormonal changes that occur during menstrual cycles can cause acne outbreaks, particularly cysts on the chin or jaw line, a day or two before menstruation begins. These cysts are not dangerous, but they can be annoying and may last for several weeks. Some women take oral antibiotics to prevent their occurrence. At menopause, lower estrogen levels may cause skin to thin, lose collagen, and replace its cells more slowly. Although hormone therapy (HT) can reduce these effects, skin condition alone is not a good reason to take HT because of its risks.

Alcohol intake. Here is another reason not to drink in excess. Heavy drinkers are at much greater risk for spider veins on the face, along with ruddy noses and cheeks.

MAINTAINING NATURAL SKIN HEALTH

Keeping your skin healthy and beautiful is not rocket science. But because women's skin is thinner and drier than men's skin, it's more vulnerable to damage caused by sun exposure and smoking and so requires some extra protection. Following a few simple guidelines, such as improving your nutrition and learning basic techniques for good skin care, can go a long way toward improving your skin's appearance.

One healthy skin habit I consider vital is wearing sunscreen. Both of my parents had melanomas. Though these were easily treated through removal, they have left scars on my parents' faces and bodies. Knowing that I'm probably vulnerable to these melanomas compels me to be even more cautious about sun exposure. I try to be vigilant by applying each morning a 30 SPF face cream containing broad-spectrum protection against both UVB and UVA rays. I'm still not as good about this as I'd like to be. But I am very diligent about applying sunscreen on days when I know I'm going to be out in the sun for a long time. Here are some basic steps for the care and maintenance of your skin throughout your lifetime:

- If you smoke, stop.
- Avoid sunbathing and tanning salons.
- In midsummer, if you're outside for long stretches of time between 10 a.m. and 4 p.m., dress to protect your skin, with a wide-brimmed hat and long-sleeved shirt.
- Wear sunscreen (for recommendations, see pages 85–86).
- Eat a healthy, balanced diet, as described in Chapter 26.
- Avoid dehydration by drinking plenty of water.

- Avoid excessive alcohol consumption.
- Try to maintain a healthy weight and avoid rapid and frequent weight fluctuations.
- Get enough sleep. We all know that bags under the eyes can be unsightly.
- Check skin often for changes: The best time is after you shower or bathe. Use a full-length mirror and examine yourself from head to toe for any new moles or skin marks or changes in the size, shape, color, or feel of moles, which may signal melanoma. Check also for sores that don't heal and persistent red, scaly spots, which are signs of basal cell carcinoma and squamous cell carcinoma. If you have any cause for concern, see a dermatologist.

YOUR SKIN CARE ROUTINE

In shaping your skin care routine, it's useful to pay attention to your skin condition, which is partly shaped by your genes, and partly by environment and other factors.

Remember that no one's skin is perfect, and the range that's considered "normal" is wide indeed. You may have different types of skin in different areas of your body and even on your face—and these may change from week to week or month to month as hormones fluctuate and weather changes. For instance, some women have oily skin around their nose and dry patches around their eyes. I tend to have dry skin in the winter and oily skin in the summer. Be aware that you may have to use different skin care products on different areas of your skin—a heavier, hydrating cream on your legs and hands, for instance, and perhaps a mild cleanser and oil-free moisturizer on your face. But don't fall into the trap of buying a slew of expensive skin products. Try to accept your skin and its tiny blemishes and flaws and be realistic about what you can expect. Avoid overcleansing or overexfoliating, which can deplete your skin's natural oils.

I find it unsettling that so much marketing of skin and hair products is directed at teenagers and young adults—hence those beauty potions filling the shelves in my daughters' bathroom. I try to reason with them, but often give up and let them have their way (parents must pick their battles!). However, I firmly believe that beyond general cleaning and hydration (and treatment for acne), there is little need for these products.

Dr. Anna Magee, a board-certified practitioner of general and cosmetic dermatology, says that women can keep their skin healthy and vibrant with just a few basic, inexpensive products. For young women who have not yet suffered much sun damage, Dr. Magee suggests using only a mild cleanser, an oil-free moisturizer to hydrate skin, and an effective sunscreen for protection from UV light during the day. Older women with some skin discoloration and sun damage may want to also use a heavier moisturizer, as well as a cream containing glycolic acid to gently exfoliate the skin, reduce fine lines, and "freshen" skin appearance. For the area around the eyes, Dr. Magee recommends an eye cream with vitamin C and antioxidants. Though there is little evidence-based data confirming the effectiveness of ingredients such as glycolic acid and antioxidants, many dermatologists do see some positive effects in their clinical practice.

WASHING

Most of us need to wash our skin only once a day, in the evening. Use a soft terrycloth washcloth or sponge, lukewarm water, and a gentle cleanser. If you have very dry skin, you may want to restrict your use of soap to the face, hands, underarms, feet, and genitals or try moisturizing soaps or beauty bars, which have a lower pH than regular soaps do. If you have oily skin, you can wash in the morning as well, even just by splashing cool water on your face and patting dry. If your skin is very oily, you may wish to use an alcohol-based cleanser. But try not to overcleanse, even if you have acne. Acne is not a surface problem and cannot be washed away.

MOISTURIZING

If you have dry skin, consider using a vaporizer or humidifier during the winter months. Although some dermatologists may tell you to avoid exposure to the cold, drying wind of winter, I say go out into the elements and enjoy your time outside! Skiing, skating, or just taking a walk or run in the cold is good for you. After you shower or bathe in the wintertime, be sure to apply moisturizer.

Many lotions, creams, and ointments help retain moisture. Most effective for very dry skin are ointments, such as Vaseline, which seal in natural skin moisture. But because they're heavy and oily, some women don't like to use them on a regular basis. Creams and some lotions made from oil and water emulsions (e.g., Lubriderm, Nivea, and Eucerin) work well for normal to dry skin. Lotions are light and easy to apply but do little to retain skin moisture except temporarily. It's best to use moisturizer immediately after showering or bathing. Use a towel to pat yourself dry and apply moisturizer while skin is still moist.

If you have very oily skin, you may want to avoid using a moisturizer.

THE 1-2-3s OF SUN EXPOSURE AND SUNSCREEN

Everyone knows that ultraviolet rays from the sun damage skin and cause premature aging, wrinkles, and skin cancer, including the sometimes lethal melanoma. But few of us are aware of the whole story behind sun exposure and sunscreen.

Dr. Magee strongly urges women to consider wearing sun-protective clothing such as lightweight, long-sleeved shirts and hats as a better alternative than sunscreens, which expose skin to an array of chemicals. However, this is not always possible, especially where face and hands are concerned, so the use of sunscreen is often essential. Sunscreens protect the skin by absorbing or reflecting radiation. Chemical sunscreens (the kind that go on invisibly) absorb UV rays and prevent them from interacting with molecules in the skin. Barrier varieties (the visible type often used by lifeguards) reflect photons away from the skin.

According to most dermatologists, all women—but especially those who are fair-skinned—should apply sunscreen every day throughout the year if they get any sun exposure at all. "You should apply full sunblock in all seasons, including winter," says Dr. Magee. How often you apply it depends on your level of outdoor exposure and activity. If you're going to be working indoors all day, it's okay to apply only once, in the morning. If you plan to be outdoors for any stretch of time, such as going for a run or a swim at the pool, you need to apply a waterproof sunscreen about 20 minutes before your sun exposure, and reapply it every 1 to 2 hours that you remain outdoors.

Not all sunscreens are created equal. It's important to look at lotions to make sure they protect against both UVB rays, which burn, and UVA rays, which can penetrate deeper and cause DNA damage in the dermis. Sun protection factor (SPF) ratings can be deceptive, because they indicate only how well a sunscreen protects skin from the sun's UVB rays. Scientists now understand that it's vital to shield yourself from UVA rays as well.

To ensure adequate protection for your skin, follow these guidelines:

Choose your sunscreen carefully. Look for products that protect against UVB rays with an SPF of 30 or higher (applied properly, an SPF 30 sunscreen filters out 98 to 99 percent of UVB) and that also protect against UVA rays with a mix of the following ingredients: avobenzone, oxybenzone, Mexoryl, zinc oxide, and titanium dioxide.

Apply early and often. Sunscreen takes about 20 minutes to absorb into the skin, so it's best to put it on 20 to 30 minutes before going out. After excessive sweating or swimming, or about 2 hours of sun exposure, most sunscreens break down and should be reapplied. Sunblocks with titanium dioxide or zinc oxide last longer, as do some new products with avobenzone, oxybenzone, and Mexoryl, which last about 4 hours.

Protect your lips by using lip balm with an SPF of 15 to 30. Applying sunblock to your lips year-round also helps prevent chapping and cold sores.

Fortunately, gone are the days when sunscreen felt heavy, unpleasant, and sticky. Most of today's lotions and sprays are easily absorbed and light enough to allow the skin to breathe, and many are unscented. It's no longer necessary to walk around smelling like coconut oil or sporting a white mask of zinc oxide to protect against UVA rays. Sunscreen products with UVA-blocking Mexoryl SX or avobenzone are much less visible on the skin.

Sun Exposure and Vitamin D

In my view, limited unprotected sun exposure is a good thing for the body, helping to sustain healthy levels of vitamin D. However, you shouldn't rely on sun exposure alone to provide your body with the vitamin D it needs. Most people will need to take supplements as well. (See Chapter 26.)

Approximately 5 to 15 minutes of sun exposure to the arms, legs, or back without sunscreen between 10 a.m. and 3 p.m. a few times a week during the spring, summer, and fall helps boost vitamin D levels for most people. I will say that it's difficult to provide general guidelines for sun exposure because suggested safe exposure times depend on a variety of factors, among them the time of year, the latitude at which you live, and your skin coloring. For instance, if you live in the northern parts of the United States, your skin can't make any vitamin D from about October to April. If you live in the South, on the other hand, you may be putting yourself at risk for skin cancer with even this little bit of exposure. "This is a tough issue," says Dr. Magee. "If you're fair and you live in, say, Virginia or Maryland or somewhere in the Southwest, and you expose yourself to 20 minutes of unprotected sun exposure on a regular basis, you're likely to get skin cancer."

If your arms and legs get a limited amount of sun exposure from time to time, don't panic. This is healthy for your vitamin D stores. But try never to expose your face to the sun without sunscreen. And if you are outside for extended periods of time, wear a hat and long sleeves or put sunscreen on all exposed areas.

COSMETICS

Cosmetic products are manufactured by a multibillion dollar industry that profits from making you feel as if you are flawed in some way and need cosmetic help. (It relentlessly pursues an "antiaging" message. I prefer to think of the measures we take to stay healthy as we grow older as "pro-aging.") Remember this, and don't be driven to buy something that you really don't need. Some cosmetics can irritate sensitive skin and clog pores; others contain ingredients such as stabilizers and fragrances that cause allergic reactions in some people. Be sure to test products on a small area of skin before applying them generally to avoid an allergic reaction. Some companies, such as Aveda and Aveeno, specialize in beauty products that are free of the more common allergenic ingredients.

If you enjoy cosmetics and find that they make you feel good about yourself, it's fine to use them. Just be aware that some of them contain toxins, and many of the claims made by manufacturers of some cosmetic products—that they can slow down or reverse the effects of aging—are grossly exaggerated.

SWEATING AND ANTIPERSPIRANTS AND DEODORANTS

Sweating is good and healthy! Sweat is our natural coolant. When we exercise or experience excess heat, temperature-sensitive nerves in the skin and body respond by signaling the brain to trigger a flow of sweat, which is released by some two million to four million glands. This liquid spreads across the surface of the skin and evaporates to cool down our body temperature. Recent research suggests that it also contains molecules important for skin surface immunity.

Sweat glands come in two varieties. Eccrine glands produce a clear fluid and are active from birth. They abound everywhere in the body but are especially dense in our foreheads, underarms, palms, and soles. Apocrine glands cluster under the arms and around the nipples and genitals and begin working at puberty. The oily sweat produced by both of these glands is odorless until it draws bacteria, which metabolize the compounds, sometimes generating a pungent odor.

Antiperspirants are designed to prevent the release of sweat by plugging sweat ducts. Deodorants mask odor temporarily with perfumes and antiseptics but do not reduce sweating or eliminate odor. Many women choose to use products that combine both an antiperspirant and a deodorant. Strong antiperspirants usually contain 10 to 15 percent aluminum chloride hexahydrate, which effectively reduces sweat in most people. If you feel you sweat excessively, see your physician. Medications containing higher doses of aluminum chloride are available by prescription.

I don't know why people are so uptight about sweating. I love the feeling of breaking a sweat when I exercise. I also think that our fear of offensive body odor is overblown and that we've been sold a bill of goods by the manufacturers of antiperspirants and deodorants. For most people, washing daily, wearing clean clothes, and shaving underarms will minimize body odor and eliminate the need for deodorants. Shaving does not affect perspiration but it can reduce odor in the short term by preventing pungent sweat from collecting in underarm hair. However, if body odor is a severe problem for you, try washing with an antibacterial soap or using a topical antibiotic on your underarms.

There's an argument to be made for letting alone your body's natural odors. Science is just beginning to understand the subtle chemical communication that may go on between humans through odor production and reception. There may be important signals conveyed in those underarm smells we seem so set on abolishing.

ACNE AND ACNE TREATMENT

Acne—the presence of small pimples, blackheads or whiteheads, or large cysts or nodules on the skin of the face, chest, or back—is not the result of dirt or overconsumption of chocolate or greasy foods, as some suggest. It occurs when the pores or hair follicles become clogged with plugs made from dead skin cells and the oily substance known as sebum. When microorganisms invade, the skin may become red and inflamed.

The condition is most common in women and in adolescents, especially at puberty, when hormonal changes spur the sebaceous glands to make more sebum. In some women, it often pops up during the week before a menstrual period and may worsen around menopause. Severe acne is caused primarily by genetic influences and tends to run in families.

Squeezing pimples to drain them may cause scarring. It's best to wash your face gently with a mild facial soap and avoid using cosmetics that clog pores. For blackheads and whiteheads, you can try using a lotion, cream, or gel with the active ingredient benzoyl peroxide once a day, which dries the skin and unclogs pores. For more serious conditions, you should consult your physician, who may prescribe oral antibiotics or special creams, such as Retin-A or Avita—stronger drying agents containing a form of vitamin A.

FACIALS AND ANTIWRINKLE CREAMS

Wrinkles and loose skin are part of the normal aging process (worsened by overexposure to the sun). In the hopes of defying the normal effects of age and sun exposure on the skin, many women turn to one or more of the hundreds of expensive creams, lotions, and facial treatments marketed as the secret to younger skin.

If you want to sample one of these products, be discriminating and try to evaluate the product's results objectively. Try it out for 6 months. If it seems to help, that's fine. But if you notice little difference, go back to the more inexpensive lotions.

Among the categories of available products are:

Facial masks made of clay, oatmeal, avocado oil, and other substances. Facial masks primarily cleanse the skin and may boost bloodflow temporarily but do little to address the issue of wrinkles or dry skin. Exfoliating or abrasive masks and body scrubs can actually create more problems than they solve. They may irritate skin, and by increasing the rate at which skin sheds dead cells, they can create scaly patches and graying skin.

AHAs (alpha hydroxy acids), also known as "fruit acids." These are compounds derived from dairy products, fruit, or sugarcane. A common AHA is glycolic acid. The prescription creams containing a 4 to 12 percent concentration of AHAs may smooth out dry skin, reduce skin discoloration and superficial wrinkles, and even improve elasticity when used daily over a period of several months. Over-the-counter preparations do little to improve wrinkles. Use of AHAs, however, can lead to redness, irritation, and sun sensitivity.

Retinoids (Renova and Retin-A). Topical retinoic acid, also known as tretinoin, was first used to treat acne. Prescription medications containing retinoids appear to eliminate fine and coarse surface wrinkles by smoothing them out and rejuvenating the outer layer of skin. They must be used daily for months before skin shows improvement and the effects last only as long as the cream is used. Some products may irritate skin and increase sun sensitivity, so it's important to wear sunscreen and protective clothing while using them. Women who are pregnant or planning a pregnancy should avoid them altogether.

COSMETIC PROCEDURES

The options for changing our faces have expanded in recent years, and range from laser resurfacing to full-blown face-lifts and other forms of invasive cosmetic surgery. Far too many of these procedures are performed because women are not happy with some aspect of their lives. They feel that a "new" face would change things for them or would please a partner or someone else. If you are considering these sorts of treatments, make sure that you understand your motives and the full scope of risks and side effects, which may include loss of facial expressiveness and serious discomfort, scarring, or illness.

Here's how I look at it: Wrinkles do not interfere with my work or my family life or with my love of running and mountain climbing. This doesn't mean that I don't sometimes wish them away, but simply that I like my face the way it is and I'm not willing to chase after a more youthful look with surgery. You may have a different take on the matter. But I feel that it's important for women to realize that we are the subjects of aggressive marketing campaigns and advertising dollars for these procedures.

If your face has been disfigured in some way or if aging eyelid skin interferes with your vision, you should not hesitate to explore treatment that would improve your quality of life with a reputable professional dermatologist or board-certified plastic surgeon. Otherwise, I urge you to consider accepting your face as it is, enjoying the individuality, character, and wisdom revealed in its lines and contours.

The following is a breakdown of what is entailed in some of the most common cosmetic procedures.

WRINKLE FILLERS

Several injectable fillers designed to rid the face of wrinkles have been approved by the FDA for use by prescription, including bovine collagen, hyaluronic acid gels, and other products. Injections of collagen—the fibrous protein found naturally in skin, bone, and connective tissue—"plumps up" skin, smoothing out superficial wrinkles for months at a time. Collagen may come from cow skin, a person's own skin, or the skin of a donor. After about 6 months, it is absorbed by the skin. In rare cases, collagen injections can cause allergic reactions. Hyaluronic acid gels are inert gels used to fill and reduce wrinkles and carry no risk of allergic reaction.

LASER RESURFACING

This new procedure uses an intense beam of laser light to remove skin damaged by age, sun, or acne so that smoother skin can grow in its place. The laser beam destroys the epidermis and heats the dermis beneath it, stimulating the growth of collagen, the protein that gives skin its smooth texture and elasticity. As the burn heals, the skin grows back smoother and tighter. The treatment can diminish fine lines around the eyes and mouth and minimize discolored or scarred areas, but it is not effective for deep wrinkles.

Treatment can be more or less aggressive depending on the type of laser used. The deeper the laser penetrates, the more dramatic the results and the greater the risks. Side effects may include scarring, swelling, itching, a burning sensation, pigment changes, development of herpes virus infections, acne flares, and dermatitis (inflammation of the skin).

BOTOX

The active ingredient in Botox is botulinum toxin type A. When used in facial treatments, small amounts of a purified and sterile form of the toxin are injected into facial muscles. This temporarily paralyzes them so they can't contract to form furrows between the eyes or in the brow. FDA guidelines recommend the use of the lowest effective dose only once every 3 months. Side effects include headache, flu syndrome, nausea, droopy eyelids, respiratory infection, and rarely, facial pain, redness, and muscle weakening.

FACE-LIFTS AND OTHER COSMETIC PLASTIC SURGERIES

Once available only to the very wealthy, cosmetic surgery is now much less expensive and widely undergone by many women at younger and younger ages. In face-lift surgery, a physician removes excess or loose skin from the neck and jowl to "lift" the face and make it look more youthful. It is not used for removing fine wrinkles. Face-lifts are most commonly performed on people ages 40 to 70 who have loose skin and fatty tissue around the neck, an ill-defined jawline with excess skin, and/or a deep crease extending from the corner of the mouth to the nose.

In some people, aging causes eyelids to sag and brows to furrow deeply. Removing skin or fat from the eyelids requires eyelid surgery, a procedure known as blepharoplasty. A brow lift is used to raise the skin on the forehead and the eyebrows to diminish creases. Side effects and risks of cosmetic surgery include problems with anesthesia, infection, numbness, skin discoloration, scarring, and blood clots.

CELLULITE TREATMENTS

Cellulite refers to deposits of fat that press against connective tissue beneath the skin and cause the skin surface to distort, dimple, or pucker. Its presence and appearance is influenced by heredity, the thickness of skin, the amount and distribution of body fat, and age. It is a normal variant in human skin. However, some women find it so unattractive that they feel they must address it. Though dozens of products purport to remove cellulite, ranging from loofah sponges to body wraps, vibrating contraptions, and toning lotions, there is no guaranteed way of eliminating it. Some women resort to liposuction (surgery to remove fat) or mesotherapy (the injection of drugs). These are not effective treatments. In fact, liposuction may make the problem worse. Experts agree that the best weapon against cellulite is a regular routine of aerobic exercise and strength training to keep muscles toned, coupled with healthy eating and weight loss if overweight is contributing to the problem.

REMOVING VARICOSE VEINS AND SPIDER VEINS

One in four American women develops varicose veins—swollen, bulging, and twisted veins that are raised above the surface of the skin. They develop when valves in the veins malfunction, causing blood to pool there. They occur most frequently during pregnancy, in the elderly, in women who stand for long periods of time during the day, and in women who are obese.

To prevent varicose veins from worsening, it helps to exercise and lose weight. It's also a good idea to avoid crossing your legs when you're sitting and to elevate them when you're resting. If varicose veins become painful or unsightly, some women opt to have them removed by a doctor—if they're large, by traditional surgery; if they're smaller, by sclerotherapy (a procedure in which the vein is injected with a chemical solution) or by the new technique of laser treatments.

Spider veins are small, superficial veins similar to varicose veins that often occur in women, especially post-pregnancy and after sun exposure. Alcoholics also are at high risk for developing spider veins on the face. Small to medium veins are most commonly treated with laser therapy; larger veins are treated with sclerotherapy.

WHAT'S ON THE HORIZON FOR SKIN TREATMENT?

With better understanding of the skin's innate protective mechanisms, researchers are working on new treatments designed to prevent photoaging. These may not only allow for improved appearance of skin in middle age and beyond, but they may also reduce the risk of skin cancer. Among them are topical antioxidants that may decrease the detrimental effects of ultraviolet light on skin and a possible oral sunscreen—an oral supplement to protect your skin against sun damage.

7

Teeth

A smile has been called the shortest distance between two people, the light in the window of your face, the least expensive way to improve your looks. It's true that a smiling face is a beautiful face, especially with a mouth full of healthy teeth—not necessarily perfectly white or perfectly straight, but *healthy*.

Recent research at Tufts University and elsewhere shows that oral health can seriously affect overall health, and vice versa. Poor health resulting from poor nutrition and eating habits affects teeth and gums even before it affects the rest of the body. Infections often enter through the mouth, for instance, and spread to other parts of the body. For this reason, it's important to view your dentist as you view your primary care doctor—as a vital part of your overall health maintenance strategy—and schedule regular visits, from infancy through old age. The route to a bright smile and lifelong oral health involves good hygiene and regular dental checkups.

My early experience with dentists was pretty grim. When I was growing up, our dentist was a family friend, an older man with shaking hands and stubby, clumsy fingers that caused great pain. As a result, I now yearn for general anesthesia for any dental procedure. I could even see using Novocaine for regular teeth cleanings! Despite this "trauma," I see the dentist twice a year for hygiene and checkups because I know it's a major part of maintaining good health. In fact, because my dentist sees me so often (twice a year) and can spot health problems, I think of him as a critical part of my primary care.

TOOTH FACTS

Adults have 32 teeth—8 flat-topped incisors and 4 pointed canines for tearing and cutting food into bite-size chunks, and 16 flat bicuspids and molars for grinding and crushing the chunks into pulp we can swallow. Most people also have 4 extra molars known as wisdom teeth.

A tooth consists of the crown (the part that's visible above the gums), the neck (at the gum line), and the root (the part beneath the gum that attaches to the jawbone). The tough outer layer of the crown is formed by hard white enamel. Inside this is a layer of softer dentine, which encloses the pulp cavity. This contains blood vessels that nourish the tooth and nerves that are sensitive to heat, cold, and pressure—but the only sensation we feel when there's a problem is pain. As my dentist says, tooth pain is nature's built-in warning that something is seriously wrong. Tooth problems can lead to lethal infections, so nature has given us the toothache—a type of pain nearly impossible to ignore—as a message to get help.

WHAT AFFECTS THE HEALTH OF YOUR TEETH?

- **Dental hygiene.** As the saying goes, "You don't have to brush your teeth—just the ones you want to keep." Brushing your teeth at least twice a day, flossing at least once a day, and seeing your dentist once or twice a year will help ensure good oral health. Brushing and flossing remove plaque (the layer of bacteria that coats teeth and causes cavities) and help keep gums healthy.
- **Smoking.** Not only does smoking discolor teeth, it also increases the risk of gum disease and oral cancer. Statistics show that smokers are up to six times more likely to develop gum disease than nonsmokers and twice as likely to lose all their teeth by age 65. Some 75 percent of those diagnosed with oral cancer are tobacco users.
- **Age.** As we age, our teeth may darken slightly and our gums may recede. We generate less saliva to wash away bacteria, so our teeth and gums become a little more susceptible to decay and infection.
- **Hormones.** Hormonal changes may trigger gingivitis, or inflammation of the gums. It often appears in women using oral contraceptives or during pregnancy. After menopause, the loss of estrogen can boost the risk of serious gum disease and tooth loss.

- **Nutrition.** What you eat affects your teeth, so it's important to make healthy food choices:
  - Eat plenty of fresh fruits and vegetables with a high water content, such as melons, pears, cucumbers, and celery.
  - Eat aged cheeses such as cheddar and Swiss, which trigger the flow of saliva that helps wash food particles from teeth.
  - Limit your consumption of sugary treats and eat them with meals, not as snacks. The longer carbohydrates remain on your teeth before brushing, the more likely they are to cause cavities. Saliva produced during meals helps wash away food particles and neutralizes harmful acids.
  - Avoid sugary foods that linger on and coat teeth, such as cough drops, hard candies, and mints. Eating excessive amounts of chewy fruit such as dates or raisins can also coat teeth.
- **Fluoride.** It's important to get sufficient fluoride, a natural chemical that strengthens tooth enamel and helps repair damage to teeth when you're young. You can check with your local water department to find out the fluoride content of your water supply. Consult your dentist to see whether you need to supplement with additional fluoride in drop or tablet form. This is especially true if your water is supplied from a well or spring.
- **Sugar-free gum.** There is some evidence that chewing sugar-free gum after eating can help clean teeth between brushings.

HOW DOES THE HEALTH OF YOUR TEETH AFFECT YOUR OVERALL HEALTH?

Not only is your smile a light in the window of your face, it's also a window to your body's health. For one thing, the early signs of diseases such as osteoporosis, syphilis, gonorrhea, eating disorders, and certain cancers first occur in the mouth. Medicine has only lately discovered that your oral health is intimately linked to your general health in other fundamental ways—another great reason to practice good oral hygiene. Mouth troubles such as gum disease, or periodontitis, may trigger other health problems. Your mouth is packed with bacteria, which normally cause no trouble. But some researchers suspect that gum disease may allow bacteria to find their way into the bloodstream, increasing the risk of cardiovascular disease, premature birth, and other health problems. Keeping your teeth clean and free of plaque prevents microorganisms from invading and triggering inflammation in your gums. When gum tissue is not inflamed, it is tighter and less leaky, preventing microorganisms from entering the bloodstream. This, in turn, relieves the body of responding systemically to bacterial assault, thereby reducing the chance of cardiovascular disease.

If you develop any of the following symptoms, contact your dentist:

- Inflammation in your gums (swelling and tenderness), which may be painless but causes bleeding even with light touch
- Loose teeth
- A bad taste in your mouth
- A shift in your bite—the way your top and bottom teeth touch
- Tooth sensitivity to hot and cold, which may indicate the presence of a cavity or nerve inflammation

BEST BRUSHING PRACTICES

According to dentists, you should spend at least 2 minutes twice a day brushing your teeth. Follow these tips for proper brushing:

- Most dentists recommend using an electric brush over a hand brush. Electric brushes clean teeth well without causing trauma to teeth and gums and are better at removing plaque because of the rotation or vibration of the bristles. Children often find them more fun to use, as well, and thus are more apt to brush regularly.
- Select a toothpaste containing fluoride. If you have a tendency to accumulate tartar—hardened plaque—use an antitartar toothpaste and brush especially well the area of your teeth near your salivary glands (inside your lower front teeth and outside the upper back teeth). If your teeth are sensitive to heat or cold, try using toothpaste for sensitive teeth.
- Hold your brush at a 45-degree angle against your teeth and use short, gentle strokes upward from where the teeth and gum meet to the tops of your teeth. Brush both outside and inside surfaces. For chewing surfaces, use short strokes and tip bristles into crevices. Gently brush your tongue and the roof of your mouth to remove bacteria.
- If you use a regular toothbrush, choose one that has soft bristles and replace it every 3 or 4 months.

TIPS FOR FINE FLOSSING

"You know, sometimes a man just can't satisfy all of a woman's desires. Which is why God invented dental floss." —Anonymous

I'm a huge fan of floss. I can go without brushing for a day, but never without flossing. It's an essential part of the teeth-cleaning process because it removes plaque from between the teeth and at the gum line, where gum (periodontal) disease often starts. If you don't floss, plaque builds up and can inflame the gum, causing bleeding and eventually periodontal disease. To floss properly:

- Use the type of floss you prefer, waxed or unwaxed.
- Carefully ease floss between teeth with a back-and-forth pulling motion and slide it down just below the gum line to the "sulcus," where plaque tends to collect and cause gum disease. Pull the floss into a C shape around the tooth and pull from below the gum line to the top of the tooth to remove attached plaque.
- Use a fresh stretch of floss as you progress methodically through your teeth.
- Remember to floss the back sides of your rear molars, top and bottom.
- Improper brushing and flossing can traumatize your gum tissue, making it bleed, so be sure to use proper technique when cleaning your teeth.

KEEPING YOUR BREATH FRESH

We're all aware that sweet breath can lead to more pleasant interactions with others. The opposite can be an embarrassment far worse than body odor. The technical term for bad breath is *halitosis*, and it can be caused by a number of factors:

- **Dieting or fasting.** Infrequent eating means that there's less saliva to wash away dead cells and decomposing matter, which can cause unpleasant odor.
- **What you eat and drink.** Along with the usual culprits, such as garlic and onions, many other types of food and drink can cause bad breath even well after they're consumed, including cheese, pastrami, orange juice, alcohol, and soda. When food is broken down and enters the bloodstream, it can reach the lungs, where its aromatic constituents are exhaled with breath.
- **Poor hygiene.** Inadequate brushing and flossing can result in deposits of food collecting in the mouth and drawing bacteria that emit hydrogen sulfide vapors.

- **Smoking or chewing tobacco.**
- **Dry mouth (xerostomia).** This condition sometimes occurs with certain medications or salivary problems.
- **Disease.** Diseases such as chronic sinusitis or bronchitis, kidney or liver ailments, diabetes, and gastrointestinal disorders can cause bad breath.

The best way to avoid halitosis is to maintain good oral health, including regular dental visits for professional cleaning and daily brushing and flossing. You can also try using mouthwashes, but their effects are generally temporary. If these measures don't work, see your dentist.

WHITENING THOSE PEARLIES

Over time, many of us experience tooth discoloration that dims our grin. Because teeth are porous, they often stain as a result of exposure to red wine, coffee, tea, soda, and other food and drink. Smoking and medications such as the antibiotic tetracycline can also cause teeth discoloration.

Teeth whitening—the process of making teeth appear whiter by removing discoloration and stains—can be performed in a dentist's office or at home. Whitening gels contain peroxide, which kills bacteria, so they may help diminish periodontal disease as well. However, it's not clear how healthy the process is over the long term. It's definitely not recommended for women who are pregnant or breastfeeding or for people with gum disease, worn tooth enamel, sensitive teeth, or an allergy to peroxide.

Teeth whitening is purely a cosmetic issue. In my opinion, most people's teeth are just fine. My dentist recently asked me if I'd like to have my teeth whitened, but I think my teeth are perfectly acceptable and healthy just as they are.

If you choose to have your teeth whitened, here is an overview of your options:

- **Bleaching at the dentist's office.** The dentist applies a bleaching agent, sometimes with a special light to enhance the bleaching action. A protective gel or rubber shield protects your gum and other soft tissues. The treatment, which may require more than one office visit lasting from 30 minutes to 1 hour, can be expensive and is not covered by insurance. How long these treatments last depends on your personal habits—whether you use tobacco; whether you drink large amounts of coffee, tea, cola, or red wine; and how often you visit your dentist for teeth cleaning.

- **Over-the-counter whiteners or bleaching agents.** These products, available in the form of gels or strips, typically contain peroxide that bleaches tooth enamel and changes the intrinsic color of teeth, removing deep and surface stains. Some require twice-daily treatment for 2 weeks; others are used overnight for 1 to 2 weeks. New versions can be used daily. Side effects include sensitive teeth and gum irritation. Dental experts suggest that keeping teeth white with at-home products requires repeated use every 4 to 6 months. It's optimal to start at-home treatment immediately after a dental cleaning, which removes any plaque that may interfere with the bleaching process.
- **Whitening toothpastes.** Although all toothpastes contain gentle abrasives that help scrub away surface stains, some whitening formulas also have chemical agents that lighten teeth slightly. This is the least expensive option for whitening. However, its effects are usually minimal, because toothpastes cannot change the natural color of your teeth.

COSMETIC DENTISTRY

Some women may opt to make cosmetic changes in their teeth to boost self-confidence or improve appearance, such as repairing chips and cracks, remolding shape, closing gaps, and moving crooked or crowded teeth with braces. Among these choices are:

- Bonding to repair teeth that are broken, cracked, chipped, or set too far apart
- Enamel shaping, which modifies teeth by contouring the enamel
- Braces
- Veneers, or thin shells that cover the front of your teeth to conceal chips, stains, poor shapes, and spacing problems

DENTAL PROBLEMS

If you have a serious overbite or other abnormal alignment of your teeth, see your dentist as soon as possible so that you can have the problem corrected with braces. There are many options for corrective appliances available now in modern dentistry.

A relatively common dental problem is grinding or clenching teeth, known as bruxism. Most often it is mild, but severe cases can cause serious damage to teeth and can lead to headaches and jaw disorders. If you have worn teeth or pain in your jaw, ear, or face, see your doctor or dentist. Treatment often consists of wearing a mouth guard at night to protect teeth from damage and sometimes stress-management or behavioral modification techniques.

8

Hair and Nails

The journalist Shana Alexander once called hair "a tangle of mysterious prejudices." It's true. Your hair is what it is—shiny or dull, dry or oily, frizzy or limp, tangled or sleek, flaming red or dark brunette or soft gray—thanks in large part to a puzzling mix of genes and environment. All too often, women wish they were born with a different hair type. We want it straighter or wavier, thicker or thinner, and we seek hair treatments that will give us what we don't naturally possess.

But whether the locks you were born with are thick and curly or thin and straight, the best thing you can do to keep hair healthy is to accept its natural state and avoid damaging it with excessive sunlight, heat, poor nutrition, and chemicals. Hair is resilient—but only to a certain point. Because it's made of dead cells, it cannot repair itself once damaged. The more it is subjected to heat and harsh chemicals, the more it will suffer.

My hair routine is nearly as minimal as my facial care. I color my hair every 3 months or so to keep the gray at bay. I'm lucky to have thick, healthy hair that's resilient to this regular use of chemicals. Before you start down this path, take measure of your own hair and its resiliency. Be selective about the dye that is used on your hair. These days there are many natural products available that do not contain harsh chemicals like peroxide or ammonia. Talk to your stylist about what kind of dye your salon uses before you undergo this often costly treatment, especially if you have short hair.

A GROWING STORY

As most of us know, hair is made of dead cells that grow out of little pockets, or follicles, in the dermis. These follicles are fed by tiny blood vessels and sebaceous glands that give hair its shine. Most women have an average of about 100,000 hairs, though the number varies with hair color. Speaking as a brunette, I have to doubt that blondes have more fun—but they do have more hair, an extra 40,000 strands or so. Redheads have fewer strands, about 90,000.

Some 85 percent of your scalp hairs are actively growing at any one time. They grow at about one-half inch a month for about 2 years or so, then enter a resting phase, and later fall out at a rate of about 50 to 100 per day. If the follicles they grow from are healthy, they will be replaced by new hair.

Each strand of hair consists of three layers, from inside out:

- **Inner medulla.** The core of hair strands reflects light, giving hair a different tone in sunlight than in shade.
- **Middle cortex.** The cortex makes up the bulk of the hair and determines both its color and its texture—straight or curly. If the cross-section of your cortex is round, your hair is straight; if it's oval, your hair is curly. The cortex also contains melanin, the pigment responsible for hair color. Eumelanin makes hair brown or black; pheomelanin yields red hair; very low amounts of melanin give rise to blonde hair; and lack of pigment results in gray.
- **Outer cuticle.** This thin, colorless layer made of overlapping scales arranged like shingles protects the middle cortex. When the scales of the cuticle lie flat and overlap tightly, they protect the inner layers from sun, heat, and chemicals, and hair looks shiny and reflects light. However, when hair is damaged, scales can separate and stand up. This allows moisture to escape, making hair brittle and dull.

WHAT AFFECTS THE HEALTH OF YOUR HAIR?

- **Your hair type.** Your hair type is intimately linked to your skin condition. If you have dry skin, chances are good that your hair will be dry, too. The same goes for oily skin. But dry hair can also be caused by overexposure to heat, sunlight, and chemicals, such as perms or hair coloring.

As with skin, some women have a combination of hair types (for instance, an oily scalp with dry ends).

- **Diet.** To keep your locks healthy, make sure you eat well. Good nutrition makes a difference in how your hair looks and feels. Poor nutrition, on the other hand, can damage hair.
- **Hormones.** Many women notice changes in their hair during pregnancy, postpartum, and around menopause. This is because hormones have an impact on hair. During puberty, hormones may boost oil secretion by the sebaceous glands, making hair feel oily. Pregnancy sometimes causes women's hair to become more difficult or more manageable. The hormonal changes that accompany menopause may exacerbate hair loss.
- **Sun exposure.** Like skin, hair is vulnerable to overexposure to sunlight. Both UVA and UVB rays can damage hair, causing it to become dry and brittle and stripping away color. Protect hair from sun exposure by wearing a hat, scarf, or bandanna, or use a hair product containing hair sunscreen.
- **Heat.** Hair dryers on high heat, flat irons, and curling irons can seriously damage hair, causing split ends and rough texture. I can't emphasize this enough. If possible, avoid blow-drying or using a flat iron or curling iron on your hair every day.
- **Harsh chemicals.** Chlorine can damage hair. So can hair colors, permanents, and relaxers, which strip away natural oils. It's best to leave straightening and waving to the experts.
- **Excessive brushing** or brushing while your hair is wet may cause split ends.
- **Age.** As we age, hair sometimes thins or turns gray as hair pigment cells lose their ability to renew themselves.

KEEPING YOUR HAIR NATURALLY BEAUTIFUL

To maintain a healthy and manageable head of hair, here are a few general rules:

- Use only those hair products you absolutely need.
- Wash with a gentle shampoo and warm water and lather downward from the scalp.
- Use a cream rinse or conditioner to hydrate and minimize damage.
- Towel dry hair and use a hair dryer as little as possible.

- Comb hair rather than brush it.
- Avoid tight braiding or buns, which can put too much pressure on hair roots and skin.
- Get your hair trimmed regularly. Haircuts help eliminate and prevent split ends.
- Minimize your exposure to sun, wind, and chlorine.

PERSONALIZING YOUR HAIR ROUTINE

Although few products can affect the health of your hair, many conditioning and styling products can make different hair types more manageable and attractive.

DRY HAIR

Dry hair often looks dull, frizzy, or rough because the cuticles on the hair shaft, which should lie flat and smooth to retain moisture, are instead raised. If you have dry hair, consider following these steps:

- Protect your hair from strong sunlight.
- Try washing your hair only once every couple of days, and use a shampoo and a conditioner labeled "hydrating" or "moisturizing."
- Let your hair air-dry when you can. Use a hair dryer only on its lowest temperature setting and point the nozzle down, away from your scalp.
- For very dry hair, some experts recommend using a few drops of safflower or olive oil after drying hair or between washings.

OILY HAIR

Remember that oily hair results from an oily scalp, so your goal is to minimize oil buildup.

- Wash your hair daily with a gentle cleansing or clarifying shampoo, which will help remove excess oil. If you have dry ends, lather the shampoo only on your scalp. You can also try a dry shampoo, a powder-based spray product that absorbs the oil and provides some volume.
- Use a light conditioner for oily hair, but apply it only on the ends of your hair. (If you have dry ends, apply a conditioner for dry hair.)
- Try not to brush your hair excessively, because this spreads the oil.

FINE HAIR

Fine hair breaks and damages much more easily than medium or coarse hair does, so it's important to be gentle with it.

- Use a volumizing shampoo and a good, lightweight conditioner.
- Avoid trying to boost volume by coloring or heat treatments. Instead, try using a volumizing product, such as styling gels and mousses.

COLORED HAIR

Some 50 percent of American women color their hair with either permanent or semi-permanent dyes.

Permanent dyes raise the scales on the cuticle so the chemicals can bleach away the natural pigment and replace it with color that remains on hair until new hair grows out. Overuse of these products can damage hair by causing the scales to separate. They can also cause hair loss, skin irritation, burning, redness, and allergic reactions.

Semipermanent dyes, which essentially coat hairs with new color, are often used to cover up gray. Their active ingredients, henna or lead acetate, are gentler, but the treatments often fade within 6 weeks. Some people experience an allergic reaction to semi-permanent dyes, so it's important to do a patch test before use.

Some studies have linked the frequent use of hair dyes with increased risk of certain cancers, including non-Hodgkin's lymphoma, leukemia, and ovarian cancer. Others, including the Nurses' Health Study conducted by the Harvard School of Public Health, found no higher risk of cancer among women who dye their hair. As with any lifestyle choice, it's important to weigh the low risk of using hair dye with the benefits you gain. However, most experts urge pregnant women to avoid dyeing their hair and advise those women who use dark dyes to pick products containing henna or lead acetate.

To minimize your risks, follow these tips:

- Never mix hair dyes.
- Follow directions carefully.
- Do a patch test to make sure you're not allergic to the dye.
- Wear gloves when applying dye.
- Leave dye on head for the minimum time needed.
- Rinse your head and scalp thoroughly with water.
- Never dye eyebrows or eyelashes unless you absolutely have to.
- Consider going to a professional.

Because coloring tends to damage hair, your hair care routine should focus on repairing or minimizing further damage.

- Try to wash and rinse your hair in cool water, which helps close your cuticles and retain moisture and color. Use a shampoo for colored hair and a nourishing conditioner.
- Protect your hair from the sun and alternate your part.
- Wear a swimming cap in chlorinated or saltwater pools and rinse thoroughly—then wash hair afterward.

DANDRUFF

Contrary to popular belief, dandruff is not caused by dry skin but by inflammation of the scalp—possibly caused by a fungus. Tiny scales build up and then fall off as visible flakes. Over-the-counter shampoos containing zinc, salicylic acid, selenium sulfide, or tars can reduce the flaking. When shampooing, rub your scalp gently and allow the shampoo to sit for 3 to 5 minutes before rinsing. For more persistent dandruff, your doctor may recommend a prescription shampoo.

HAIR LOSS (ALOPECIA)

A certain amount of hair loss is normal and expected, as old hairs fall out to be replaced by new ones. However, some women experience hair thinning and loss that exceeds the rate of replacement. This may result in bald patches, especially over the top and sides of the head. Hair loss is most common after menopause, but sometimes begins as early as puberty. The loss may be temporary, as is often the case in the months after childbirth, during periods of extreme stress, dieting, or illness, or with the use of some prescription drugs. Perms, color, and other hairstyle changes can lend hair a fuller appearance. If this doesn't help, a clinician may prescribe a drug such as Rogaine to slow or stop hair loss and to help hair grow.

REMOVING UNWANTED HAIR

Unwanted female hair is a touchy subject. Almost your entire body is covered with hair—most of it so fine it's invisible to the naked eye. However, coarser, darker hair often appears on the legs, underarms, and pubic area. Though unwanted body hair is no threat to health, many women elect to remove it for cosmetic reasons. If unwanted hair is bothering you, how much or how little hair you choose to remove is a highly personal decision. Existing methods for achieving smooth, hairless skin vary in cost, comfort, and speed, but—with the exception of electrolysis—all are temporary.

SHAVING

An easy, inexpensive option for removing hair from legs and underarms, shaving requires only a razor, warm water, and soap or shaving gel or cream. However, it lasts only 1 to 3 days and sometimes causes nicks, razor burn, and ingrown hairs—when hair is cut below the level of the skin surface and regrows into surrounding tissue, causing irritation and redness. To avoid these problems, it's best to use a sharp razor and shave after a shower, when pores are open and hair is softened by heat and water. Lather with shaving soap, gel, or cream, and shave in the direction of hair growth. To remove ingrown hairs, try exfoliating with a loofah sponge and plucking out hair with a pair of sterilized tweezers.

TWEEZING

Easy and inexpensive, tweezing is often used for removing unwanted facial hair, especially in the eyebrows, upper lip, and chin. Sterilize tweezers with rubbing alcohol. Wash the skin around the hair follicle and dab with alcohol. Pull skin tight, and use tweezers to extract hair close to the root. To keep an area clean by tweezing, it's best to pluck on a weekly basis—but the treatment can be painful.

WAXING

Waxing works like tweezing, but is generally used over a broad area to remove unwanted hair on legs, bikini regions, and eyebrows. Sticky melted wax is spread over skin and allowed to cool. Then a cloth strip is applied to the wax and quickly stripped off, taking the hairs and hair roots with it—sometimes a very painful process. Because waxing can cause skin irritation and, sometimes, infection of the hair follicles, it's a good idea to have the procedure done by an expert at a salon. Best performed when hair is at least a ¼ inch long, the procedure leaves the area smooth for 3 to 6 weeks. A common side effect of waxing is redness or inflammation, especially in women with sensitive skin. To minimize or prevent these effects, make sure that your wax product doesn't contain any ingredients to which you may be allergic. To soothe skin after waxing, apply an after-wax cooling or aloe-based product.

DEPILATORIES

Depilatories are chemicals in the form of creams, foams, or lotions that are used to remove hair on the legs, underarms, or bikini area. Special varieties may also be used on the face. The chemicals are left on the skin for a short time—usually about 10 minutes—and work by dissolving the proteins in hairs so the unwanted hair may be wiped or washed away. The treatment is inexpensive and lasts for up to 2 weeks. But it's important to test a small area of skin before using it widely, because these chemicals can irritate and even burn.

LASER REMOVAL

Though not permanent, laser hair removal lasts for up to 6 months and works on large areas of skin on any part of the face or body. A laser beam is directed into the hair follicle, where it halts growth. The treatment is expensive and sometimes causes inflammation. It can also cause significant pain.

VANISHING PUBIC HAIR

Not long ago, I was surprised to learn from my colleague Hope Ricciotti that more and more young women are shaving or waxing all of their pubic hair. This may result from efforts to create a clean bikini line for bathing suits that are diminishing drastically in size, revealing far more of the pubic area. Or it may just be a fad. In any case, it should be noted that removing hair from the pubic area can be demanding, uncomfortable, and unsafe.

The pubic area is highly sensitive, and shaving, waxing, tweezing, or clipping pubic hair can have health consequences, such as itching, bumps, blistering, genital infections, and folliculitis—an infection of the hair follicle caused by ingrown hairs. Also, keeping your pubic area hairless requires almost daily care. Given the risks, I encourage women to leave their pubic hair in its natural state.

ELECTROLYSIS

The only permanent form of hair removal, electrolysis is an expensive procedure performed by a professional electrologist over a series of appointments. It is usually used for small areas such as the upper lip or eyebrows, which may take several visits to complete. The electrologist inserts a fine needle into individual hair follicles and sends a jolt of electricity into the hair root, destroying it. Some people find the process painful, and occasionally it results in scabbing, scarring, or inflammation of the surrounding skin, as well as infections of the hair follicles if instruments are not sterile.

CARING FOR YOUR NAILS

You may think of your nails as mere opportunities for decoration; in fact they're also vital organs of the hand, important for manipulating fine objects, for fingertip sensitivity, and as an immunologic protective barrier. They're also "biomarkers" for health and nutritional deficiencies, not unlike the rings on a tree, which reveal periodic droughts and good growing seasons. In fact, in the 19th and early 20th centuries, physicians relied on the appearance of nails for signs of nutritional deficiencies. Nails also reflect the aging process. Beginning around age 50, they begin to develop ridges and some brittleness.

Most nail flaws—ridges, splits, discoloration—are not signs of health concerns. However, some nail conditions may signal other health issues, from anemia to diseases of the liver or thyroid. You may wish to consult a physician if your nails look pale or concave, bluish, opaque and whitish, ridged with horizontal lines, brittle and separated from the nail bed, or extremely rounded, like the back of a spoon.

I've had only four or five manicures in my life—the first one at age 32 in preparation for a friend's wedding. (My daughters, on the other hand, go for manicures periodically, often together as a way of socializing.) I tend to keep my nails clean and very short because I rock climb.

NAIL BASICS

The nail plate—the part of the nail that looks translucent, smooth, and shiny—is made of dead skin cells hardened by keratin, the same protein found in hair. The nail plate grows out of the living skin, called the matrix. This is located in the nail bed just beneath the cuticle, that thin flap of skin at the base of the nails. In healthy nails, the nail plate is smooth, not ridged or grooved, and looks pink because of the network of blood vessels that run through the nail bed beneath it.

Nails grow at a rate of about 0.1 millimeter a day, or 2 to 4 millimeters a month. If a nail is torn off but the nail bed is not injured, the nail will regrow completely in 4 to 6 months. Like hair, nails grow more quickly in summer than in winter. Fingernails grow roughly four times faster than toenails, which only need to be clipped about once a month. As we age, our nails grow at about half the pace they do when we're young.

WHAT AFFECTS THE HEALTH OF YOUR NAILS?

Injury to the fingertip and nail is a common occurrence—from slammed car doors or use of hammers, saws, machines, and chains. If the nail bed is severely affected, there may be permanent deformity of the nail.

Overexposure to strong detergents (for example, during dishwashing) and chemicals can cause nails to become brittle and split easily.

Poor nutrition may also result in brittle nails. The process of building nails involves protein, so it's a good idea to make sure that your diet includes plenty of protein-rich foods.

High-heeled or tight shoes can cause painful ingrown toenails, when the edges or corners of a toenail curl down and grow into the skin. Even running shoes can cause problems. If you're running in a long-distance race, and your running shoes don't fit well, you may end up losing a toenail or two. Make sure your shoes fit as well as possible and that your toenails are clipped. During a race, your feet may swell, so you need to make sure that you have a large "toe box" in your running shoes to accommodate the swelling.

Infection. When a cut or hangnail allows microorganisms to infect the skin around a nail, infection of the nail bed may result. Fungal infections may persist over long periods of time and can result in discolored and deformed nails. Because over-the-counter topical medications are rarely effective against fungal infections, treatment may require oral antifungal drugs.

Age. As we age, the integrity of the nail may change and become more prone to cracking or splitting. At this stage in life, it may be a good idea to apply a few layers of strengthening lacquer or polish to keep brittle nails from breaking.

NAIL CARE

Women in this country spend billions of dollars each year on products and services designed to care for and beautify our nails. But most experts agree that the best route to healthy nails is a simple three-step process:

Keep nails clean, trimmed, and moisturized. For fingernails, use a sharp manicure scissors and an emery board to smooth edges. When moisturizing your hands, rub lotion into your nails. Cut toenails straight across to avoid ingrown nails.

Avoid abusing your nails. This includes biting them, injuring them, or exposing them to harsh detergents and chemicals. Never pick at your cuticles or pull off hangnails, which may cause bleeding and infection. When using harsh chemicals, protect your hands with cotton-lined rubber gloves.

Eat a healthy diet. Though ingesting gelatin and calcium have no effect on the strength of nails, a balanced, healthy diet does.

MANICURES AND PEDICURES

If you like to have manicures and pedicures to enhance the appearance of your nails, keep in mind the following suggestions:

- Make sure your nail technician sterilizes all tools used during your manicure and do not have your cuticles cut. You can also bring your own kit to a nail salon and request that they use your tools.
- Use nail hardeners, which can help with brittle or weak nails, but avoid products containing formaldehyde or toluene sulfonamide.
- To make polish last longer, use several thin coats of polish rather than one heavy layer. Touch up polish when needed rather than repainting.
- Try not to extend the polish to the living tissue at the base of the nail.
- Avoid using nail polish remover with acetone more than once or twice a month, because it dries and weakens nails.

productive Choices Fertility and Preg
enopause Sexual Abuse and Sexual A
in Teeth Hair and Nails Body Weigh
etabolism Blood Sugar Eating and Exc
uscles Bones JointsHeart and Blood
d Respiration Common Infectious Dis
utoimmune Disease Cancer Vision He
hell, Taste, and Touch Mental Health
nce Abuse Making Change Managing
d Sleeping Well Shifting Your Food En
ent Getting Active Screenings and H
aintenance Reproduction Sexuality an
l Health Reproductive Choices Fertilit
egnancy Menopause Sexual Abuse and
l Assault Skin Teeth Hair and Nails
eight and Metabolism Blood Sugar E
d Excreting Muscles Bones JointsHea
ood Lungs and Respiration Common
us Diseases Autoimmune Disease C

PART III

Keeping in Balance

Your body is a metabolic wonder. It takes in energy in the form of calories from food and drink and expends those calories doing what it needs to do over the course of a day, keeping your heart and digestive system going, your muscles pumping, your brain working. So finely built is the body for balancing its energy intake and expenditure that an average adult can eat something like 10 million calories over a decade and experience only a slight change in weight.

If this is so, why do so many of us struggle to keep off those creeping pounds—even when we feel like we're eating less and exerting our willpower and self-discipline?

Obesity: It's the gorilla in the room, the consuming worry for millions of women. Am I carrying too many extra pounds? Is that unsightly tire around my waist an inevitable consequence of age? Will I get diabetes? Will I ever again look decent in a swimsuit? For many of us, these concerns, driven by advertising and public health messages, overwhelm most other health considerations.

I've been fortunate in this: Apart from my freshman year in college and my three pregnancies, maintaining a healthy weight has been relatively easy for me. My love of being physically active helps a lot. I'm also lucky to have a well-functioning satiety center that tells me when I've had enough to eat. Now that I'm entering midlife, however, I find I have to work harder to hold my weight steady. In fact, I've already put on a few extra pounds. I know I'll have to shift my habits, eat fewer snacks, smaller portions, less dessert. (As a huge fan of my after-dinner ice cream, for instance, I know I'll have to shrink my scoop!) I'm prepared to gain a little, but only as much as is reasonable and healthy—no more than 10 pounds or so. And I'm certain that I'm up to that challenge.

If you've been at your ideal body weight when you enter midlife, you should expect to gain some weight. That's okay: Embrace it, but don't let it get out of hand—you don't want to gain 30, 40, 50 pounds. If you're already overweight or obese when you enter your middle years, you'll need to work harder to maintain your weight or even shed some pounds.

It's essential to have realistic expectations of what your body will look like in your older years. It's even more important to emphasize strength and fitness over appearance. Difficult as it may sometimes be, try to focus on what your body can *do* rather than how it *looks.*

This part of the book will help you understand your energy balance and how best to manage it to achieve and maintain a healthy weight. It also explains blood sugar, or glucose, and the importance of controlling it to avoid or manage diabetes. Finally, it explores some of the health issues that may arise in digestion and excretion.

To keep in balance and maintain a healthy digestive system, be **S.M.A.R.T.:**

1. Create a healthy food environment to eat a little less, and to eat better.
2. Minimize sedentary behavior and increase physical activity.
3. Manage your body weight.
4. Get screened for diabetes and control your blood sugar levels.
5. Manage stress to minimize digestive problems.
6. Consume plenty of plant-based foods for regularity.

9

Body Weight and Metabolism

We've heard a lot lately about the worsening problem of overweight and obesity in this country. It's true that the number of women and men who weigh more than what is considered healthy for their height is growing at a disturbing pace.

In the talks I give, I often show a sequence of maps from the Centers for Disease Control and Prevention on weight trends among adults in the United States from 1985 to the present. These maps highlight in blue those states that have a rate of less than 20 percent obesity and in pink those states with higher than 20 percent obesity. As I project the series of maps for each year, the blue starts to dwindle, and pink spreads across the map—until 2001, when the pink darkens to red in some states, showing obesity rates of 25 percent or more. This red rapidly swells, and then in 2005, many states move to yellow to show rates of obesity of 30 percent or more.

These slides make a powerful impression. The recent maps look like the profile of a landslide political race or the spread of some terrible epidemic—which in fact it is. We are facing a major epidemic of overweight and obesity in this country (and many other places in the world). Today only four states have obesity rates of less than 20 percent; 22 states have greater than 25 percent; and two—Mississippi and West Virginia—have 30 percent or greater. (That's one out of three residents of those states.) The latest estimates suggest that two-thirds of US women—about 65 million—are overweight or obese. The problem affects people of all ages, all racial and ethnic groups, and all educational backgrounds.

Not too long ago, my husband came to a talk I was giving. He saw the slides and statistics and on the ride home he asked me, "I know you have been working hard for the past two decades, but what the heck have you been doing? Things seem to be getting worse."

This is a really good point, and something I think about a lot. In fact, it's what drives me professionally these days. Over the past decade, our research at Tufts has shifted. We used to focus on very controlled research in which women came to our laboratory and participated in studies under tight supervision. Then several of my colleagues and I

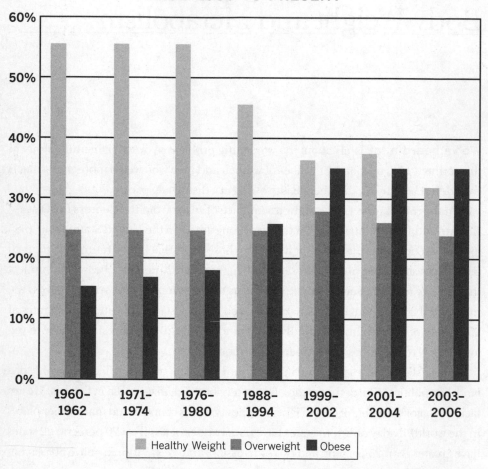

WEIGHT TRENDS AMONG AMERICAN WOMEN FROM 1960 TO PRESENT

Source: Centers for Disease Control and Prevention

This graph shows how body weight has shifted for women in this country over the 40-year period 1960–2006. In 1960, 55 percent of women were a healthy weight; 23 percent were overweight; only 15 percent were obese. Weight categories remained stable until 1980, when a major shift occurred for a constellation of reasons. Now less than 32 percent of women are a healthy body weight; 26 percent are overweight; and 33 percent are obese. For the first time in history, there are now more women in the obese category than in any other. Very few women are underweight.

grew restless with this type of research. We felt that although we were conducting excellent studies, our work wasn't having an impact in the real world. The real world—the place you and I live—is not a controlled laboratory.

In response, we launched the John Hancock Research Center on Physical Activity, Nutrition, and Obesity Prevention at Tufts, which focuses on creating behavioral and environmental interventions to prevent obesity. We've had great success with the interventions we've developed. In our Shape-Up Somerville program, led by my close colleague Christina Economos, we got the entire population of the city of Somerville, Massachusetts, to get in better shape. Our StrongWomen program has been testing body-weight interventions in the rural United States, helping women change their personal environment so that they can more easily lose weight by eating healthfully and being more active.

FACTORS THAT CONTRIBUTE TO OBESITY

From our research at Tufts and the work of other scientists around the country, we believe the reason for the growing epidemic of overweight in this country is a complicated stew of factors, among them:

- **Our food environment.** Our food supply has changed radically in the past 30 years. (See Chapter 26 for more detail.) We get more of our foods in prepackaged form at grocery stores, gas stations, and pharmacies, and at fast-food restaurants everywhere. Most of these foods don't even resemble real food. They are cheap and convenient, but they tend to be devoid of nutritional value and high in calories. Good foods are harder and harder to find. Research shows that limited access to fresh fruits and vegetables, as well as a preponderance of fast-food restaurants in low-income, ethnic minority neighborhoods, may contribute to the increasing prevalence of obesity in these populations.

- **Portion sizes.** Part of the change in our food environment is the growth of portion sizes. In the past 20 years, portion sizes have doubled, and many portions are now "supersize." A typical bagel was once 140 calories, now it's 350 calories. A serving of french fries used to have 210 calories; today's portion has 610 calories. Even salads aren't safe: An average Caesar salad once had 390 calories; now it's often 790. Research shows that when we are served more, we eat more. With the growth of portion sizes comes expanded waistlines and higher body weight.

- **Sedentary lifestyles.** Most Americans get very little physical activity throughout the day—thanks in part to technology. We drive instead of biking or walking to run short errands; we use dishwashers to wash our dishes; we take elevators instead of stairs; we spend hours a day sitting and watching TV or using the computer. Moreover, the design of our environment often does not encourage walking; many of our communities lack sidewalks.
- **Our eating habits.** Finally, our habits of eating have changed dramatically over the past 30 years. Hardly any of us cook as much as we used to, so we eat more prepared foods. Families eat fewer meals together at night. Many people watch television while they eat, or consume their meals in the car or at their desks. Because they are not "mindful" when they eat, they do not heed normal satiety cues.

Although I believe that the main forces contributing to the obesity epidemic are outlined above, I keep an open mind about the possibility that other factors may be involved. For instance, there is interesting new research suggesting that infection with a common virus, human adenovirus-36 (Ad-36), may be partially responsible for the rise in obesity. One study suggests that the virus is present in 30 percent of people who are obese and in only 11 percent of those who aren't. The virus appears to play a role in changing preexisting stem cells into fat cells to increase fat storage. This is fascinating research, but still highly speculative and much work remains to be done to confirm the link.

THE RISKS OF OBESITY

Obesity can create or contribute to a number of health concerns, including:

- Insulin sensitivity and diabetes
- Hypertension
- Coronary heart disease
- Stroke
- High blood cholesterol
- Osteoarthritis
- Gallbladder disease
- Sleep apnea and other respiratory problems
- Cancers of the breast, colorectum, endometrium, and kidney
- Menstrual irregularities
- Complications of pregnancy

- Incontinence
- Hirsutism (excessive body and facial hair)
- Psychological disorders such as depression
- Increased surgical risk
- Increased mortality

In addition, people who are overweight and obese also have the cluster of risk factors known as metabolic syndrome (see the box Metabolic Syndrome on page 132) and are at increased risk of coronary heart disease and other vascular diseases, as well as type 2 diabetes. The risks of these ailments jump dramatically the more obese you are. The good news is this: Even small weight reductions are very beneficial. If you're overweight or obese, losing just 5 percent of your body weight can significantly reduce your chances of developing these health problems.

If you are overweight, you may or may not be at greater risk for the above conditions. It depends on whether you are sedentary or have a genetic predisposition to chronic disease, both of which are indicators of elevated risk. If you are overweight but physically fit (by being active), most likely you are not at elevated risk.

HOW MUCH SHOULD I WEIGH?

I'm constantly surprised by the expectations many women have for their own weight. "I'm 45 with three children, but I believe I should weigh the same as I did when I was 20. I should weigh what my daughter weighs because we're the same height. I should be a size 6."

Determining the body weight that's right for you should not be driven by unrealistic expectations or even by a number on your scale. As you may recall from the Smart Woman's Health Assessment at the beginning of the book, among the best measures of healthy weight is body mass index, or BMI—the measure of your weight in relation to your height. If you haven't already done so, go to the chart on page xxi to determine your BMI. This calculation is a more accurate indicator of overweight and obesity than weight alone is. A BMI of less than 18.4 is considered underweight; 18.5 to 24.9 is considered healthy; 25 through 29.9 is overweight; 30 to 39.9 is obese; and 40 and above is extremely obese.

Here are some general rules of thumb for weight goals. If you are:

Underweight
- Bring your BMI up to 18.5 through good nutrition and strength-training exercise.

Ideal body weight

- If you have maintained an ideal body weight for years, keep up the good work!
- If you are ideal weight but gaining, work to stabilize your weight.

Overweight

- If you are overweight and healthy and have been for years (i.e., you have no elevated cholesterol, blood glucose, or other markers of chronic disease), focus on your fitness.
- If you are overweight and gaining, try to stabilize your weight.
- If you are overweight with health conditions that would improve by losing weight, then slowly work toward an ideal body weight.

Obese

- Work slowly to bring your weight down to the overweight category.
- Begin or maintain a fitness program to improve your health and reduce your risk of chronic disease.

Extremely obese

- Seek medical assistance to determine the safest and most effective way for you to reduce your weight.

Maintaining weight after weight loss

- Be vigilant about maintaining healthy behaviors—eat well and stay active.

In all cases, focus on fitness and good nutrition to improve your overall health.

WHAT FACTORS CONTRIBUTE TO MY BODY WEIGHT?

There's no question that some people possess a combination of genes that make them more susceptible to overweight and obesity. But genes always interact with other factors, including the amount and quality of the food you eat and the frequency and intensity of your physical activity. Genes probably account for 60 percent of the tendency toward overweight; the other 40 percent is determined by our behaviors and environment.

In rare instances, a medical condition such as an underactive thyroid gland or very low metabolism can cause significant weight gain. If you suspect that you have an underlying condition of this type, you should seek a medical evaluation.

In the end, most overweight results from an energy imbalance. Our daily energy balance is like one of those old-fashioned scales. On one side sit the calories we consume;

on the other, the calories we use. It's a fairly delicate balance. We gain weight when the calories we consume exceed those we use, day after day, over a long period of time. So sensitive are our bodies to excess energy intake over extended periods of time that only 10 extra calories a day—the equivalent of an extra cracker or chip—can result in the gain of 1 pound over the course of a year.

However, the other side of the equation—the energy expenditure that comes with physical activity—can be helpful in tipping the scale in the direction of weight loss and fitness. When people think of physical activity, they often think only of vigorous exercise or sports. But physical activity does not have to be strenuous to offer health benefits. Any bodily movement that expends energy—household chores such as vacuuming and window washing, yard work, climbing stairs, walking, dancing, throwing a Frisbee with your dog—contributes to your overall good health and to your efforts to lose weight or maintain it at a healthy level. (See Chapter 27.) Ideally, women should engage in a combination of light, moderate, and vigorous activities throughout the week to help with maintaining body weight. In the end, the more physical activity you participate in, the easier it is to maintain a healthy weight throughout life.

WHAT DOES MY METABOLISM HAVE TO DO WITH MY WEIGHT?

"I have a friend who seems to eat freely and never gain an ounce, while I just *look* at a piece of pie and put on three pounds!"

I hear this lament again and again. Does the difference come down to metabolism? Many people believe that lean people are lean because they have a high metabolism and heavy people are heavy because they have a low one. This is only part of the story. It's true that metabolism influences your energy needs, and that genes help determine your metabolic rate. But metabolism alone does not dictate weight; diet and lifestyle can make a huge difference in your energy equation. And physical activity is the best and most efficient way to actually rev up your metabolism.

Just how many calories you burn every day is determined by three factors:

- **Your resting metabolic rate (RMR).** This is the energy you use to fuel all the basic needs of your body—for the smooth functioning of your vital organs, blood circulation, respiration, and cell growth and repair. RMR consumes the biggest wedge of the calorie pie, some two-thirds to three-quarters of your total energy expenditure. It typically slows as we get older, reducing our calorie needs. Dieting by drastically reducing your calorie intake can also slow metabolism, ironically making it harder to lose weight. Fortunately, you can boost RMR by as much as 5 to 10 percent with physical activity. When you are physically active, your muscles are more metabolically active. Moreover, physical activity builds muscle, and muscle burns more energy than fat does. So the more active you are and the more muscle you have, the higher your RMR. This ratio of muscle to body fat is why men, who tend to have more muscle, often have a higher RMR than do women, who tend to have more fat.

- **Digesting and processing your food (thermic effect of food).** Eating takes energy. About 10 percent of your total energy expenditure is consumed by digesting, absorbing, transporting, and storing the food you eat. This energy requirement is consistent and not easily changed; there's very little evidence that special combinations of food step up the energy expended in digestion.

- **All physical activity.** This is the final wedge of the energy pie, and the one that varies most from person to person and has the most elasticity. The variability in energy expenditure from overall activity during the day can range from as low as 200 calories to more than 2,000 calories and even higher in elite endurance athletes. The number of calories you burn depends on the amount and the intensity of the physical activity you pack into a day. This includes not just planned exercise, which is a great way to burn calories, but also just moving more each day—walking your dog, climbing the stairs to your office, gardening, parking at a distance from the stores where you shop, even washing your car yourself rather than taking it to a car wash. Boosting this incidental physical activity can make a real difference in maintaining a healthy weight. Even fidgeting can burn calories!

MANAGING YOUR WEIGHT

In thinking about how to manage your weight, it's important to ask yourself where you are with your weight control. Do you want to maintain your current weight? Lose weight? Keep your weight where it is after having lost pounds? Each of these categories of weight management requires a different approach:

- **Weight maintenance.** If you're at your ideal body weight, you've probably been doing a lot of great work to keep from putting on the pounds. To continue maintaining your weight as you grow older, good nutrition and exercise are of equal importance. You can follow these guidelines:
  - Eat healthy foods and control your portion sizes.
  - Be active. (See Chapter 27 for details.)

THE THREE COMPONENTS OF TOTAL ENERGY EXPENDITURE

Resting Metabollic Rate (RMR)
900 to 1,400 calories

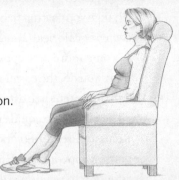

RMR is the energy needed to maintain body function during rest and sleep. It is largely dependent upon body size and body composition.

Formula to estimate RMR for women:
RMR = 655 + (4.35 × weight in pounds) + (4.7 height in inches) − (4.7 × age in years)

Thermic Effect of Food (TEF)
150 to 300 calories

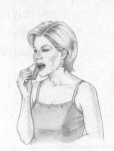

TEF is the energy needed to digest and metabolize food. It is dependent upon how many calories you eat.

Approximately 10 percent of all calories consumed is needed for TEF (e.g., if you consume 2,000 calories per day, 200 calories will be expended as TEF).

All Activity
150 to 2,000 calories and up

Every time you move a muscle you expend energy. This includes activities of daily living such as carrying groceries to going for a long run. The greater the intensity and duration of the activity the more energy you expend.

Estimate your expenditure due to activity (all estimates approximate):

Sedentary = RMR × 1.2

Lightly active (1–3 exercise sessions per week) = RMR × 1.375

Moderately active (3–5 exercise sessions per week) = RMR × 1.55

Very active (6–7 exercise sessions per week) = RMR × 1.725

Total energy expenditure—the number of calories you burn every day—is made up of three parts. Resting metabolic rate accounts for the majority of the total in sedentary people. A small proportion is expended by the thermic effect of food—the energy used in digesting and processing food. By far the most elastic part of energy expenditure consists of physical activity of all types, from fidgeting to folding laundry or vacuuming, from walking or biking to running a marathon.

- **Weight loss.** If you need to lose weight, diet will contribute about 75 percent to your weight loss; physical activity, about 25 percent. You should:
  - Change your eating habits to embrace healthful, nutritious food choices and eat fewer calories.
  - Become more active; exercise vigorously for at least 30 minutes a day (the more you do, the easier it gets) and increase your everyday physical activity.
- **Weight maintenance after weight loss.** To keep off the weight that you've lost, you'll need to place equal emphasis on nutrition and physical activity.
  - Remain disciplined about your diet. You cannot assume that your body's natural appetite regulation will maintain your weight. You need to pay close attention to portion size and avoid tempting foods and situations that you know may trigger overeating.
  - Studies show that people who maintain weight loss most successfully exercise for at least 60 minutes a day.

HOW CAN I LOSE WEIGHT AND KEEP IT OFF?

So many women fight to lose weight with one diet or another and then to keep off the pounds. It can seem like an unending uphill struggle, and statistics suggest that it gets harder as we age. Only one in five women in her twenties is overweight or obese. By ages 30 to 49, it's one in three; and by the mid-fifties, it's more than 67 percent. But the truth is, women of all ages succeed in losing weight and not regaining it. I find that women who are most successful at losing weight are motivated mainly by a desire to become fit and healthy.

The key is finding a long-term plan for eating and exercise that you enjoy so that you'll stick with it. Research from the National Weight Control Registry (NWCR) at Brown Medical School confirms that the secret to successful weight loss is finding new eating and exercise patterns that will last you a lifetime. The NWCR has tracked more than 5,000 individuals who have lost from 30 to 300 pounds and kept off the weight for at least a year. Eighty percent of the registered members are women. Nearly all reported that they lost weight by modifying their food intake in some way and increasing their physical activity—most often by walking. A little more than half lost weight with the help of a program; the rest accomplished the weight loss on their own. Although the participants used different methods to lose weight, they depended on similar strategies to maintain their weight loss. Among them:

- Consuming a healthy diet of nutritious foods, with fewer calories
- Being consistent in their day-to-day pattern of eating
- Eating breakfast

- Limiting consumption of fast food and other foods eaten away from home
- Maintaining a high level of physical activity; about 90 percent of the NWCR registrants exercise, on average, about an hour a day
- Spending a minimal amount of time watching TV; two-thirds of NWCR participants watch fewer than 10 hours of TV a week
- Weighing themselves regularly

THE MOST EFFECTIVE DIET

Calories are what count!

Which diet is most effective in aiding weight loss and weight maintenance? Is it a low-carbohydrate/high-fat/high-protein diet? Or one with high carbohydrates/low fats/moderate proteins? A large study published in 2009 in the *New England Journal of Medicine* helps clear up some of the confusion. Researchers at Harvard University and Louisiana State University studied a pool of more than 800 men and women in midlife who were overweight or obese. The volunteers were randomized to one of four different heart-healthy diets, which they consumed for 2 years: 1) 20 percent fat, 15 percent protein, 65 percent carbohydrate; 2) 20 percent fat, 25 percent protein, 55 percent carbohydrate; 3) 40 percent fat, 15 percent protein, 45 percent carbohydrate; 4) 40 percent fat, 25 percent protein, 35 percent carbohydrate.

The results of the study showed that there was little difference among the diets. Men and women in all groups lost weight and there was no difference among the groups in terms of weight loss or hunger, satiety, and satisfaction. The important factor was how many calories the volunteers took in and whether they stuck with their diets. Volunteers in all groups lost an average of 19 pounds in the first 6 months and kept off an average of 8 pounds after 2 years. All of the diets also improved lipid-related risk factors and fasting insulin levels, thereby reducing overall risk of heart disease, diabetes, and metabolic syndrome.

This study shows us that it doesn't matter which type of diet you go on. What matters is reducing calories! A wide range of options work, provided they are heart-healthy—low in saturated fat, with plenty of fruits, vegetables, whole grains, nuts, and legumes, and a reasonable amount of protein.

Changing lifelong eating habits is difficult, but you can do it. The key is changing your microenvironment. (See Chapters 24, 26, and 28.)

Here are 10 guidelines that will help you achieve sensible weight loss and maintain a healthy weight as you get older:

1. **Start now.** Life is always busy. Now is a good time to set aside excuses and get going. Focus on changing your behavior and reevaluating how you approach food and exercise. This is perhaps the most difficult change you'll ever make in your life.

2. **Set realistic goals.**
   - Try to take a fresh look at your weight. Many of us have in our minds an ideal weight that is outmoded or unrealistic, based on a preconception or something we once heard or saw in a magazine.
   - If you're seriously overweight or obese, a realistic overall goal is to lose 10 percent of your body weight. If you can maintain your new weight for a year and you wish to lose more, you can set another goal.
   - Start by setting smaller goals of one unit of BMI at a time. That's about 5 to 7 pounds, depending on your height, so plan on 5 to 7 weeks to bring your BMI down by one unit.
   - Don't expect to lose weight overnight. Healthy weight loss is gradual weight loss, about a pound a week. Crash dieting lowers your metabolic rate, which makes it harder to lose weight.

3. **Surround yourself with supporters** who also practice these behaviors. Healthy habits really are contagious!

4. **Change your food environment to eat more healthfully.** Chapter 26, "Shifting Your Food Environment," targets how to change your food environment to help you eat more healthfully. I encourage you to read that chapter to help give you the tools you need.

5. **Be more active and less sedentary.** Chapter 27, "Getting Active," is a comprehensive program to help you become more active and maintain that activity in the weeks, months, and years ahead.

6. **Establish good eating habits.**
   - Eat regular meals, including a healthy breakfast. Studies indicate that people who take in more of their overall daily calories at breakfast consume fewer calories during the day.
   - Eat at a leisurely pace. When you eat too quickly, your brain doesn't have time to register satiety signals from the stomach. Also, when you eat slowly

and mindfully, you can better enjoy the taste of food and find it more satisfying.

- Eat only at the dining table and not in front of the television. Studies show that when we watch TV, our brains can't keep track of our food intake, and we easily overeat.
- Avoid late-evening eating (from 8 p.m. to midnight), which is highly correlated with obesity.
- Get back into cooking. Even simple meals that you cook at home are healthier than those you pick up on the fly. Baked potatoes, steamed asparagus, and fish on the grill: simple, delicious, and healthy!

7. **Monitor your food consumption.** Write down everything you eat in a food journal or diary. In one weight-loss study, people who kept scrupulous records of what they ate lost more weight than those who did not. Writing down what you eat makes it easier to recognize problematic eating patterns and address them, and it makes it harder to deny overeating. It also helps you keep your focus on your weight-loss effort and boosts your commitment and motivation. (See the Food Log and discussion of self-monitoring in Chapter 24.)

8. **Believe in yourself.**
   - Like any arduous personal challenge, weight loss requires sustaining motivation and focus. It requires picturing your own success and acting as your own coach to urge yourself on. This was affirmed in a study at the University of Maryland in 1996. Women in the study who believed they would lose weight, did—about 30 percent more weight than the women who lacked faith in themselves. (See the section on self-efficacy in Chapter 24.)
   - Watch how you talk to yourself. Many women are overly critical of themselves when it comes to body weight. This does not help your efforts to make positive change. Try to give yourself a more supportive message, focusing on self-acceptance and on appreciating your progress, whether it's eating more vegetables or taking the stairs instead of the elevator. When you nurture yourself emotionally, you're better at nurturing your body.

9. **Keep track of your progress.** By weighing yourself regularly, you'll know whether your efforts are working. Even if you don't shed pounds right away, you may well notice other benefits—that you look better, feel better, and have more energy.

10. **Reward your successes!** Losing weight is a major triumph, and you should celebrate your accomplishments! If your muscles are sore from exercise, treat yourself to a massage. If you dropped a clothing size, buy yourself something new. Or just plan some fun, such as an evening out with friends.

10

Blood Sugar

We hear a lot about the critical importance of keeping your blood sugar, or glucose, at a healthy level. But what does this mean?

We all carry glucose in our bloodstream. When the body digests food, glucose moves into the blood. Too much is toxic, while too little hampers brain functioning and may cause confusion, visual disturbances, and even seizures. To keep glucose levels at a healthy balance, the body has two mechanisms—hunger and insulin: If blood sugar is low, we feel hungry, which makes us eat food that is absorbed and converted into glucose, raising the level of sugar in our blood. When blood sugar is high, the body signals the pancreas to release insulin, a hormone that regulates glucose. The insulin dispenses the glucose to body cells, and our blood sugar levels fall back to lower, fasting levels.

DIABETES

The condition known as diabetes arises when the body has a shortage of insulin or a weakened ability to use the hormone, resulting in excess glucose in the blood. If diabetes is not treated and controlled, both glucose and fat remain in the blood at high levels and can damage vital organs. The result may be:

- Heart disease (death rates from heart disease are two to four times higher in people with diabetes)

- Stroke
- Blindness
- Kidney failure
- Pregnancy complications
- Toe, foot, and leg amputations
- Death related to flu or pneumonia

It's critical to become aware of your risk factors for this serious disease. When you undergo your annual physical, ask your doctor to perform the following tests and measurements:

- Fasting blood glucose
- Blood lipids, including triglycerides
- Blood pressure
- Body mass index
- Waist circumference

In the past decade or so, the number of Americans diagnosed with diabetes has more than doubled, reaching 24 million in 2007—8 percent of the population. In addition, some 57 million adults age 20 or older have prediabetes (also called impaired glucose tolerance), a condition of elevated blood sugar, which puts them at increased risk of developing full-blown diabetes.

There are three forms of the disease:

- **Type 1 diabetes**, which arises most often during childhood or adolescence, accounts for 5 to 10 percent of cases. In type 1 diabetes, the body can't make enough insulin. The immune cells of the body destroy the "beta" cells in the pancreas that make the hormone. Risk factors include genetic, autoimmune, and environmental issues. Treatment involves insulin delivery by injections or a pump.
- **Type 2 diabetes**, which is linked to obesity and physical inactivity, is by far the most common form. It used to be that this condition was seen only in older people. Now it occurs in people of all ages, including children and adolescents. In type 2 diabetes, the body makes insulin but can't use it properly. The condition

often begins with insulin resistance, in which insulin becomes less effective in transporting glucose into cells. Initially, the pancreas responds by boosting its production of insulin. But if the pancreas can't keep making high levels of insulin or the cells are not responsive to insulin, blood sugar levels begin to rise, resulting in diabetes.

Type 2 diabetes has its most severe impact on older adults, women, and members of certain racial and ethnic groups. African Americans, Latin Americans, American Indians, and Alaska Natives are twice as likely as Caucasian adults to suffer from the disease.

• **Gestational diabetes**, a third form of the disease, occurs in some women during pregnancy. It is most common among the ethnic risk groups mentioned above and among women who are obese or who have a family history of diabetes. The disorder requires treatment to normalize maternal blood levels of glucose during pregnancy. Women with gestational diabetes during pregnancy have a 20 to 50 percent chance of developing diabetes in the following 5 to 10 years.

ARE YOU AT RISK FOR DIABETES?

Your chances of developing type 2 diabetes are greater if:

• You are overweight or obese.
• You are 40 years or older.
• You have a parent or sibling with the disease.
• Your ethnic background is African American, Latin American, American Indian, Asian American, or Pacific Islander.
• You've had gestational diabetes or given birth to a baby weighing more than 9 pounds.
• Your blood pressure is 140/90 or higher.
• Your HDL, or "good," cholesterol level is 35 or lower, or your triglyceride level is 250 or higher.
• You are sedentary, or you exercise fewer than three times a week.
• You have polycystic ovary syndrome (PCOS).
• You've tested positive for impaired glucose tolerance (IGT) or impaired fasting glucose (IFG).
• You have a history of cardiovascular disease.

HOW IS DIABETES DIAGNOSED?

A variety of tests are available to diagnose diabetes, among them:

- **Fasting blood glucose test.** If you are not pregnant, this is the preferred method of testing. It is usually done in the morning, after an overnight (8-hour) fast. A fasting blood glucose level of 70 to 99 milligrams per deciliter (mg/dL) is considered normal. A level of 126 mg/dL or higher indicates diabetes.
- **Random blood sugar test.** In this test, a blood sample is taken at any time of day, regardless of the timing of your last meal. A blood sugar level of 200 mg/dL or greater, coupled with the presence of diabetes symptoms, suggests diabetes.
- **Oral glucose tolerance test (OGTT).** This test involves drinking a beverage containing 75 grams of glucose dissolved in water. After 2 hours, if your blood glucose level reaches 200 mg/dL or higher, you will be diagnosed with diabetes.

    The OGTT test is used to diagnose gestational diabetes. Blood glucose levels are checked after 1, 2, and 3 hours. Because glucose levels are lower during pregnancy, levels considered indicative of diabetes are also lower. A pregnant woman is diagnosed with gestational diabetes if she has two blood glucose levels that meet or exceed the following:
    - ○ Fasting blood glucose level of 95 mg/dL
    - ○ 1-hour level of 180 mg/dL
    - ○ 2-hour level of 155 mg/dL
    - ○ 3-hour level of 140 mg/dL

WHAT IS PREDIABETES?

Being prediabetic means having blood glucose levels that are higher than normal but not high enough to be diagnosed as type 2 diabetes. Some 57 million adults in this country have the condition. Prediabetes is a red flag, indicating an increased risk of developing full-blown diabetes within 10 years if steps are not taken to prevent or delay it. The condition also raises the risk of heart disease and stroke. Prediabetes is diagnosed using one of two measurements:

- **Impaired fasting glucose (IFG).** Blood glucose level is high—100 to 125 mg/dL—after an overnight fast.
- **Impaired glucose tolerance (IGT).** Blood glucose level is high—140 to 199 mg/dL—after a 2-hour OGTT.

METABOLIC SYNDROME

Metabolic syndrome is a collection of conditions linked to overweight and obesity—among them, excess abdominal fat, elevated blood pressure, high fasting blood glucose levels, and abnormal cholesterol levels—which occur together and may especially boost your risk of diabetes and heart disease. More than 50 million people in this country have metabolic syndrome, and the condition is becoming increasingly common.

To determine whether you have metabolic syndrome, answer the following questions:

1. Do you have a waistline that is 35 inches or larger? ☐ Yes ☐ No
2. Do you have a higher than normal triglyceride level (150 mg/dL or higher), or are you on medicine to treat high triglycerides? ☐ Yes ☐ No
3. Do you have a lower than normal level of HDL cholesterol (less than 50 mg/dL), or are you on medicine to treat low HDL? ☐ Yes ☐ No
4. Do you have higher than normal blood pressure (130/85 or higher), or are you on medicine to treat high blood pressure? ☐ Yes ☐ No
5. Do you have higher than normal fasting blood sugar (100 mg/dL or higher), or are you on medicine to treat high blood sugar? ☐ Yes ☐ No

If you answered YES to three or more of the questions, you have metabolic syndrome and are at high risk of developing heart disease, type 2 diabetes, and stroke. If you have type 2 diabetes and metabolic syndrome, you are at much higher risk for heart disease than if you have type 2 diabetes without the syndrome.

Once you have metabolic syndrome, it's difficult to revert to a normal state. However, it is possible. All of the factors that contribute to the syndrome (waist circumference, triglycerides, HDL, blood pressure, and fasting blood glucose levels) are related to your physical fitness, body weight, and diet. If you modify these factors, you can manage, or sometimes even eliminate, metabolic syndrome.

Fortunately, there is a great deal you can do to prevent the progression from pre-diabetes to type 2 diabetes. Studies show that you can bring your blood glucose levels back to normal and lower your risk of developing diabetes by losing just 5 to 7 percent of your body weight through healthy eating and physical activity.

PREVENTING TYPE 2 DIABETES

Although some people have a strong genetic predisposition to type 2 diabetes, most people can prevent the development of this disease if they are active, eat well, and maintain a healthy body weight. It is far easier to prevent type 2 diabetes if you are not prediabetic. But hopeful new research suggests that we have the ability to prevent or delay diabetes even in prediabetics through healthy lifestyle measures.

A major clinical trial known as the Diabetes Prevention Program has shown that people who are prediabetic (the most at risk for developing type 2 diabetes) can sharply lower their risk of developing the disease through diet and exercise. In this study, over-weight people who lost just 5 percent of their body weight by exercising moderately for 150 minutes a week and eating well reduced their risk of developing type 2 diabetes by 58 percent. This held true across all participating ethnic groups and for both men and women. A small amount of weight loss achieved through healthy eating habits and exercise appears to reduce the risk of diabetes by helping the body use insulin and process glucose more efficiently. The study also showed that the physical activity and nutrition intervention were much more successful than treatment with a diabetes-prevention drug (metformin), which reduced the risk of developing diabetes by only 31 percent.

In an ongoing follow-up study, participants are being evaluated for the long-term effects of these lifestyle interventions, including the impact on cardiovascular disease. The data collected so far suggests that lifestyle changes are particularly effective at reducing the risk of health conditions linked with diabetes, such as high blood pressure and metabolic syndrome.

PHYSICAL ACTIVITY

Exercise is a potent weapon in the fight against high blood glucose levels. After aerobic exercise or strength training, blood glucose can stay low for hours, even a day or more. Over time, exercise helps control blood glucose. Exercise causes cells to be more sensitive to insulin, so you don't need as much to get the glucose from the blood into the cells. Exercise also stimulates the production of special glucose "carriers" called non-insulin-dependent glucose transporters, which can help get glucose out of the blood and into cells.

Research has shown that physical activity can lower your blood glucose and your blood pressure, reduce your bad cholesterol and raise your good cholesterol, and improve your body's ability to use insulin. One study conducted at Tufts University by my colleague Dr. Carmen Castaneda-Sceppa showed that women and men with type 2 diabetes who participated in a strength-training program for 4 months experienced substantial improvements in the control of their blood sugar levels. They also had reductions in abdominal body fat and lower blood pressure. Some 70 percent of the men and women were able to reduce their diabetes medication.

MANAGING PREDIABETES AND DIABETES

If you have prediabetes or diabetes, work with your health care providers to keep your blood glucose levels under control. This will help you feel better on a day-to-day basis and may well prevent or delay complications of diabetes, such as nerve, eye, kidney, and blood vessel damage. You can keep track of your blood sugar levels at home with a glucose monitoring device. To see how well you're controlling your blood sugar levels over the long term, your health care provider can give you a glycosylated hemoglobin test, or hemoglobin A1C test.

You can help manage the disease effectively, delay its progression, and prevent complications by following some lifestyle guidelines:

- Monitor your blood glucose.
- Periodically measure your hemoglobin A1C.
- Lose a small amount of weight (10 pounds or more), and keep the weight off.
- Engage in regular exercise.
- Eat a healthy diet.
- Minimize your stress levels.

TAKE THE HEMOGLOBIN A1C TEST

The glycosylated hemoglobin test, or hemoglobin A1C test, indicates your average blood glucose levels over the past 2 or 3 months. In this sense, it reflects your overall success in managing your diabetes.

When you have too much sugar in your bloodstream, the extra sugar attaches to (or glycosylates) molecules of hemoglobin, the oxygen-carrying protein in your blood. The hemoglobin A1C test works by measuring how much blood glucose is attached to hemoglobin. The protein carries a "memory" of the blood sugar levels over weeks and months. In a person without diabetes, the hemoglobin A1C is normally 5 percent or less. If you have diabetes or prediabetes, your hemoglobin A1C levels will normally be higher, around 6 percent. However, if your blood sugar is badly out of control over a long period of time, the level can rise to as high as 25 percent. It's best to take action if the level rises above 7 percent.

If you're prediabetic or diabetic, you should have your hemoglobin A1C level measured about three times a year (or no more than once every 3 months). The test can help you confirm the results of your self-monitoring and determine whether your management plan is working.

LOSE WEIGHT

People who are obese are four times more likely to develop type 2 diabetes than people of a healthy weight. In fact, the rapid rise in the incidence of the disease is due in large part to the growing epidemic of obesity and overweight in this country. For every 2 pounds of excess body weight you carry, your risk of diabetes increases 4.5 percent. Because fat cells are more insulin resistant than muscle cells are, extra body weight puts added pressure on the body's ability to maintain insulin levels essential to properly control blood sugar. Central obesity, or excess fat around the waist, heightens the risk of diabetes and high blood pressure. However, losing even small amounts of weight—in the range of 5 to 10 percent of overall body weight—can greatly reduce your risk of developing the disease.

EXERCISE REGULARLY

If you have diabetes, you need to plan your physical activity carefully—what type of exercise you engage in, when, and for how long. It's best to exercise after a snack or light lunch so that your blood glucose doesn't drop too quickly. If you have very high or very low blood glucose levels, it's not safe to exercise.

To establish a safe and pleasurable exercise routine, follow these steps:

- Talk to your health care provider about which activities are safe for you, given the condition of your heart, blood vessels, nervous system, eyes, kidneys, and feet.

- Establish a regular exercise plan. The more consistent you are with your exercise each day, the easier it is for your body to develop a routine that helps you maintain safe blood sugar levels. (See Chapters 24 and 27.)
- Wear a medical identification bracelet or ID tag indicating your condition.
- Keep water and a carbohydrate-based snack, such as a granola bar, handy during exercise.
- Monitor your blood glucose response to exercise. This will offer concrete evidence of the benefits and also safeguard against letting your glucose drop too low. Excessively low blood glucose (hypoglycemia) can occur during or after physical activity, especially if you take insulin or a diabetes pill. It can also occur when you skip a meal or when you exercise strenuously or for a long period of time. If you feel hungry, nervous, or shaky while exercising, be sure to check your blood glucose level. If it measures 70 or below, eat a sugary snack or drink ½ cup (4 ounces) of either fruit juice or a soft drink. If your glucose does not rise, have one more serving until it measures at least 70.

EAT A HEALTHY DIET

There are two main components of the diet that affect blood sugar levels: the number of calories you consume and the types of foods. Calorie intake in excess of expenditure puts you at risk for elevated blood glucose levels and type 2 diabetes.

To fuel its metabolic functions, your body converts the carbohydrates from the food you eat into glucose. Simple carbohydrates break down especially rapidly in the stomach and small intestine, increasing glucose levels quickly (in less than half an hour). Complex carbohydrates are broken down more slowly and converted into glucose in about 2 hours. Fibrous carbohydrates, which resist digestion, make their way through the intestinal tract without conversion into glucose and actually slow down the digestion of other carbohydrates.

You can determine how quickly different carbohydrate-rich foods convert into glucose and boost your blood sugar levels by knowing a food's glycemic index. The glycemic index is a scale used to determine how quickly carbohydrates are broken down into blood sugar, or glucose. Foods with a high glycemic index, such as high-fructose corn syrup, white rice, white bread, or anything with refined flours or grains, quickly convert into glucose. Low-glycemic foods, such as most vegetables, fruits, legumes, nuts, and seeds, take longer to convert into glucose.

Eating too many high-glycemic carbohydrates, which are quickly metabolized into glucose, can cause a sugar spike that triggers the release of large amounts of insulin. Over time, the high levels of insulin may cause the insulin receptors in your cells to become less sensitive to the hormone, so it can't do its job properly. As the receptors lose their sensitivity to insulin, they accept less glucose, so more of the sugar remains in the blood, overflows into the urine, and passes out of your body—without doing its job as a fuel source. In response to high blood sugar levels, your pancreas labors to make even more insulin and can burn out in what may become a vicious cycle.

Eating low-glycemic foods, which are converted into glucose more slowly, can reduce insulin production. The most important factor, however, is keeping your calorie intake in check—this is what makes the biggest difference.

11

Eating and Excreting

When you eat, your body accomplishes a kind of miraculous alchemy, transforming food into flesh and blood. Just the sight or smell of that fresh-baked whole-grain bread or peach pie launches a cascade of events in your body. And once you ingest such foods, an incredible transformation takes place.

It all begins in your mouth, where your salivary glands release saliva—a mixture of water, mucins, and enzymes that breaks down carbohydrates and moistens food. Your teeth help grind down harder food particles mechanically, and your tongue rolls the moistened and transformed food into a soft, smooth "bolus" that easily slides down your throat. Muscles in your esophagus propel the food down toward the stomach in a wave-like movement called peristalsis.

At the opening of the stomach is a ringlike valve or sphincter that prevents backflow into the esophagus while still admitting food. The stomach, a J-shaped sac, can expand to hold nearly a quart of food. Its job is to further break down food by kneading and mixing it with powerful digestive juices such as pepsin and hydrochloric acid. The latter also serves to kill most bacteria that enter with food.

Once thoroughly mixed and liquefied in the stomach, the food moves into the small intestine, a 15- to 20-foot tubular passageway where the food particles are further dissolved with the help of juices from the pancreas, gallbladder, liver, and intestine before being absorbed through the intestinal walls into the bloodstream. The waste products from this process, including undigested parts of food, such as fiber, then pass into the colon, where they remain for a day or two before moving into the rectum for temporary storage. Two sphincter muscles work to keep the anus—the opening to the rectum—closed and prevent leakage before the waste is expelled in a bowel movement.

All of this occurs with the help of ingenious hormones such as gastrin, secretin, and cholecystokinin, as well as a network of nerves throughout the intestinal tract, which control and coordinate digestion.

GOOD GASTROINTESTINAL (GI) BUGS

Some women jump in alarm or cringe in dismay when they hear that they carry within them a full 2 pounds of microorganisms—bacteria, viruses, and other microbes. It's true: By the time we're adults, we possess 10 times more microbial cells than we have human cells, most of them living in our digestive tracts. (Their small size relative to our own cells means that we don't look more like germs.)

Whatever you think of your resident microbes, you couldn't live without them: They are utterly essential to your health and well-being. Some of these friendly bugs help you digest and absorb your food and extract otherwise inaccessible nutrients or even produce them (such as vitamin K and biotin, a B vitamin); others fine-tune your immune system and prevent harmful pathogens from multiplying in your GI tract.

It's important to keep in mind this ecosystem within when you consider taking antibiotics. Some antibiotics may kill friendly bacteria in the gut along with the unfriendly varieties, shifting the balance of populations in your digestive tract. This can allow pathogenic microbes to take over and cause gastrointestinal symptoms or disease. Make sure that you consult with your health care provider about the possible side effects of antibiotics and follow directions carefully.

Probiotics are foods that naturally contain or include additives of live beneficial microorganisms like those typically found in your gut. Foods with probiotics include yogurt, miso, tempeh, and some juices and soy drinks. Although you don't need to take probiotics to be healthy, some people find them beneficial, especially in counteracting side effects from antibiotics, such as cramps, diarrhea, or yeast infections.

COMMON DIGESTIVE PROBLEMS

DRY MOUTH

Also called xerostomia, dry mouth occurs when the salivary glands do not produce sufficient saliva to keep your mouth moist. Among the causes are:

- Certain diseases, such as diabetes, Sjögren's syndrome, Parkinson's disease, and HIV/AIDS
- Some 400 medications, including drugs for high blood pressure and depression
- Certain medical treatments, such as radiation therapy and chemotherapy
- Nerve damage to the head or neck

If you think you have dry mouth, see your dentist or physician. Without treatment, the disorder can cause problems with chewing, swallowing, and speaking, and can increase dental decay and other mouth infections. Depending on the cause of the condition, your dentist or physician may adjust your medication, treat you with medicine that stimulates the salivary glands, or recommend that you use artificial saliva to keep your mouth moist. To improve symptoms:

- Sip water often, especially during meals, which will make chewing and swallowing easier.
- To stimulate saliva flow, suck on sugarless candy or chew sugarless gum, especially citrus-flavored candy or gum.
- Avoid tobacco, alcohol, and drinks with caffeine, all of which can aggravate dry mouth.
- Avoid spicy or salty foods, because they may cause pain.
- Use a humidifier in your bedroom at night.
- Keep your teeth healthy. Brush at least twice a day with a fluoride-containing toothpaste, floss every other day, avoid sticky, sugary foods, and get a dental checkup at least twice a year.

HEARTBURN

Also known as indigestion, heartburn is often caused by gastroesophageal reflux disease (GERD). This condition occurs when stomach acids flow back into the esophagus through the sphincter, causing burning pain in the stomach or chest, bloating, nausea, burping, and vomiting. Among the causes are overweight or obesity, pregnancy, stress, and poor posture and eating habits. However, genes can also play a role, as I've learned from personal experience.

When I was growing up, my dad suffered from severe heartburn. It was a constant struggle for him. I assumed it was because he was overweight and because he drank and smoked. (Fortunately, he is fit and healthy now, and takes much better care of himself.) My brother began to suffer from GERD as well when he reached midlife. I got on my high horse and told him he had to look closely at his lifestyle. However, I got my comeuppance when I entered my late forties. One Christmas after I ate a heavy holiday meal late at night, I felt severe, debilitating pain in my chest. I was convinced it was stress, probably an ulcer. Or worse, a heart attack. But when I went to see a doctor, it was diagnosed as GERD. I have a pretty healthy lifestyle, so clearly age and genetics were at work here. Slowly, over time, I was able to pinpoint the triggers for me: cooked tomato or tomato sauces, wine, chili and other spicy foods, and ibuprofen. So now I stay away from these, and I try to eat my meals well before I go to bed.

To minimize symptoms of heartburn and GERD:

- Reduce the size of your meals and eat more frequently.
- Relax when you eat and try to minimize stress throughout your day.
- Pay attention to good posture while eating and remain upright after eating.
- Leave at least 3 hours between eating and going to bed.
- Lose excess weight.
- Learn your trigger foods and avoid them. (Common trigger foods include high-fat/fried foods, caffeine, spicy foods, tomatoes, citrus, and chocolate.)
- Wait 2 hours after a meal before exercising.
- Reduce consumption of alcohol.
- Stop smoking.
- Raise the head of your bed at night.
- Check with your doctor about any medications you're taking.

Physicians often treat GERD with techniques to manage weight and stress and to improve posture and diet. Medications, many of them over-the-counter, may also help.

BLOATING, BURPING, AND INTESTINAL GAS

We're all familiar with the consequences of intestinal gas: bloating, burping, and flatulence. Intestinal gas is a perfectly normal by-product of digestion, but it can be annoying and embarrassing. It's most often caused by swallowing excessive air and by the natural process of digestion and fermentation of foods in our digestive tract. Eating or drinking too fast can make you swallow excess air. So can drinking carbonated drinks, talking while you eat, and sucking on hard candy or chewing gum.

Bloating is the buildup of gas in the intestinal tract, producing discomfort and sometimes gas pains, which may be relieved by belching or passing gas. Burping is your body's way of getting rid of excess gas. Some burping is normal, but if it's excessive, it may be a symptom of GERD (see above) or gastritis.

Flatulence is most often caused by the fermentation of undigested food by bacteria in the colon or by the incomplete breakdown of certain food components. However, it may also be the result of shifts in the composition of your gut microbes due to antibiotics or other medications. (See the box Good Gastrointestinal (GI) Bugs on page 139.)

It's normal to have some gas and gas pains (most adults pass gas 14 to 23 times a day). If you're troubled by excessive gas, you can try modifying your diet. You can also try avoiding certain foods and drinks that contribute to the problem, including fatty foods, which slow digestion; carbonated beverages; and carbohydrates that contain indigestible starches, fibers, and sugars (especially fructose, sorbitol, raffinose, and, for some, lactose). Among the most common culprits are:

- Broccoli, Brussels sprouts, onions, cabbage
- Beans and lentils
- Foods containing the sugar lactose (for those who are lactose intolerant), including dairy products, as well as certain processed foods, such as breads and salad dressings. Many women become more lactose intolerant as they grow older. To minimize discomfort, consume dairy products that naturally contain less lactose, such as yogurt; eat only very small portions; or use products that have reduced lactose, such as Lactaid milk.

If you feel that excessive gas is interfering with your quality of life or if gas is accompanied by chronic heartburn, nausea or vomiting, diarrhea, weight loss, rectal pain, blood in stools, or fever, you should see your health care provider.

CELIAC DISEASE

Sometimes known as gluten intolerance, celiac disease is an autoimmune disorder characterized by an inability to tolerate gluten, a protein found in wheat. When someone with celiac disease consumes gluten, the protein damages the lining of the small intestine. Among the symptoms are diarrhea, abdominal bloating and discomfort, and fatigue. Treatment for celiac disease most often involves eliminating from your diet any products containing wheat gluten and using nutrient supplements as necessary.

BLADDER AND BOWEL CONTROL

After your body has extracted nutrients from the food and drink you consume, the waste products that are left behind remain in the blood and bowel.

Your urinary system (together with the lungs, skin, and intestines) works hard to keep in balance the total volume of water in your body and the concentration of substances dissolved in it—and to remove unwanted waste. The organs that largely manage this water balance and waste removal are your kidneys, two small bean-shaped organs about 4 inches long, tucked in your abdominal cavity behind the lower portion of your ribs. Your kidneys filter the water molecules from your blood and expel the unwanted waste in urine. Included in this waste is urea, a compound produced when protein-containing foods are broken down in the body.

Over a 24-hour period, kidneys filter some 50 gallons of water via the blood, returning most of it back to circulation, and expelling only about 3 pints a day as urine. The urine is sent through two thin ducts called ureters to the bladder, a hollow, muscular organ perched in your pelvis, for temporary storage. A healthy bladder can hold up to 2 cups of urine for about 2 to 5 hours.

When nerves in the bladder signal your brain that it's full and needs to be emptied, the brain in turn sends a message to the muscles around the bladder to release urine. It passes out of your body through another duct, the urethra. The opening between the bladder and the urethra is controlled by two circular muscles known as sphincters. Muscles in the pelvic floor, beneath the bladder, also help control urine flow and prevent leaking.

Contrary to what some beverage companies would like you to believe, there is no evidence that women are chronically dehydrated. The recommendation to drink 8 cups of water a day was largely fabricated by a beverage industry following Europe's trend to bottle and sell water. Our thirst centers are good at sending signals that stimulate us to drink when needed. Regular fluid consumption from a variety of sources, especially water and non-sugar-sweetened beverages, keeps us well hydrated. The only time we need to increase our fluid intake is when we are ill, exposed to hot temperatures, or exercising. So let your thirst center guide you to drink what you need to stay hydrated.

URINARY INCONTINENCE

Good bladder control is an important part of leading a healthy, active life. However, many of us experience some loss of control and leakage, or involuntary release of urine, after childbirth or with advancing age. More women than men suffer from the problem, including some 10 percent of women over the age of 65.

Childbearing is hard on the bladder. In pregnancy, the added weight and pressure from the uterus can temporarily weaken our pelvic floor muscles. Soon after I had my third child, I was leading an exercise group made up of my neighbors. When I leapt into a set of jumping jacks, I felt my bladder go and thought, *whoa!*

Bladder control problems sometimes emerge after menopause, when the body stops making estrogen. Some evidence suggests that estrogen keeps the lining of the bladder and urethra robust; lack of the hormone may exacerbate weakness in the muscles that control the bladder. In addition, as we age, the muscles in our ureters, bladder, and urethra may lose strength.

Incontinence occurs when the bladder muscles contract without warning, squeezing urine out of the bladder, or when the sphincter muscles surrounding the urethra relax. If muscles are weakened, coughing, sneezing, laughing, exercising, or lifting heavy objects can create leakage known as stress incontinence. This is most common among young and middle-age women, though it sometimes begins at menopause.

Fortunately, loss of bladder control after childbirth or because of age or menopause can be prevented or alleviated by training the pelvic floor muscles with Kegel exercises. This involves squeezing and holding the muscles of the pelvic floor and then relaxing them multiple times. This process is repeated several times a day. (See the box Kegeling at right.)

Urge incontinence—when you can't control your bladder long enough to reach the toilet—can be caused by infections, medications, Alzheimer's disease, Parkinson's disease, and nerve damage from diabetes or stroke. But for most women, the cause is bladder irritants, aggravated by thinning of the bladder lining and urethra during menopause, which makes the bladder more sensitive to irritants. Bladder irritants vary from person to person, but for many, the culprit is coffee, even decaffeinated coffee. Other common irritants include diet sodas, alcohol, spicy foods, citrus, and tomatoes. If you have urge incontinence infrequently, do a quick survey of what you had to eat or drink over the past 24 hours, and see whether you can identify the irritant. Too much or too little water can also contribute to the problem. Most experts recommend 4 to 6 glasses a day.

Kegels can help with urge incontinence, but they're not as effective as they are for stress incontinence. Most women note that part of the trigger for leakage is know-

KEGELING

Kegel exercises strengthen your pelvic floor muscles, the group of muscles that stretch like a shallow bowl between your pubic bone and your tailbone, supporting your uterus, bladder, and bowel. These are the same muscles you would use to stop your flow of urine if you were going to the bathroom. Try to do a set of 10 Kegels two or three times a day: Focus on lifting your pelvic floor muscles, counting for 5 to 10 seconds while contracting and holding the muscle, then release while counting for 5 to 10 seconds. At the beginning, you may want to start with just a 3-second hold and gradually work up to 10 seconds.

ing that relief is imminent. It may help to focus on breathing and calmness—on slowing down rather than hurrying up—so that mental urgency does not contribute to physical urgency. It's worth trying this technique before turning to medications.

If you're having difficulty with bladder control, contact your physician or gynecologist or other health care provider, who can:

- Determine whether you have stress or urge incontinence or both
- Assess whether you are able to Kegel effectively
- Consider whether low-dose vaginal/topical estrogen might be helpful
- Offer referrals to physical therapists or urologists who specialize in the treatment of women's incontinence, including: bladder training, biofeedback, and electrical stimulation

If the above measures are not successful, your health care provider may also refer you for a fitting with a vaginal device (called a pessary) or for surgery, both of which may be effective in supporting the bladder.

KIDNEY STONES

Stones, or calculi, made of substances in urine such as calcium, can form in the kidney or elsewhere in the urinary system. Sometimes they are the source of significant pain and infection. Symptoms include severe and persistent pain in your back or side, blood in your urine, fever and chills, vomiting, cloudy or foul-smelling urine, and a burning sensation when you urinate. Treatment involves removing the stones through surgical or nonsurgical means. Some women are more prone to developing certain kinds of kidney stones when they take calcium supplements.

URINARY TRACT INFECTION (UTI)

More common among women than men, infections of the urinary tract are caused by bacteria. If the infection occurs in the bladder, it's referred to as cystitis; if it's the more serious variety, in the kidney, it's called pyelonephritis. Symptoms include a painful, burning sensation while urinating, the feeling of an urge to urinate frequently, and sometimes blood or pus in the urine. If you experience any of these symptoms, you should seek medical help. Physicians usually prescribe antibiotics to treat infections.

To prevent UTIs, it helps to:

- Empty the bladder before and after sexual intercourse.
- Change sanitary napkins frequently.
- Always wipe from front to back after a bowel movement.

If you are prone to UTIs consider drinking unsweetened cranberry juice regularly. There is some evidence that antioxidants called anthocyanins in cranberry juice reduce bacterial adherence to the bladder wall, thus reducing UTIs.

HEALTHY BOWEL HABITS

The solid waste generated by our bodies is stored in the rectum before being expelled as a bowel movement. Having regular bowel movements is an important part of your overall health. Keep in mind that the normal number of bowel movements ranges from three times a day to three times a week. But if you're irregular, the following tips can help:

- Eat plenty of plant-based foods and fewer animal-based foods.
- Drink enough water and avoid alcoholic or caffeinated beverages.
- When you feel the need to use the bathroom, respond promptly. The best time is 20 to 30 minutes after a meal or a warm drink.
- Exercise regularly to stimulate muscle activity and aid peristalsis.

COMMON BOWEL PROBLEMS

Constipation

Difficulty moving your bowels, or constipation, is most often caused by hard stools that move too slowly through your intestines. Common causes include insufficient fluid, fiber, or exercise; suppressing the urge to have a bowel movement; and regularly using laxatives. If you suffer from constipation, try drinking more fluids and eating more fiber. In addition, most doctors recommend a stool softener such as docusate sodium (Colace) or a fiber supplement such as psyllium (Metamucil) or methylcellulose (Citrucel). (If you take a fiber supplement, make sure you drink plenty of water.) The added fiber helps soften the stool. Increasing your physical activity also helps constipation. It is generally not a good idea to use laxatives, because they can lead to dependency and reduced bowel function. If the problem persists, talk to your health care provider.

Diarrhea

Diarrhea refers to the passage of frequent loose, watery stools more than three times a day. The most common form of diarrhea is temporary or acute diarrhea, lasting a day or two before going away on its own without treatment. The cause is most often bacterial, viral, or parasitic infection.

If diarrhea persists for 3 days or more, you should see a doctor. Chronic diarrhea poses a risk of dehydration and can indicate a more serious problem, such as an adverse reaction to a medication or intestinal diseases such as celiac disease or inflammatory bowel syndrome.

To alleviate temporary diarrhea, try to avoid foods that worsen the condition, which include dairy products; caffeine; and greasy, high-fiber, or sugary foods. As your diarrhea improves, add only soft, bland foods to your diet, such as white rice, bananas, toast, crackers, and boiled potatoes.

If you think your diet may be contributing to periodic diarrhea, keep a journal to figure out which foods might be acting as a trigger. You can try removing the likely culprits—such as raisins, dried fruits, coffee, beans, lentils, artificial sweeteners, milk, or wheat—for a week or so. Reintroduce problem foods slowly.

Diverticular Disease

A common cause of pelvic or abdominal pain, diverticular disease takes two forms. The mild form, known as diverticulosis, arises when small pouches in the colon called diverticula bulge outward through weak spots in the colon. Roughly one in 10

Americans over the age of 40 has diverticulosis, which is thought to result when slow-moving stools raise pressure inside the colon. Most of the time, diverticulosis causes no symptoms.

The more severe form, called diverticulitis, occurs when the diverticula become infected or inflamed. Symptoms of diverticulitis may include abdominal cramps and tenderness (especially near the left side of the lower abdomen), bloating, and constipation. Fever, nausea, vomiting, and chills may also occur.

Most cases of diverticulosis are treated with a high-fiber diet, which prevents complications such as diverticulitis. If diverticulitis develops, it may be treated with "bowel rest"—a diet of clear liquids—and antibiotics to fight infection. Most doctors will counsel their patients who have diverticulosis to avoid seeds, fruits that contain small seeds, and small nuts. These foods can get stuck in the pouches and cause a flare-up of the disease.

Although the cause of diverticular disease is unknown, for some people a low-fiber diet is to blame. Too little dietary fiber often causes constipation, which makes muscles in the intestinal tract strain and increases pressure in the colon. This pressure may make the weak spots in the colon bulge out. To stave off the disease, the American Dietetic Association recommends 20 to 35 grams of fiber daily from high-fiber foods.

Fecal Incontinence or Loss of Bowel Control

One out of every 100 adults is affected by fecal incontinence, the accidental release of waste from the rectum. The condition can be the source of much embarrassment and anxiety. It is most commonly caused by:

- Damage to the anal sphincter muscles from childbirth, injury, surgical procedures, or rectal prolapse
- Diarrhea due to infection or irritable bowel syndrome
- Constipation caused by immobility or illness
- Nerve injury or disease such as stroke, multiple sclerosis, or spinal injury

If you have a problem with fecal incontinence, you should seek the help of a health care professional, who may recommend drug therapy, sphincter exercises to improve bowel control, devices to prevent leakage, or surgery. Specialists in the field include colorectal surgeons and gastroenterologists.

Hemorrhoids

Hemorrhoids—inflamed and swollen veins around the anus or lower rectum—often result from straining during a bowel movement, chronic constipation or diarrhea, pregnancy, or aging. To relieve the symptoms of pain and itching:

- Bathe several times a day in warm, clear water for about 10 minutes.
- Apply a hemorrhoidal cream or suppository to the affected area.
- After every bowel movement, clean the anus well with pads soaked in witch hazel (such as Tucks).

To prevent hemorrhoids, physicians recommend reducing the strain of constipation by increasing the amount of fiber and fluids in your diet. Drink 6 to 8 cups of non-alcoholic fluid a day and consume fiber in the form of fruits, vegetables, and whole grains. In addition, some doctors recommend a stool softener such as psyllium (Metamucil) or a fiber supplement such as methylcellulose (Citrucel).

For serious cases of hemorrhoids, doctors may suggest endoscopic or surgical treatment to shrink or destroy hemorrhoidal tissue.

Inflammatory Bowel Disease

Also referred to as Crohn's disease, inflammatory bowel disease is a serious condition of chronic inflammation of the gastrointestinal tract that can eventually cause the lining of the tract to tear. Symptoms include cramping, rectal bleeding, fever, weight loss, nausea and vomiting, and persistent diarrhea. Scientists suspect that the disease is an autoimmune disorder. (See Chapter 18.) However, genetic and environmental factors may also play a part. Physicians treat the disease with medications and/or surgery. But patients can help manage their symptoms by modifying their diet—eating small, frequent meals, drinking plenty of fluids, and avoiding irritating foods—and preventing excessive weight loss.

Irritable Bowel Syndrome (IBS)

Irritable bowel syndrome affects as many as 25 million Americans, nearly three-quarters of them women. But sadly, only 10 to 20 percent of those with the syndrome seek medical help. IBS is characterized by inflammation and spasms of the gastrointestinal tract, especially the colon, causing abdominal pain and bloating, nausea, constipation, and diarrhea. Symptoms include abdominal pain or discomfort for at least 12 weeks in the past year. This pain or discomfort has two of the following features:

- Relief when you have a bowel movement
- With onset of pain or discomfort, either a change in bowel movement frequency OR
- A change in the appearance of your stool

Other symptoms include feelings of urgency, difficulty passing stool, mucus in the stool, or abdominal bloating.

Many women with the syndrome think it's just something they have to live with. It's important to understand that IBS is not "all in your mind"; it's a real disease with real symptoms, which can often be treated. Though the cause is still unclear, IBS has been linked with heightened sensitivity in the GI tract, disrupted communication between the colon and the brain, and bacterial or viral infection. Symptoms are aggravated by stress, anxiety, or menstruation.

Trigger foods and beverages include:

- Large meals loaded with fat and calories
- Alcohol
- Carbonated drinks
- Milk products
- Candy and chocolate

- Beverages with caffeine
- Baked goods made with white flour or refined sugar
- Red meat
- Dried beans and lentils
- Cruciferous vegetables

If you think you may have IBS, see your doctor. Treatments include lifestyle measures (see below) and medications, including laxatives, antidiarrheals, antispasmodics, and antidepressants. In addition, two prescription drugs designed specifically for women are available, tegaserod (for constipation with IBS) and alosetron (for diarrhea with IBS).

Making lifestyle changes may help ease symptoms of IBS.

Minimize stress, get sufficient sleep, exercise regularly, keep a food diary, reduce your meal sizes, drink plenty of fluids, and eat high fiber foods. Probiotics may also be helpful.

Exercise and Bowel Trouble

As cocaptain of the President's Marathon Challenge at Tufts University, I am often asked about the problem of bowel movements during a long run. Marathoner Bill Rodgers is said to have warned a group of runners: "More marathons are won or lost in the porta-toilets than at the dinner table."

Indeed, for many people, exercise can cause intestinal problems—abdominal cramps, bloating, diarrhea, and other concerns. Women are more likely than men to experience these troubles, especially if they're dieting. And those in running and high-intensity sports are particularly susceptible.

To ease the problem, do a little light exercise before a big athletic event to help stimulate your GI system to empty your bowels, train at different times of day to see what works best for you, and before exercising, minimize your intake of high-fiber foods.

roductive Choices Fertility and Pregr
enopause Sexual Abuse and Sexual A
in Teeth Hair and Nails Body Weigh
etabolism Blood Sugar Eating and Excr
scles Bones JointsHeart and Blood
d Respiration Common Infectious Dis
toimmune Disease Cancer Vision He
ell, Taste, and Touch Mental Health
ce Abuse Making Change Managing
d Sleeping Well Shifting Your Food Env
t Getting Active Screenings and H
intenance Reproduction Sexuality and
l Health Reproductive Choices Fertilit
gnancy Menopause Sexual Abuse and
l Assault Skin Teeth Hair and Nails
ight and Metabolism Blood Sugar E
d Excreting Muscles Bones Joints Hear
od Lungs and Respiration Common
us Diseases Autoimmune Disease C

PART IV

Standing Strong:
Our Living Framework

Perhaps because of the messages sent to us by society, women often underestimate their own strength and athletic prowess. I've spent most of my professional life conducting research that shows how women's muscles and bones have fantastic potential for strength. We are the proud owners of a physical framework that's stronger pound for pound than steel, yet light, alive, and skilled at self-repair. This bony scaffolding is moved by a meshwork of flexible, responsive, and shapely fibers capable of rapid change and reformation. If this makes you sound like some kind of superwoman, that's because you are. Your 206 living bones, linked at more than 100 bendable joints, provide not only amazing strength and support, but also suppleness and agility. Your hundreds of muscles cushion the bone; they lift, lower, twist, turn, and stabilize it; and they make it grow.

My fascination with muscles and bones probably arises from my lifelong interest in physical activity and sports (or perhaps, from the many broken bones I suffered in my youth). My first scientific study focused on the importance of muscles in the aging process. Since then, I've conducted several studies on both muscles and bones and have written three books on the topic.

As I've learned in my research, our musculoskeletal system is vulnerable. Muscles and bones are living tissues that may suffer damage or diminish with age as a result of shifting hormone levels, metabolism, and especially, inactivity. But the good news is that exercise at any age can boost both the strength and the quality of muscles and bones.

Women begin adult life with less muscle than men have and with lighter bones. So although both sexes tend to lose these tissues at about the same rate, women may experience more problems from muscle loss in the long run. When researchers looked at the factors that most affect women's ability to perform the basic activities of daily life, they found that the health of our muscles and bones is vital. The Women's Health and Aging Study, which included 1,000 women 65 and older, showed that a third of American women over the age of 70 have trouble performing basic self-care activities, primarily because of musculoskeletal weakness or pain.

Keeping your musculoskeletal system healthy is essential for the kind of active, engaged lifestyle most of us want for ourselves at any age. To keep your skeleton upright and your muscles working well, you need to build robust bone and muscle mass early in life, during adolescence, and in adulthood by eating right (plenty of fruits, vegetables, and calcium) and getting adequate vigorous exercise.

These **S.M.A.R.T.** strategies will help you maintain healthy muscles, bones, and joints throughout life:

1. Engage in a program of regular physical activity that includes strength training (i.e., lifting weights) as well as weight-bearing exercise, such as walking and jogging.
2. Avoid extremes of body weight.
3. Limit alcohol intake.
4. Get sufficient calcium and vitamin D.
5. Train wisely to avoid injuries.
6. Take measures to prevent falls.

12

Muscles
_____

When you look at a woman with a beautiful quintessentially "feminine" figure such as Marilyn Monroe or Kate Winslet, what you're seeing is musculature. The size, shape, and proportion of muscles define the contours of our bodies, our arms and legs, abdomen, back, and butt. Muscles not only give us a beautiful body shape, they also make us physically strong, allowing us to maintain our energy, vitality, and ability to live independently as we grow older.

Whether you think of yourself as strapping strong or not, your body likely has the same 600 or so muscles possessed by even the beefiest bodybuilder. Those muscles make up some 30 to 50 percent of your body weight. It's hard to overstate their importance. They power every move you make, from striding toward a movie theater to focusing your eye lens once inside the darkened room. Never-resting muscles in the walls of your internal organs power everything from the beating of your heart (called cardiac muscles) to your breathing, the movement of food through your digestive tract, and the pressure of your blood streaming along inside your vessels (all controlled by involuntary smooth muscles).

Skeletal muscles—the kind that move your bones—are what give Marilyn and Kate their contoured arms and shoulders. But they have countless benefits beyond shapeliness. Muscles give us all the ability to do the kinds of daily activities we depend on to keep life going. They improve our balance and flexibility. They raise our energy level and boost our metabolism, which helps us burn calories faster. They protect us from bone loss and reduce our risk of many diseases, from depression to obesity, heart disease, and adult-onset diabetes. And finally, they help maintain a healthy immune system.

As we grow older, we want to maintain both muscle strength and muscle mass. We want our muscles strong so that we can be independent and enjoy an active lifestyle. We want to preserve muscle mass because it helps keep up our resting metabolism and sustain healthy glucose levels, reducing our chance of developing type 2 diabetes. It also serves as a repository of proteins that are important for our overall health.

Unfortunately, as we age, we tend to lose muscle and gain fat. Beginning at about age 40, a woman may lose about ¼ pound of muscle a year, or some 5 percent of her muscle mass every decade—most of it replaced by fat. By the time she reaches the age of 70, she may have lost as much as 25 percent of her total muscle mass, putting her at an increased risk for falls and resulting fractures.

This wasting process, called sarcopenia (from the Greek *sarco* for "flesh" and *penia* for "loss"), is not an inevitable result of aging. Being severely underweight, having a disease such as rheumatoid arthritis, or taking steroids or other medications may cause this sort of muscle loss. But more often, the culprit is inactivity. Remain sedentary, and your muscles will atrophy. Get active, and they will grow strong.

When we stimulate our muscles through exercise, we boost muscle mass, strength, and quality. In the past two decades, I've learned firsthand by working with thousands of women in their mid-forties to mid-nineties that no matter how old you are, you can defy sarcopenia and regain the youthfulness of your muscles through physical activity and

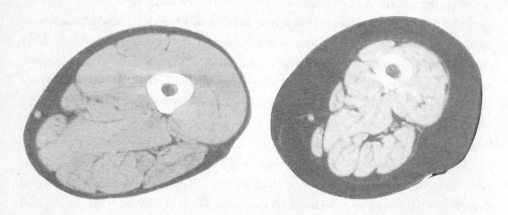

These CT scans show a cross section of two women's thighs. In both scans, the white areas are bone; the light gray area is muscle; and the dark gray area is a thin layer of fat. The scan on the left is the thigh of 23-year-old woman; muscle takes up about 90 percent of her thigh area. The scan on the right belongs to a 67-year-old sedentary woman; only 50 percent of her thigh area consists of muscle. While age affects muscle mass, activity is a bigger factor. With regular strength training, an older woman can retain much of her muscle mass.

regular strength training. My research has taught me never to underestimate the ability of someone to grow stronger just because of gender, age, or existing health condition!

A REAL FOUNTAIN OF YOUTH

In the late 1980s, my colleagues at the Tufts USDA Human Nutrition Research Center on Aging launched a study to see how strength training might benefit the elderly. They selected six women and four men who lived in a nursing home. These were frail, sedentary people, ranging in age from 86 to 96, some of whom had arthritis and osteoporosis and struggled to get out of a chair by themselves. The researchers set up a training program for them lifting weights three times a week. After only 2 months in the program, these elderly men and women gained an astounding amount of strength—double, even triple what they had before. Their balance and walking speed rose by an average of 48 percent. They found they could more easily get in and out of their chairs. Some discarded their canes.

This innovative research inspired me, and shortly after it began, I launched my own study with colleagues on the effects of strength training on 40 sedentary postmenopausal women, ages 50 to 70, which showed equally exciting results. We asked half of our volunteers to act as controls by simply maintaining their usual sedentary lifestyle. The other half we asked to lift weights twice a week.

The remarkable results were published in the *Journal of the American Medical Association* in 1994. After a year of strength training, the muscles and bones of the women in the control group had aged, and the women were more sedentary than ever, with a 25 percent drop in activity. The weight lifters, on the other hand, had muscles that looked 15 to 20 years more youthful than they had a year before; the women had gained about 3 pounds of muscle and lost that much fat. In addition, the women who didn't exercise had lost about 2 percent of their bone density, while those who strength trained *gained* an average of 1 percent. Moreover, the strength-training women had become more active, trim, and happy. Some said they were in better health than they had ever been in their lives, and their muscles were evidence of that.

In the years since, we've learned that another important benefit of strength training is improving balance and reducing the risk of falls. For older women especially, falling is a serious risk and the leading cause of injury and injury-related deaths. After age 70, your chance of taking a fall is about one in three over the course of a year. (See the box Better Your Balance on page 158.) Boosting the strength of your ankles, legs, and lower body through strength training will give you better balance, mobility, and speed of movement—all of which will reduce your risk of falling if you lose your footing.

BETTER YOUR BALANCE

Our sense of balance is sometimes called our "sixth sense." It's actually an exquisite and complex process involving vision, sense of touch (especially from the touch and pressure sensors in our feet), proprioceptive sense (our awareness of where we are in space and the positions of our limbs), the muscles of our legs and torso, and our vestibular system, minute, fluid-filled tubules in our inner ears. All of these sensory and motor parts interact to help us keep our bodies balanced and upright.

Maintaining good balance is vital, especially as we grow older. Otherwise we risk losing our balance and taking a hard fall, which can lead to fractures. According to the Centers for Disease Control and Prevention, an older adult is treated in an emergency department for a fall every 18 seconds. In 2008, more than 430,000 people were hospitalized for fall-related injuries. Many of us have older friends or relatives who have fallen, with devastating consequences. More than 90 percent of hip fractures are precipitated by a fall.

But falling is not an inevitable consequence of aging. An important underlying cause is compromised physical fitness—specifically, strength and balance. The key to maintaining balance as we age, then, is keeping up our muscle strength, aerobic fitness, and balance-training exercises. I encourage you to build into your physical activity routine the simple at-home balance exercises suggested in Chapter 27, "Getting Active." Activities such as tai chi and yoga are also excellent ways of boosting steadiness.

Maintaining your bone density and balance is the one-two punch that will help you reduce your overall risk of fracture as you age. Other strategies for avoiding falls include:

- Getting your eyes checked regularly, at least once a year
- Improving lighting throughout your house
- Keeping your floors and hallways free of clutter
- Installing a banister or railing along stairs and in the bathroom

IMPROVING MUSCLE HEALTH: BUILDING QUANTITY AND QUALITY

Now we know that a progressive program of strength training can boost strength and build muscles in women of all ages. To see how strength training affects muscle, let's linger for a minute on the mechanics.

Muscles are masterpieces of natural engineering. Each muscle is basically a biological puller. It works by shortening, or contracting, and pulling the bone to which it's attached through tough, cordlike tendons.

Muscles tend to work in pairs, performing complementary actions so that your bones remain aligned and stabilized throughout any action. Take, for example, your biceps, the muscle in the front of your upper arm. This muscle originates in your shoulder and inserts into your forearm. When you pick up a dumbbell, the biceps contracts, shortening and pulling up the bone, and bringing up your forearm. This is called a concentric contraction. As you lower the dumbbell in a controlled manner, your biceps relaxes and lengthens (called an eccentric contraction), while your triceps, the muscle at the back of your upper arm, contracts to straighten your arm. Oddly enough, it's the eccentric action—the lowering of the weight—that most stimulates the growth of muscles.

Strength training boosts muscle mass by stimulating hypertrophy, or enlargement of the muscle cells (myofibrils). This happens when eccentric contractions cause microstructural damage to the cells, which causes them to make more proteins that build more myofibrils. The additional proteins not only repair the damage to the fibers, but they also enlarge them, building muscle mass.

This does not mean that you'll "bulk up" as a result of the training. In fact, my study and other studies show that although women who strength train may gain about 50 to 100 percent in muscle strength, their muscles don't grow all that much, only by a few pounds, with an equivalent loss in fat mass; their muscle contours are just more visible, better defined because of this youthful shift in body composition.

In just the first few weeks of strength training, you can get noticeably stronger without even increasing your muscle mass. Muscle strength can increase through the reinforcement of nerve pathways that stimulate the motor units in the muscle. Every movement—lifting a dumbbell, brushing your hair, swinging a tennis racket—begins with a signal from the brain that initiates a sequence of events. The nerve signal travels along motor nerves to the motor unit in the muscle. When it arrives there, it "fires" the

FIBROMYALGIA

Fibromyalgia is a condition that is still poorly understood. What we know is that it's a cluster of chronic symptoms marked by fatigue, mood, and sleep disturbances, and especially, pain in the muscles, ligaments, and tendons in many areas of the body. Although it can cause debilitating pain and depression, it's not progressive and does not cripple or deform joints. Some physicians believe that the condition arises as a result of increased sensitivity in the brain to pain signals. it is more common in women than in men and often runs in families, so there may be a genetic component. Symptoms sometimes start after an infection or an emotional or physical trauma, but may also occur without a precipitating event. In some cases, underlying medical issues, such as depression, may exacerbate the condition.

If you think you may have fibromyalgia, see your health care provider. Although there is not much evidence that medication works for the condition, several self-care measures can help, including reducing stress, getting sufficient sleep, and exercising. In the first 6 weeks or so, exercise may worsen pain, but after this, regular walking, swimming, or biking often diminishes symptoms.

muscle fibers, causing them to contract for a split second. Strength training recruits more muscle fibers into the motor unit that responds to the nerve signal—in essence, giving them a wake-up call!

It's also important to maintain the *quality* of your muscles. Good muscle tissue is surrounded by the tiny vessels known as capillaries, which infuse the tissue with blood so nutrients can reach the cells. It also possesses abundant enzymes and mitochondria, the little energy "powerhouses" inside cells. And it stores sugar in the form of glycogen to aid in blood glucose control and to supply energy for exercise and for the brain. Both strengthening exercises and aerobic activity are great ways to build quality muscle tissue.

13

Bones

Why worry about the health of your bones?

The answer may seem obvious: Bones support our bodies and give them structure, anchoring our muscles and allowing us to stand and move. They also shelter our internal organs, swaddling the brain, shielding the heart, lungs, and intestines, and armoring the spinal cord. But bones are far more than a simple system of load-bearing, protective struts. They're living, growing tissues that provide the body with a vital storehouse of calcium, phosphorus, and other minerals that are essential to the function of all of its organs, but particularly to the nerves and muscles. These minerals are carried via the bloodstream wherever they're needed. In essence, bone fulfills two competing functions—bearing weight, which requires strength and ample supplies of calcium and phosphorus, and at the same time, serving as a ready supplier of these same elements when they're in short supply and needed for vital function in the rest of the body. Our bones, then, are not unlike a bank, where we deposit calcium or phosphorus in our early years to use later in life. Too few deposits or too many withdrawals may lead to osteoporosis, a disorder in which bones weaken and break more easily.

In short, our bones are organs like any others: To remain strong and in good health, they need nurturing and care.

BONING UP ON BONES

Some fun facts: When you're a child, you have some 300 bones; as you grow, several bones fuse together so that by the time you're a woman, you have only 206. The ends of most bones are enveloped in cartilage, a strong, resilient protective tissue more bendable than bone, which acts as a shock absorber and reduces friction. Although both sexes have bones of the same shape, women's bones are generally smaller than men's.

The weight of your skeleton? For a 145-pound woman, about 17.5 pounds, or 12 percent of your total body weight. Though the word *skeleton* comes from the Greek word *skeletos*, meaning "dried up," your skeleton is a living, growing organ. Throughout your life, your bones are constantly breaking down and rebuilding themselves, and generating cells that transport oxygen and fight infection.

Bones may feel as tough as a two-by-four, but beneath that sturdy exterior is a latticelike, porous network of little struts and rods called trabeculae. The hard, dense outer layer, known as cortical bone, makes up about 80 percent of your bone mass. The remaining 20 percent consists of the inner trabecular layer. It is within the spaces of this spongy trabecular layer that calcium and other minerals are stored. A network of nerve fibers runs through the bone and also blood vessels, which supply it with nutrients and transport its minerals around the body.

Although all bones contain both types of tissue, the amount of each type varies from bone to bone. The big bones in our legs are made mostly of the cortical material, capped at both ends by trabecular bone. The bones of the spine, pelvis, and wrist, on the other hand, are largely trabecular, with just a veneer of cortical bone. You can develop osteoporosis in any of your bones, but the disease is most common in sites where trabecular bone dominates.

BONE GROWTH AND MAINTENANCE

Most bone growth takes place in the first 25 years of life. But even after you've stopped growing, your bone continues to remodel, with old bone breaking down to be replaced with new bone. Remodeling is a fascinating process of demolition and rebuilding that goes on throughout life. Distinct squads of bone cells partake in the process: Osteoclasts ("bone breakers") dissolve old bone, creating little pits and cavities, and releasing calcium and other minerals into the bloodstream. When these cells receive signals from your body that it needs calcium, they dissolve more bone. That's why it's so important to take in sufficient calcium through diet or supplements to replenish this supply.

After osteoclasts have created a tiny depression or deformity in the bone's surface, a second squad of cells called osteoblasts ("bone builders") assembles to lay down new bone in the cavity. These cells line the hole with matrix, a material rich in the protein collagen. Then they pull from the bloodstream calcium and other minerals, which fill the matrix. Eventually, the collagen and minerals mature and harden, forming new bone, but the process takes as long as 3 to 6 months. This is one reason bone fractures take a long time to heal.

These specialized bone cells, osteoblasts and osteoclasts, are constantly communicating, forming new bone at one site and removing old bone from another. The balance between the destruction and rebuilding of bone determines our bone mass and density. When the activity of the bone-demolishing osteoclasts outpaces the bone-building osteoblasts, as happens with age, we start to lose bone. How much bone we maintain depends on several factors, including our age, sex, hormones, genes, health, diet, and physical activity.

BEYOND OUR GENES, WHAT DETERMINES BONE MASS?

- **Estrogen.** This hormone packs a powerful punch when it comes to bone mass. Estrogen curbs the bone-munching activity of osteoclasts and kindles the bone-building activity of osteoblasts. It helps our bodies absorb calcium from dietary sources and hold on to it in our kidneys. It also boosts the activity of vitamin D, which is essential for calcium metabolism. So when our estrogen levels fall, so usually does our bone mass.
- **Physical activity.** Exercise stimulates bone growth in two ways: First, by direct stimulation to the bone cells; second, through the force of muscle pulling on bones (which comes mainly with weight-bearing exercise). The more powerful your muscles, the more they boost the activity of bone-building osteoclasts. Moreover, exercise of all kinds boosts the secretion of hormones that stimulate bone and muscle growth. When the mechanical force produced by muscle is reduced, bone mass and strength are also lost. In other words, it's the same as with muscle: "Use it or lose it."
- **Nutrition.** A healthy, well-balanced diet that includes plenty of calcium-rich dairy foods, and fruits and vegetables, is vital to maintaining bone health throughout life. Although calcium and vitamin D play especially important roles in building and maintaining bone, other nutrients are also important, including minerals such as magnesium, potassium, and zinc, as well as vitamins C and K.

VITAMIN D AND CALCIUM

The raw material of bones

Bones are made of a rich mix of proteins and minerals, especially calcium, phosphorus, and magnesium. If the body doesn't have these raw materials, it cannot build and maintain strong bones as we grow older. We actually get too much phosphorus from processed foods and grains. As for magnesium, a good diet supplies all we need; there's no evidence that supplements help.

In general, I don't advise women to take vitamin and mineral supplements as long as they're eating a good diet. The exceptions are vitamin D and calcium, the two nutrients most important to bone health—and often in short supply. Unless you are eating an abundance of calcium-rich foods, working outside a good portion of the day, or drinking cod liver oil, you most likely need both calcium and vitamin D supplements for optimal health.

Calcium

The recommended daily calcium requirements for women are as follows:

- **Girls age 9 to 18:** 1,300 mg/day
- **Women age 19 to 50:** 1,000 mg/day
- **Women age 51 and older:** 1,200 mg/day

Although foods such as green leafy vegetables, salmon, and sardines contain calcium, dairy foods are by far the most concentrated source of the mineral, with each serving (1 cup of yogurt or milk) providing approximately 300 mg. For women age 19 to 50, getting enough calcium from diet requires eating at least three servings of low- or fat-free dairy foods per day. For women younger than 19 or older than 50, the requirement is at least four servings per day. In other words, if you eat three servings of dairy foods each day (900 mg), you would only need about 100 to 300 mg of supplementation per day.

At least half of American women do not get sufficient calcium from their diet. For this reason I encourage all women over the age of 16 to assess their calcium intake through diet. If they are not meeting the recommended levels, I suggest they increase their intake of calcium-rich foods *and* take a calcium supplement.

There are two main types of calcium supplements: calcium carbonate and calcium citrate. They usually come in the form of pills or chewable tablets or candies. Both benefit bone growth and maintenance. Calcium carbonate is less expensive but must be taken with a meal and may cause gas. Calcium citrate is a little more expensive but can be taken at any time of day, with or without a meal, and is better absorbed and usually better tolerated than calcium carbonate.

Vitamin D

As you may remember, I encourage you to get your vitamin D blood levels checked at the beginning of this book. It's vital to know your D levels: New research shows that the vitamin not only reduces risk of fractures and improves bone density but also boosts immunity. It reduces rates of certain infectious diseases and may reduce your risk of cancers, including breast cancer. In addition, it also lowers hypertension and reduces the risk of type 1 diabetes.

We get vitamin D in three ways: exposure to sunlight (our skin makes the vitamin in response to UV rays), through diet, and from supplements. Right now more than a third of adults in this country have suboptimal blood levels of vitamin D. This is in part because they do not get sufficient exposure to sunlight. Dietary sources of vitamin D include fatty fish, such as salmon, tuna, and mackerel, and to a lesser degree egg yolks and cheese. But it is nearly impossible to get sufficient vitamin D from diet alone. Supplements often come in units of 200 IU, 400 IU, and 1,000 IU. You can take them at any time of day, with calcium or without.

How much vitamin D you need to take, if any, depends on the season and on your current blood levels of the nutrient. If it is not summer, I encourage you to take supplements. If your blood levels are low or marginal, then you need to take supplements all year round. Here are my recommendations based on my review of the most recent research:

- Women up to the age of 70 need at least 1,000 IU/day.
- Women over 70 may need 1,500 IU/day.

Vitamin D is the only supplement that I take on a regular basis because I work inside all day and live in a northern climate.

BONES THROUGH THE AGES

Building strong bones at an early age—during childhood and adolescence—is our best defense against developing osteoporosis later in life. But no matter how old you are, it is never too late to start taking care of your bones.

CHILDHOOD AND ADOLESCENCE

Between the ages of 10 and 20, our bone mass doubles, growing especially quickly during puberty and our adolescent growth spurt, as the legs and torso lengthen and the hips and chest widen. In early puberty, the upsurge in bone mass arises from growth in bone length; in late puberty, the increase reflects a boost in density. During the spurt of rapid growth in early puberty, fractures are not uncommon, perhaps because the bone is weakened when growth in length exceeds the pace of mineralization. In their early years, growing girls tend to build up their trabeculae to create a store of calcium for pregnancy and lactation, while boys beef up their cortical bone.

During their preteen and teen years, girls build toward their peak bone mass. The more bone they create during these critical growth years, the more robust and resilient their skeletons will be later in life. In other words, puberty is a window when girls can make major deposits in their "bone bank." To build strong bones during these years, teenage girls need weight-bearing physical activity and plenty of calcium and vitamin D, especially in the wintertime. (See the box Vitamin D and Calcium on pages 164–165.) Unfortunately, studies show that as little as 2 percent of American girls get adequate amounts of calcium and probably 25 percent have suboptimal vitamin D status, especially in the winter and spring.

Osteoporosis really is a disease that begins in childhood, so it's important for parents to encourage girls to adopt lifelong bone-healthy eating and exercise habits.

ADULTHOOD

Bone mass generally peaks in our early to mid-twenties and holds steady through our thirties. Bone building and breakdown are in balance during these young- to mid-adult years. An abrupt turnabout comes in our mid-forties and we start to lose more bone than we make. Bone mass tends to decrease by about ½ to 1 percent during the year or two before menopause. During the 5 years surrounding menopause, women can lose from 2 to 5 percent of bone mass each year. This is in part because of falling levels of estrogen. Five years after menopause, bone loss slows to about 1 or 2 percent a year until about age 70. During the three decades from 40 to 70, we may lose a total of 25 percent of our bone. After age 70, bone loss continues, but diminishes to a lesser rate.

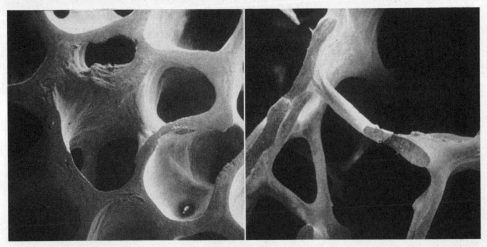

These photos show bone biopsies. The photo on the left is normal bone; the one on the right is osteoporotic.

OSTEOPOROSIS

Osteoporosis is a weakening of bones that can lead to fractures. Age-related osteoporosis is by far the most common bone disease. Women are four times more likely than men to develop the disorder. But osteoporosis is not just a disease of old women. Some young women develop the disorder because of prolonged use of steroids or inadequate nutrition. Fixation on slenderness may lead to eating disorders or diets with insufficient amounts of calories, calcium, and protein. Young women who have stopped menstruating because of disordered patterns of eating have as much as 20 to 30 percent lower bone density than their peers. Even young women who are not underweight but frequently diet to lose weight tend to have lower bone density. That's because when they lose weight, they're losing not just fat but also bone and muscle. However, it is typically not until later in life that loss of bone strength begins.

Osteoporosis is a silent disease. It has no signs or symptoms, so you may not know that your bones are weakening until you actually break one. Roughly half of all women age 50 and older will have an osteoporosis-related fracture in their lifetime. In the United States alone, osteoporosis plays a part in more than 1.5 million fractures each year. These fractures may cause not only pain but also disability and depression.

ARE YOU AT RISK?

Gender, age, genetics, ethnic background, and lifestyle all play into the risk of osteoporosis. Women are at greater risk than men. Older women have a higher risk than younger women do. In the highest risk group are women who weigh less than 127 pounds, with fair skin and blue eyes. To determine your risks, ask yourself a few basic questions:

- *Do you have a close relative with osteoporosis or a history of bone fractures? Have you suffered any bone or spinal fractures yourself?*

  A family or personal history of osteoporosis or fracture can be a red flag. Genetic factors determine some 50 to 90 percent of our bone mass and quality. If any of your immediate family members have (or had) osteoporosis, this increases your risk. If your mother broke her hip when she was in her sixties or seventies, you have double the normal risk. If you yourself have broken a bone or suffered spinal fracture after the age of 40, you have a higher risk—even if the bone broke as a result of an accident or trauma. A personal history of fracture may triple your risk.

  Our genes set limits on how much bone we acquire to begin with, the rate at which we lose it, and its response to nutrients and exercise. One gene known as the vitamin D receptor gene, for instance, comes in several different variants and influences bone density. Whatever variation you carry is thought to affect how much bone you gain during your teen years (rather than how much—or how quickly—you lose it after menopause). But no single gene bears full responsibility for your bone mass; rather, many genetic elements combine to determine its density and strength.

- *What is your racial heritage?*

  Race also plays into the bone density picture. Lighter skin color increases your risk for osteoporosis. Among women over 50, those who are African American have only a 10 percent risk for osteoporosis, while white and Asian women have a 30 percent risk. Asian women have a 25 percent lower incidence of hip fractures than do white women. Nonetheless, African American and Hispanic women are still at risk and, like all women, need to be vigilant about bone health.

- *What is your menstrual history?*

  Women who begin menstruating relatively late—at age 15 or older—have a greater risk of osteoporosis. This is because of estrogen's important role in bone formation. The more estrogen you're exposed to, the stronger your bones will be. Amenorrhea, the cessation of menstrual periods after the onset of puberty and before menopause, is dangerous to bone health.

- *What is your body type?*

  If you weigh less than 127 pounds, your risk of developing osteoporosis is greater. Slender women have less bone mass than heavier women do, so they're more vulnerable to bone breaks. They also typically have lower estrogen levels. If you're slender, being physically active helps reduce your risk.

- *What is your medical history?*

    Certain medical problems can have an impact on bone, including rheumatoid arthritis, disorders of the thyroid and parathyroid, type 1 diabetes, lactose intolerance, chronic digestive problems such as colitis or Crohn's disease, and food allergies. In addition, some common medications weaken bones, among them steroids, thyroid hormone, anticonvulsants, certain diuretics, gonadotrophin-releasing hormone agonists, and antacids containing aluminum.

HOW TO IMPROVE BONE HEALTH

Some factors that affect your bone health, such as age, sex, and genes, are beyond your control. But there is much you can do to keep your bones strong. The lifestyle choices you make, especially diet and physical activity, are responsible for up to 50 percent of bone mass and structure. Even small gains in bone density made through lifestyle changes can have a huge impact on your risk of fracture from osteoporosis.

Here are several steps you can take to maintain healthy bones:

1. **Eat right and get sufficient calcium and vitamin D every day.** (See the box Vitamin D and Calcium on pages 164–165.) Healthy bones also depend on a range of nutrients, such as vitamins A, K, and C, potassium, zinc, and magnesium, found in foods such as fish, lean meats, green leafy vegetables, and oranges. Protein is also very important. We used to think that protein was damaging to our bones. Although it's true that extreme high-protein diets such as the Atkins Diet are not good for your bones, diets rich in protein do promote good bone health.

2. **Get moving.** Physical activity builds bone density when you're young and slows bone loss when you're older. Although all types of exercise contribute to bone health, activities that are weight bearing or involve impact are especially good for improving bone mass and strength. These include any activities in which the body works against gravity, so it supports or carries the body's weight, such as;

- Strength training
- Stair climbing
- Brief sessions of high-impact activity
- Working in the garden
- Playing sports such as basketball, tennis, or soccer
- Dancing
- Running, jogging, or speedwalking
- Tai chi

(See Chapter 27 for more information on physical activity.)

3. **Maintain a healthy body weight.** Being underweight puts you at risk for fractures and bone loss. When a woman's body weight is beneath healthy levels because of overexercise or undereating, her estrogen levels may drop, negatively affecting her bone mass. Yo-yo dieting is also associated with bone loss.

4. **Reduce your risk of falls.** Fractures are commonly caused by falls. To reduce the risk of falling, work on balance training. (See the box Better Your Balance on page 158.) When possible, eliminate medications that cause dizziness, confusion, or low blood pressure. Make your environment safer by clearing clutter from your floors, removing throw rugs that may cause you to slip or trip, using a rubber bath mat in your shower, attaching phone cords and wires to the wall, installing night-lights, installing stair railings, placing grab bars in the shower, and wearing rubber-soled shoes and slippers.

5. **Don't smoke.** Smoking can damage your bones by mechanisms that are poorly understood. Numerous studies have linked smoking to a higher risk of hip fracture.

6. **Drink alcohol in moderation.** Limit your alcohol intake to no more than one drink a day. (A single drink is defined as a 12-ounce bottle of beer, a 5-ounce glass of wine, or 1.5 ounces of hard liquor.) Alcohol use can create multiple problems for bones. It inhibits bone remodeling, possibly by affecting vitamin D or by reducing bone formation; it may contribute to the loss of calcium and magnesium from the body; and finally, it affects balance, heightening the risk of falls and fractures.

7. **Drink coffee in moderation.** Most studies show that drinking more than five cups of coffee a day has a negative effect on bone health, although the reason for this is not well understood.

8. **Discuss your medical history and medications with your doctor.** Be sure to ask whether any chronic medical conditions you have or any medications you're taking might affect your bones.

9. **Get your bones tested (see below).**

BONE MINERAL DENSITY TEST

A bone mineral density (BMD) test uses a special x-ray machine to measure the density of various bones in your body, such as your spine, hip, forearm, or wrist. Safe and painless, the test provides important information about the minerals in your bones, and thus, their health. The higher the mineral content of your bones, the denser they are. Lower bone mineral density can mean a greater risk of osteoporosis and fracture.

There is some controversy over who should have a BMD test and when they should have it. I deviate a little from the national testing guidelines. I recommend that all women have a BMD test at around the age of 50, when they are on the verge of menopause or have just gone through it. The test will give women a baseline measurement—a kind of reference point—that their health care provider can use in determining future recommendations for bone treatment.

Here are the standard guidelines. You should get a BMD test if you:

- Are age 65 or older
- Are under age 65 and postmenopausal, with one or more risk factors for osteoporosis
- Are age 50 or over and have broken a bone after age 40
- Are going through menopause with certain risk factors, such as having experienced years of amenorrhea as a younger adult
- Are postmenopausal and you have stopped hormone replacement therapy
- Are under age 65 and planning to start taking certain medications such as anticonvulsants or steroids (such as prednisone or cortisone to treat rheumatoid arthritis) that may affect your bone mass
- Are receiving treatment for breast cancer
- Have an overactive thyroid or parathyroid gland or are taking thyroid hormone medication
- Have experienced back pain, possibly due to fracture
- Have lost considerable height
- Have gone through early menopause
- Have rheumatoid arthritis or other conditions that may affect your bones

For the test, a diagnostic machine called a DEXA scanner (dual energy x-ray absorptiometry) is used to measure bone density in the hip, spine, and sometimes the forearm. You lie down on a padded table, and the device scans your body for about 5 to 15 minutes. Although the equipment emits radiation, it amounts to only one-tenth the amount of radiation in a chest x-ray. The test will result in a "T-score," which suggests whether your bone density is above or below normal, as compared with the bone density in a healthy 30-year-old with peak bone density. A T-score:

- Above -1 is normal bone density
- Between -1 and -2.5 indicates low bone density or osteopenia
- Of -2.5 or lower indicates osteoporosis

DO I NEED TREATMENT?

Knowing your bone density can be very helpful in motivating you to take the best possible care of your bones through lifestyle measures. If the results of your test suggest that you may need to consider taking medications to help prevent or treat osteoporosis, you should consult with your health care provider. My treatment guidelines for postmenopausal women age 50 and older are as follows. If your T-score is:

- Above -1 (normal bone density), you do not need treatment. Just continue taking good care of your bones through lifestyle measures.
- Between -1 and -2.5, you should talk with your doctor about your bone health. Continue caring for your bones through lifestyle measures. Only consider taking an osteoporosis medication when you also have other risk factors that put you in danger of fracture. (See the box Is Osteopenia Overblown? on page 174.)
- Below -2.5, you should discuss with your health care provider taking medication for osteoporosis. Combine medication with aggressive lifestyle measures of exercise (both strength training and aerobic activity), take calcium and vitamin D supplements, and minimize any negative lifestyle habits, such as smoking and drinking more than one alcoholic beverage a day. Review other medications you may be taking that may negatively affect bone.

CAN MEDICATION HELP?

Because medications are so often prescribed for women to preserve or boost bone density, I want to offer some more detailed information on the options available.

If you have been diagnosed with osteoporosis, you should have a thorough discussion with your health care provider to explore your options for medication. Although the ideal treatment has not yet been developed, a host of medications are available to curb bone loss, and some even help restore bone mass.

There are two main types of drugs for osteoporosis: antiresorptive and anabolic agents. Antiresorptive therapies are the most widely used agents for patients with osteoporosis. They reduce bone loss and help prevent fractures by decreasing the activity of the osteoclasts, blocking the process of bone resorption, or breakdown, and decreasing bone turnover. The antiresorptive agents include: hormone therapy (estrogen); bisphosphonates—nonhormone compounds; selective estrogen receptor modulators (SERMs); and calcitonin.

The second type of drug, anabolic agents, aims to reverse skeletal fragility by stimulating bone formation. The only FDA-approved anabolic agent is teriparatide (brand name Forteo), a synthetic form of a parathyroid hormone normally found in the body.

Hormone Therapy (HT)

For several years, postmenopausal hormone therapy was the top choice for the prevention and treatment of osteoporosis. In studies carried out by the Women's Health Initiative, HT was shown to have consistently favorable effects on bone density in the spine, hip, and other bones and to reduce the risk of osteoporotic fractures. Hip and spine fractures were reduced by at least a third, and total fractures fell by 24 to 30 percent.

However, in 2002, the WHI discontinued its trials because of the harmful effects found in women taking HT, including increased risk of stroke, cognitive impairment, breast cancer, and dangerous blood clots. Although the increase in risk for these problems was small, the trials were halted.

HT may still have its place in our medical arsenal against osteoporosis, but it's clear that consideration of the benefits to the skeleton must be tempered by other safety concerns. In keeping with the FDA's recommendations, I advise that postmenopausal women who are considering HT talk to their healthcare provider.

It is generally recommended that if women choose to use HT early in menopause, they should do so at the lowest possible dose for the shortest amount of time needed to achieve treatment goals. HT provides benefits to a woman's skeleton only during the years she is taking the hormones. After therapy is terminated, she will not enjoy the reduced risk of fracture. Even women who have been on HT for more than 10 years do not have a lower risk of hip fractures just several years after the end of therapy.

Bisphosphonates

Among the more recently developed medications for preventing and treating osteoporosis, bisphosphonates limit the activity of bone-dissolving osteoclasts. These drugs may be especially useful if you've stopped using hormones and might otherwise experience rapid bone loss, if you have osteoporosis because of rheumatoid arthritis or steroid use, or if you're on HT and still suffer from severe osteoporosis.

The FDA has approved four bisphosphonates for this use: alendronate (Fosamax) and risedronate (Actonel), both of which are taken either daily or weekly, and ibandronate

IS OSTEOPENIA OVERBLOWN?

In my view, the pharmaceutical industry has exaggerated the problem of osteopenia (low bone density). As a result, osteoporosis drugs are overprescribed to women with bone density levels in the osteopenia range. Women should realize that many people have levels in this range (T-score of -2.5 to -1). Most likely, they have had this moderate bone density all of their lives as a result of genetic factors. Although there is a slightly increased risk of having a fracture when you have osteopenia, it is minimal compared with the risk that comes with osteoporosis. What is most important is that you continue to take good care of your bones so that you don't lose bone mass as you age.

A new Web-based tool called WHO FRAX, developed by the World Health Organization, can help health care providers estimate your risk of fracturing a bone over the next 10 years or so. The estimate, called "absolute fracture risk," is based on factors such as bone mineral density of the hip, age, smoking and alcohol use, steroid use, personal and family history of bone breaks, and the presence of rheumatoid arthritis. This tool is designed to help health care providers determine whether to treat patients with osteopenia. (See riskcalculator.fore.org.)

Having osteopenia is not a de facto reason to take medication. If you have osteopenia, talk with your doctor and consider your absolute risk of fracture (including your general health, activity level, nutrition, vitamin D blood levels, etc.). Consider monitoring your bones over the next year or two to see whether your bone density is stable or diminishing. If you are healthy and maintaining bone density over time, there is no need to take medication. However, if you are losing bone rapidly, then you may need to consider treatment. Your health care provider can help you make these decisions.

(Boniva), which is taken once a month, and zoledronic acid (Reclast) a once-yearly medication that is taken as an injection. Studies show that some 95 percent of postmenopausal women who take bisphosphonates such as alendronate maintain or increase their bone mass. The benefits of these drugs can be seen within a year. After 2 or 3 years of use, the drugs can raise bone density by some 5 or 6 percent. This may not seem like much, but the increase comes with major reductions—some 50 percent—in the risk for fractures of the spine, hip, and wrist. Moreover, unlike HT, bisphosphonates may continue to provide benefits for at least 30 months after treatment is discontinued.

However, because bisphosphonates require good kidney function to be cleared from the blood, you should not take these drugs if you're pregnant or have poor kidney function.

Both alendronate and risedronate may cause some side effects, including stomach or esophageal pain and difficulty swallowing. You can minimize irritation of the esophagus by remaining upright for a half hour after taking the drug. Because all bisphosphonates are poorly absorbed, you should take them first thing in the morning on an empty stomach with an 8-ounce glass of water and avoid eating food for at least 30 minutes afterward.

The most troubling and dangerous side effect of bisphosphonates is osteonecrosis of the jaw. This is a condition where the blood supply to the jaw is lost, weakening and exposing the bone. The overlying tooth usually falls out and leaves an open lesion. This is a rare condition, but worth bringing up with your doctor. If you are planning to undergo oral surgery, your doctor may advise you to stop taking bisphosphonates for several months before your surgery.

In short, these medications do provide benefit, but there are often serious side effects, and you need to follow directions carefully. New bisphosphonates that need only be administered once a year and cause fewer gastric side effects are under development but not yet approved by the FDA.

Selective Estrogen Receptor Modulators (SERMs)

These drugs interact with estrogen receptors in tissues located throughout the body and have some estrogen-like benefits, including improvement of bone density. The FDA has approved only one SERM for the prevention and treatment of postmenopausal osteoporosis, raloxifene (Evista). In studies, raloxifene was shown to increase by 3 percent the bone density in the spine and hip of postmenopausal women with osteoporosis. Spine fractures were reduced by approximately 50 percent, but the drug showed no effect on hip or other non-spine fractures.

Side effects include hot flashes, leg cramps, swelling of the hands and feet, and—in about 1 percent of users—blood clots in the legs and lungs.

Raloxifene may be a good option for postmenopausal women with an elevated risk for osteoporosis who can't or prefer not to take HT, particularly women with a family or personal history of breast cancer, because raloxifene has a modest effect on reducing the risk of breast cancer.

Calcitonin

Among the first drugs made available for the treatment of osteoporosis, calcitonin is a hormone made by the thyroid gland. Still prescribed for those who cannot take other osteoporosis drugs, it improves bone density and reduces fractures by inhibiting the activity of bone-destroying osteoclasts. It's about as effective as raloxifene at reducing fractures, but not as effective as HT and bisphosphonates. It does have one advantage: It can help ease back pain caused by recent osteoporotic fractures in the spine.

There is no oral form of calcitonin, but it's available as a nasal spray (Miacalcin) and in injectable form (Calcimar and Miacalcin). For the nasal form, some possible side effects include nosebleeds and nasal irritation. Researchers are working to develop a new form of calcitonin that can be taken orally.

Parathyroid Hormone

Teriparatide (Forteo), the only anabolic agent approved by the FDA, can be a useful option if you have severe osteoporosis and have suffered a fracture related to the disorder. Unlike the antiresorptive agents, which block bone breakdown, teriparatide actually stimulates new bone formation. Studies show that in postmenopausal, osteoporotic women, therapy with this drug actually thickens the outer layer of bones and increases the links between trabeculae of bone within the skeleton. It has been shown to decrease spine fractures by 65 percent and non-spine fractures by 53 percent.

Because the drug must be given as a daily subcutaneous injection, it is more expensive than bisphosphonates and has more severe side effects. Among the possible side effects are dizziness, leg cramps, and nausea.

Combination Therapy

In some situations, women with osteoporosis may be treated with a combination of two antiresorptive agents or with an antiresorptive and an anabolic agent, either simultaneously or sequentially.

14

Joints

Your skeleton has superb flexibility thanks to your body's 120 joints, places where two bones join to allow movement. However, every time you move, your joints are subjected to significant mechanical stress. Your hips and knees, for instance, feel 3 pounds of pressure for every pound of weight on your body. That means that if you weigh, say, 150 pounds, those joints experience 450 pounds of pressure when you walk.

Wherever bone meets bone, the body has a shock-absorbing system consisting of muscle and cartilage, as well as lubricating liquid called synovial fluid. This fluid surrounds the entire joint and is contained within a membrane known as the synovium.

In a healthy joint, muscles and cartilage cushion and absorb shock, and both cartilage and synovial fluid make the joint smooth and slippery so that it can move easily. However, over time muscle may weaken and cartilage may degenerate or become inflamed, causing arthritis (from the Greek *arthron*, for "joint," and *itis* for "inflammation"). As cartilage deteriorates, its surface grows rough; when it wears down completely, bone rubs against bone, causing damage and pain. The body cannot grow new cartilage and what cartilage it has does not repair itself well or quickly because it has no blood supply. That's why it's important to protect cartilage by building up the muscle around it.

JOINT TROUBLE: ARTHRITIS

There are 100 or so different kinds of arthritis, but by far the most common is osteoarthritis, a painful, degenerative disease that affects 21 million people in this country, and accounts for four out of five cases of arthritis worldwide. By the age of 65, more than half the U.S. population shows osteoarthritis in at least one joint.

Among the most debilitating forms of arthritis is rheumatoid arthritis, an inflammatory disease that strikes more than 2 million Americans. I know how devastating this disease can be. My sister-in-law was diagnosed with an aggressive form of rheumatoid arthritis at age 32. At the time, she had three young boys, and she struggled through daily life with a lot of pain. Finally, she decided that she had to take action to change her life. She refined her diet and, with the help of a personal trainer, began a rigorous exercise

ACL INJURIES: A JOINT PROBLEM FOR FEMALE ATHLETES

One Saturday night, at a dinner party my husband I attended with three other couples, the subject of athletic high school daughters came up. It turns out that among the four families, there were four daughters who had ruptured their anterior cruciate ligament, or ACL, by playing sports. My two daughters have escaped this injury, so far at least. The other girls have had months, if not years, of rehabilitation.

Among high school and college women, a torn or ruptured ACL is among the most common sports-related joint injuries. The ACL is one of four ligaments that link the thighbone to the shinbone and control the range of movement and stability of the knee. Sports such as basketball, soccer, gymnastics, and field hockey that require cutting, pivoting, and sudden turns place high demands on the ACL. An ACL tear occurs when the ligament is stretched too far. If you tear your ACL, you may hear a "pop" in the knee, feel the joint give out or buckle, and experience sudden swelling of the knee. The injury can be treated through nonsurgical rehabilitation or surgical reconstruction.

Women have three to eight times more ACL injuries than men do, perhaps because of differences in hormones (which affect ligament strength and stiffness), anatomy, positioning during sports (men crouch more when they play; women tend to play upright), or just insufficient strength or fitness. Good coaches of female athletes will demand a high degree of fitness in their players and require sport-specific training programs that help prevent ACL injuries by promoting strength, balance, power, and agility.

UNFANCY FOOTWORK:
KEEPING YOUR FEET HEALTHY

When it comes to footwear, women have been sold a bill of goods. Can you imagine men wearing ill-fitting shoes with 3-inch heels? The stylish, often tight, high-heeled shoes that many women wear are flat-out dangerous and unhealthy. Shoes that don't fit correctly can contribute to bunions. Heels, especially high heels, put a terrible strain on knees and the joints in the foot. An absence of padding contributes to bruising of the foot bed. The lack of support and smooth soles typical of women's shoes can contribute to falls. And yet, we continue to go for style over health at the peril of our feet.

I'm as guilty as the next woman: In the fall of 2008, I had the good fortune to be invited to the White House for the release of the inaugural Physical Activity Guidelines for Americans, which I helped develop. Needless to say, I dressed up in a nice blue suit, stockings, and a pair of modest heels. The day of the event, I walked six blocks from my hotel to the White House. When the ceremony was over, I went for a 2-mile walk around the U.S. Capitol and the Mall with my colleagues before the next gathering. By the end of the day, my feet were in such pain that I had to take off my shoes and walk through the airport in my stockings.

There's no doubt that heels are stylish. But they are not worth trashing your feet. Find the most comfortable shoes you can, with the flattest heel. Wear sneakers or flat shoes when you need to walk any distance or stand for long periods of time. Wear heels only when you feel you absolutely need to. Take care of your feet.

program. These changes made all the difference. Combining her healthy nutrition and physical activity with medications and even some surgery has allowed her to stay in the best shape possible, and she continues to be my hero.

Arthritis—osteo- or rheumatoid—is not fatal, but it can make life difficult, limiting mobility, interfering with common daily activities, and causing depression—a hallmark of the disease. Although we still have no cure, the disease can be treated and managed to minimize pain. Changes in lifestyle (especially exercise and diet) and some impressive new medications and surgical interventions can ease pain, protect your joints from further damage, and restore healthy functioning.

OSTEOARTHRITIS

Osteoarthritis may affect any joint in the body, but it tends to strike the neck, lower back, hips, knees, and feet and also the small joints of the fingers and the hand. Mechanical stress on the joints, also known as "wear and tear," causes small microfractures in the cartilage. These microfractures draw white blood cells to repair the damage. Unfortunately, the white cells become part of the problem because they produce enzymes that further break down the cartilage. The microfractures may grow and the cartilage itself may shrink, losing its precious synovial fluid and its springiness. To compensate, the bone near the joint may enlarge, forming spurs that can hinder motion and cause pain in bones, tendons, and ligaments. With pain, people tend to use their joints less, which weakens the muscle. This, in turn, causes more damage to the cartilage in the joint and more pain in what may become a vicious cycle.

The disease develops slowly and often silently, without preliminary signs or symptoms. Eventually, deteriorating cartilage may cause joints to become painful, swollen, or stiff during or after use. Bony lumps or knobs may form on the joints of the fingers or thumb.

Just what causes osteoarthritis is still largely a mystery. We do know that overweight and obesity greatly increase the risk of developing the condition. Scientists suspect that other factors may include age, heredity, muscle weakness, and joint injury or stress.

WHAT ARE THE SIGNS OF OSTEOARTHRITIS?

Symptoms of the disease range from mild joint pain and stiffness when you get out of bed to severe pain, typically in your weight-bearing joints, or in your hands, neck, and lower back. Sometimes there's a "crunchy" feeling in your joints, or a noise of bone on bone. However, as many as two out of three people who show x-ray evidence of osteoarthritis have no outward symptoms. The opposite is true as well: For many people who have symptoms, evidence of osteoarthritis does not appear on x-rays.

HOW IS THE DISEASE DIAGNOSED?

Your physician may use several tests to diagnose osteoarthritis, including x-rays and the relatively new technique of arthroscopy. In arthroscopy, a surgeon makes a small incision near your joint and inserts an arthroscope, a tubular probe with a light and a camera attached, which projects an image of the inside of your joint onto a monitor. In this way, your physician can diagnose a range of joint ailments, from bone spurs and fragments to torn cartilage and ligaments. If the joint requires surgery, a surgeon can insert instruments through the arthroscope to make repairs.

ARE YOU AT RISK?

As with osteoporosis, being female puts you at greater risk for osteoarthritis. Some 33 percent of women have the disease, compared with 25 percent of men. Although it's not clear why gender influences risk, hormones may play a role.

The most significant risk is your age. Of women aged 45 and younger, only about 15 percent show signs of osteoarthritis on x-rays. In women over 65, the number jumps to 50 percent. Other factors that increase your odds and may make you more prone to developing the disease may include:

- **Overweight.** Excess weight puts more stress on the joints of your hips and knees. Studies show that overweight women are four times more likely to develop arthritis of the knee than women of normal weight. Obese women are 10 times more likely to develop the disease. Because age is not modifiable, this may be the most important risk factor that you can control.
- **Joint injuries.** A previous injury to joints from physical activity or sports, especially contact sports such as boxing and football, may increase your risk. Running does not seem to increase a woman's risk of osteoarthritis.
- **Heredity.** Having hereditary conditions involving defective cartilage or joints and/or a family history of osteoarthritis puts you at greater risk.
- **Muscle weakness.** Weak muscles, especially thigh, or quadriceps, muscles, may raise your risk of developing osteoarthritis in your knees.

HOW TO REDUCE YOUR RISK

Keep your weight at a healthy level. As little as 20 excess pounds can place an extra burden of 60 pounds on your knees and hips. On the other hand, even small losses in weight can dramatically reduce the stress on joints and the pain and stiffness of arthritis.

Strengthen your muscles. Strong muscles, especially strong quadriceps (the large muscles on the front of the thighs that control the movement of the knee joint), reduce the stress on cartilage and can help prevent it from wearing out. A study that I conducted with colleagues at Tufts showed that simple home-based strength training in men and women with osteoarthritis of the knee reduced knee pain by more than 40 percent and improved overall functioning. (See Chapter 27 for more information on strength training.)

Avoid wearing high heels. Shoes with heels more than 2 inches high—both stiletto and chunky heels—put excessive strain on the knee joint at the back of the kneecap. For those women who already have osteoarthritis in the knee, wearing insoles or shoes with cushioning can help ease stress on the knee. (For more information, see the box Unfancy Footwork on page 179.)

Eat a diet of fruits and vegetables rich in vitamin C and take vitamin D supplements. Studies show that a diet rich in vitamin C can benefit joints. (There is no evidence that taking vitamin C through supplements is advantageous, though.) Taking extra vitamin D if your blood levels are not optimal may also improve joint health.

WHAT ARE THE TREATMENT OPTIONS FOR OSTEOARTHRITIS?

Exercise. One of the best treatments for osteoarthritis is exercise. It decreases the pain and disability of arthritis by boosting muscle strength around the joints. It can also prevent further damage and improve your ability to comfortably carry out the tasks of daily living, from putting on shoes to carrying groceries. (See Chapter 27.)

Cold or warm packs. To relieve pain or discomfort, warm towels, hot baths, or hot or cold packs can offer temporary relief for the pain and discomfort of osteoarthritis.

Medication. Several medicines are available for the treatment of osteoarthritis. It's important to discuss them thoroughly with your doctor to decide on the best options.

- **Pain-relieving drugs.** For pain relief, the usual treatment is acetaminophen (e.g., Tylenol), which has few side effects. Aspirin also helps reduce pain, but it is not usually the first choice in pain relief because it is tough on the stomach.
- **Anti-inflammatory pain-relieving drugs.** For stronger pain relief, doctors may use nonsteroidal anti-inflammatory drugs (NSAIDs) such as naproxen (Anaprox and Naprosyn) and ibuprofen (Advil, Motrin, etc.). These NSAIDs may cause side effects such as gastrointestinal discomfort, especially when used in large doses or for long periods of time, but they can help reduce inflammation. If you're over the age of 65 or have a history of ulcers or stomach bleeding, you should be cautious about using NSAIDs. Other options are COX-2 inhibitors, including celecoxib and valdecoxib, which may be less damaging to your stomach.
- **Topical pain medications.** These over-the-counter creams, gels, lotions, and patches can help ease arthritis pain temporarily during flare-ups. You should discuss these products with your doctor before using them.
- **Corticosteroids.** Some physicians may recommend injecting cortisone or other steroids in a particular joint or muscle to help numb pain. Steroids can reduce

inflammation and relieve pain for weeks or even months. However, these drugs have some serious side effects if used daily for long periods of time, including liver damage, easy bruising, weakened bones, and a heightened risk of cataracts. Corticosteroids may also be taken orally or as a topical ointment.

Surgery. When medication and other therapies do not provide sufficient pain relief, or if you have serious loss of motion or deformity of a joint from osteoarthritis, you may opt for surgery to replace joints or to fuse or reposition bones.

- **Arthroscopy.** The less invasive procedure of arthroscopy is often used to address a range of ailments, including the removal of bone spurs or fragments or scar tissue and the repair of damaged cartilage and torn ligaments.

GLUCOSAMINE AND CHONDROITIN

Do they reduce pain from osteoarthritis?

Glucosamine and chondroitin sulfate, natural compounds found in cartilage and sold in supplement form, are often touted as alternative treatments for osteoarthritis pain. In 2006, researchers at the University of Utah conducted a large-scale study to evaluate the efficacy and safety of these treatments. The study included more than 1,500 patients with painful knee osteoarthritis. Sixty-four percent of the patients were women. The researchers found that glucosamine and chondroitin alone or in combination were not significantly better than a placebo in reducing knee pain.

The investigators then looked to see whether different subgroups responded differently to the supplement. Analysis showed that research volunteers who had moderate to severe osteoarthritis of the knee may have gained some benefit from the supplement, whereas those who had mild knee pain did not. Although these results are preliminary, there may be some benefit for those who have moderate to severe knee pain from osteoarthritis.

My recommendation is this: If you decide to try glucosamine and chondroitin supplements, take the supplements for 3 or 4 months. If you find that your knee pain is reduced, then continue taking the supplements. If you don't experience any improvement, discontinue use. As always, talk with your doctor before you start taking any supplement. Some people have severe allergic reactions to glucosamine and chondroitin.

- **Joint replacement.** Four out of five surgeries for osteoarthritis are hip or knee replacements. Hip replacement surgery, called hip arthroplasty, and knee replacement, or total knee arthroplasty, can relieve pain and restore normal range of motion. Once considered feasible only for people age 60 and older, hip arthroplasty is now an option for younger, more active people, thanks to the development of stronger, more durable artificial joints. For knee replacements, many joint designs are available to match your age, weight, gender, and activity level. Made of high-grade plastics and metal alloys, they are designed to mimic the natural motion of your knee. Shoulder arthroplasty is an option for people with severe arthritis of the shoulder.

Alternative or complementary therapies. A number of complementary therapies are available. Most have not been tested. There is some evidence of pain relief with acupuncture. The most heavily promoted alternative medicines are glucosamine and chondroitin, but there's mixed evidence on whether these treatments have any effect. (See the box Glucosamine and Chondroitin on page 183.)

ON THE HORIZON

The therapies now available can relieve pain and stiffness, but they can't halt the development of osteoarthritis. Fortunately, there are some exciting new areas of research aimed at slowing or stopping progressive joint damage. New drugs under development include antibiotics that obstruct the action of proteins involved in breaking down cartilage and other drugs that block the signals that trigger inflammation. Tissue engineering (transferring cells from healthy tissue in the body to damaged areas to improve joint mobility) and gene therapy (targeting specific genes that affect cells in your joints) also offer hope. New therapies may also be developed soon to offer more pain relief to people with osteoarthritis.

RHEUMATOID ARTHRITIS

This disease is among the most aggressive and incapacitating forms of arthritis. Whereas osteoarthritis tends to affect a single joint, rheumatoid arthritis is a systemic autoimmune disease involving many body tissues and multiple joints, especially the small joints of the hands and feet. For unknown reasons, the body's white blood cells attack the synovium, the tissue lining the joints, causing pain and deformity and making simple daily activities, including sleep, difficult or impossible. It can also cause inflammation of the tear and salivary glands and the linings of the heart and lungs.

Rheumatoid arthritis strikes women two to three times more often than men, usually between the ages of 20 and 50, though it can occur even in very young children. It varies in severity, and symptoms may come and go; flare-ups of the disease may alternate with periods that are relatively symptom-free.

In rheumatoid arthritis, the synovium becomes inflamed, making the joint warm, red, swollen, and painful. Eventually the thin synovial membrane is replaced with a thick mass of cells and blood vessels that prevent nutrients from diffusing into the joint. Proteins released during the inflammation also wreak havoc on bone, cartilage, tendons, and ligaments so that the joint may grow misshapen and misaligned.

All of this misplaced immune activity has another destructive effect: It revs up the body's metabolism by about 20 percent. This may cause the fatigue that often accompanies the condition. Increased metabolism means that the body needs more calories. Unfortunately, it does not draw the extra calories from fat stores but from muscle tissue, so people with rheumatoid arthritis often lose more muscle and store more fat. Pain and muscle weakness often result in reduced physical activity, causing even more muscle atrophy.

WHAT ARE THE SIGNS OF RHEUMATOID ARTHRITIS?

If you have rheumatoid arthritis, you may experience pain and swelling in the joints, particularly those in the hands and feet; aching and stiffness in both muscles and joints, especially after rest; and limited motion or deformity in a joint. The disease often occurs in a symmetrical pattern, so if a joint on one side of your body is affected, the joint on your other side will likely be affected as well. This is one way rheumatoid arthritis is distinguished from other forms of arthritis. You may also feel sick, slightly feverish, and/or tired. Rheumatoid arthritis can interfere with sleep patterns, robbing the body of restorative REM sleep and causing fatigue.

HOW IS THE DISEASE DIAGNOSED?

Many doctors diagnose the disease with the help of blood tests. Among the most frequently used is the rheumatoid factor test. However, this test is not completely reliable: Not everyone with the disease tests positive, and some people who do test positive are free of the disease. Your doctor may also take your white blood cell count and give you an erythrocyte sedimentation rate test, which signals inflammation in the body. In addition, x-rays of affected joints can be helpful in diagnosing the disease and assessing its progression. Another diagnostic tool is arthroscopy, which allows a surgeon to take a biopsy.

WHAT ARE THE CAUSES OF RHEUMATOID ARTHRITIS?

Although the causes of this disease are still unknown, scientists believe that the disease may be triggered by a bacterium, virus, or other infection in people who are genetically susceptible. Long-term smoking may also be a factor. A woman's risk of contracting the disease goes up with age, except after age 80, when it declines.

PAIN IN THE BACK

When I was in sixth grade I was playing around during recess, doing some gymnastics tumbling with a friend. During one tumble, I fell and couldn't get my arms in position to soften the blow. I crushed several vertebrae and was in a brace for months. I recovered well, but as I've gotten older, I have back problems from time to time as a result of the injury. I'm sure that all the sitting I do at my desk job doesn't help.

I'm not alone. Sixty to 90 percent of all adults experience back pain at some point in their lives. It is no wonder when you look at what backs have to do—twist, lift, shove, heave, etc. Our backs are made up of a series of vertebrae, ligaments, tendons, and nerves. The vertebrae come together at 20 small, intricate joints.

The causes of back pain are numerous:

- Lack of strength and flexibility
- Excess body weight
- Poor posture
- Degenerative discs
- Scoliosis
- Osteoporosis
- Trauma
- Herniated disc
- Arthritis
- Spinal stenosis

WHAT CAN I DO IF I HAVE THE DISEASE?

Rheumatoid arthritis is best managed with a combination of self-care techniques and medical treatment.

Self-Care Techniques

- **Get regular exercise.** Walking, riding a stationary bicycle, and aquatic exercise are all beneficial. In addition, engage in a regular strength-training program. (See Chapter 27.) Exercise will build muscle, reduce pain, promote good sleep, and help you maintain a positive attitude.
- **Maintain a healthy body weight** to avoid putting extra stress on your joints.

Other reasons for back pain range from cancer and premenstrual symptoms to environmental issues such as a poor bed or pillow or workspace setup. Whatever the reason for your back pain, you should try to understand its causes and treat it accordingly. If the cause is a medical condition, treat the medical condition first; if the cause is environmental, create a better home or work environment to ease the pain.

A caution here about back surgery. There is something called "failed back surgery syndrome." It isn't really a syndrome; the term simply refers to the failure of many back surgeries to alleviate pain, and the persistence of pain following surgery. Before you decide to have back surgery, make sure that you have done everything you can to provide support to your back. Explore alternative practices, such as yoga, tai chi, acupuncture, and chiropractic medicine. Only after all other courses of action have been exhausted should you consider back surgery.

To maintain a pain-free back, keep it strong and flexible through exercise, maintain a healthy body weight, and make sure that your home and work environments support it. If your desk is not aligned with your chair at work, or if your bed doesn't provide adequate support, fix or replace them. Your back deserves all the help it can get. To learn more about back health, refer to my book *Strong Women, Strong Back*. (See Resources section.)

- **Eat a healthy diet** with adequate calories, protein, and calcium; plenty of fresh fruits and vegetables; whole grains; and foods rich in omega-3 fatty acids, such as coldwater fish. Try to eat at least three servings of fish per week.
- **Apply heat** to increase local bloodflow, relax tense muscles, and ease pain.
- **If you have an acute flare-up, consider applying cold** to reduce inflammation.
- **Use relaxation techniques** to help control pain.
- **Rest** when the disease is in an active phase to help reduce fatigue and inflammation in the joint.

FISH OILS AND FATTY ACIDS FOR RHEUMATOID ARTHRITIS

In recent years, we have begun to hear more and more about the health benefits of the fatty acids known as omega-3s. In the fight against rheumatoid arthritis, omega-3s are a powerful ally. Inflammation in the joints is what causes the pain and stiffness characteristic of rheumatoid arthritis. Omega-3 fatty acids contain compounds that help create anti-inflammatory substances, which suppress inflammation in and around the joints.

So what are the best sources of omega-3 fatty acids? Fish oils, found in high concentrations in such coldwater fish as salmon, tuna, and mackerel. A Danish study found that people who ate an average of 4 ounces of coldwater fish every day for 6 months had less morning stiffness and tenderness in their joints. Some studies suggest that fish oil taken in capsules can also reduce the symptoms of rheumatoid arthritis.

Other foods contain a kind of omega-3s that are less effective against arthritis but still good for joints. These include canola oil, flaxseed oil, tofu, green leafy vegetables, and nuts, especially walnuts.

Study after study shows that eating coldwater fish on a regular basis is much more effective than taking fish oil tablets as a source of omega-3s. I'm not surprised. In nearly every case, eating real food containing a nutrient is better than taking the isolated nutrient in supplement form. Some people worry about mercury and other contaminants in fish. If you're pregnant, you should avoid mercury-laden fish; otherwise, the benefit of eating coldwater fish regularly outweighs the risk.

Medical Treatment

Medical treatment may include medication for pain relief and to reduce inflammation and/or surgery to restore function or ease pain in a severely damaged joint.

Medications

Many of the medications that may help relieve the pain and stiffness caused by rheumatoid arthritis are the same as those used for osteoarthritis. These include:

- Pain relievers such as aspirin and acetaminophen
- NSAIDs such as ibuprofen and naproxen sodium (Aleve) and others available by prescription, as well as COX-2 inhibitors
- Corticosteroids such as prednisone and methylprednisolone (Medrol)

In addition, your doctor may suggest use of a disease-modifying antirheumatic drug (DMARD). Often used in combination with an NSAID or corticosteroids, DMARDs can actually slow the course of rheumatoid arthritis and limit the extent of joint damage. To combat the depression that sometimes accompanies rheumatoid arthritis, doctors may also prescribe antidepressants.

Surgery and Other Treatments

For severe cases of rheumatoid arthritis, physicians may advise surgical or other procedures. These include Prosorba column, a technique of blood filtering to remove antibodies involved in joint and muscle pain and inflammation, and joint repair or replacement surgery.

If you have any type of arthritis, give your joints the best support you can by combining medical care with good nutrition, weight control, and physical activity.

productive Choices Fertility and Preg
enopause Sexual Abuse and Sexual A
in Teeth Hair and Nails Body Weigh
etabolism Blood Sugar Eating and Exc
scles Bones JointsHeart and Blood I
d Respiration Common Infectious Dis
toimmune Disease Cancer Vision He
ell, Taste, and Touch Mental Health
nce Abuse Making Change Managing
d Sleeping Well Shifting Your Food En
nt Getting Active Screenings and H
intenance Reproduction Sexuality and
l Health Reproductive Choices Fertilit
gnancy Menopause Sexual Abuse and
Assault Skin Teeth Hair and Nails
eight and Metabolism Blood Sugar E
d Excreting Muscles Bones Joints Hear
od Lungs and Respiration Common I
us Diseases Autoimmune Disease C

PART V

Heart Smart and Breathing Easy

Women are finally getting the message about the importance of heart health, thanks in part to the American Heart Association's "Go Red for Women" national campaign to raise awareness of heart disease. Still, too many of us aren't taking the care of our hearts as seriously as we should. As the author of *Strong Women, Strong Hearts* and several studies on heart health, I often give talks on this topic to women's groups. I always ask my audience, "What is the number one killer of women?" Most women get the answer right away: heart disease. But when I ask my audience members whether they know their own risk for heart disease, only a few hands go up.

This part of the book will help you determine your risk profile for heart disease. Determining your risk is a simple matter of having a few basic measurements taken (blood pressure, lipid profile, blood glucose, and perhaps some inflammation markers). As far as tests go, these are far easier and cheaper than getting a mammogram— and yet women are not demanding them of their doctors, and doctors are not insisting on them for their patients. Just as essential as knowing your blood pressure and lipids is knowing your fitness level. This is one risk factor that your health care provider will probably not ask you about because it is not yet in the standard procedures for determining risk—but it should be.

I repeat a message from the first part of this book: Every woman should know her body's numbers. This is especially true when it comes to the numbers that affect your cardiovascular system. Once you know your risk profile, there is much you can do to diminish your chances of developing heart disease.

Just as heart health is vital to your well-being, so too is lung health. Your lungs play multiple roles in the body, defending the body against intruders (such as dust, viruses, and bacteria), removing toxins, relieving your blood of carbon dioxide, and returning to it a rich supply of oxygen—the all-important fuel for your cells and organs. It's a shock to acknowledge that roughly one out of every five women in this country puts her lungs at high risk by smoking. That statistic also holds true for teenage girls. Although the dangers of cigarette smoking are well known, and many women know that lung cancer kills more of us than breast cancer does, they still continue to smoke.

To keep your heart and lungs healthy, follow these **S.M.A.R.T.** tips:

1. Eat heart-healthy foods.
2. Be physically fit.
3. Maintain a healthy weight and waist circumference.
4. Don't smoke.
5. Manage stress.
6. Control blood cholesterol.
7. Control blood pressure.
8. Maintain positive social interactions.
9. Be assertive and seek help if you think you are having heart trouble.
10. Pay attention to air quality, and avoid exposing yourself to air pollutants and allergens.

15

Heart and Blood

Your cardiovascular system consists of your heart, the major organ of the system, along with all of your blood vessels.

Roughly the size of a clenched fist, the heart is a surprisingly sturdy and powerful little muscular pump, strong enough to withstand a lifetime of rhythmic pounding (about 2.6 billion beats) and pumping (some 4,300 gallons each day). With each beat, the heart sends blood into vessels that carry the precious liquid throughout the body, delivering oxygen and nutrients to cells everywhere. The circulating blood also removes toxins and waste products.

The muscle in your heart contracts and relaxes about 60 to 80 times a minute to push blood from the chambers of the heart into the vessels. When you exercise, your heart pumps rapidly; when you rest, it pumps more slowly. Each heartbeat is a carefully orchestrated event involving intricate coordination between cardiac muscle and nerves, which regulate the speed at which the muscle contracts.

The heart is divided into four chambers: the right atrium and right ventricle, and the left atrium and left ventricle. Oxygen-rich blood from the lungs is pushed from the left ventricle out to the strong, flexible blood vessels known as arteries, including those that nourish the muscles of the heart itself, known as coronary arteries.

Every minute, your blood cycles through the body, traveling the long double loop of the cardiovascular system—from the heart, through the lungs, and back to the heart; and then from the heart to the rest of the body and back. In both loops, arteries carry blood under high pressure away from the heart; veins carry it back again under much lower pressure.

From the arteries, blood travels to the smaller arterioles and finally seeps into the body's 10 billion or so capillaries, tiny weblike blood vessels embedded in the tissues of the body. So thin are the walls of capillaries that individual blood cells must pass through single file. Through these slender capillary walls, the vital exchange of oxygen and carbon dioxide occurs between blood and other body tissues. Blood cells deposit oxygen and nutrients to nourish the body's tissues and also pick up carbon dioxide and other waste products. Carrying its new waste-rich cargo, the blood flows from the capillaries into the small veins known as venules, then to large veins, and eventually back to the heart through the right atrium. At this point, the blood is pumped into the right ventricle and out through veins to the capillaries in the lungs, where it drops off carbon dioxide and restocks with oxygen. Then it flows back into the heart through the left atrium, and from there to the left ventricle, where the loop begins anew.

A system of valves between the heart's chambers assures that blood always flows in the right direction. The lub-dub sound of a heartbeat is actually the opening and closing of valves. If a valve does not close completely, and blood leaks backward, it's called a murmur, which can be detected with a stethoscope.

WHAT IS HEART DISEASE?

Heart disease is one of several cardiovascular diseases—a term used to describe disorders of the heart and blood vessels, including heart attack, heart failure, valvular disease, high blood pressure, and stroke.

The most common form of heart disease is coronary heart disease, a narrowing or partial blockage of the coronary arteries that supply the heart muscle, resulting in impeded bloodflow and reduced oxygen supply to the heart. This occurs when cholesterol-rich fatty and fibrous plaque accumulates inside the arteries that supply the heart muscle, a condition also known as atherosclerosis (from the Greek *athero*, meaning "gruel" or "paste," and *sclerosis*, or "hardening"). It can also result from inflammation within an atherosclerotic artery. If the interior of the artery becomes inflamed, the plaque along the lining may rupture or dislodge, spurring the formation of a blood clot, which can lead to heart attack or stroke.

When bloodflow (and thus, oxygen supply) to heart muscle is reduced, it may be experienced as angina, chest pain, squeezing, or discomfort, sometimes accompanied by pain in the back, arms, neck, or jaw. In women, it may also be felt as fatigue or simply feeling not quite right. Sometimes angina is experienced during exertion such as running to catch a bus or hurrying up a flight of steps to answer a ringing telephone; other times, its symptoms occur during resting—a more worrisome condition known as unstable angina.

When most or all bloodflow to the heart is suddenly cut off through atherosclerosis or because a blood clot triggered by inflammation lodges in the coronary arteries, the result is myocardial infarction, or heart attack. The heart muscle cells do not receive sufficient oxygen and begin to die. Without treatment to restore the bloodflow, the heart may be severely damaged, causing irregular rhythms or even cardiac arrest and death.

WOMEN AND HEART DISEASE

We've made progress in recognizing the special risks women face where heart disease is concerned. Still, there are many myths and misunderstandings. For example:

- **Myth: More women die from breast and ovarian cancer than from heart disease.** Heart disease is the leading cause of death among women in this country, killing some 500,000 women each year. More women die from heart disease than from all forms of cancer combined; even women in their thirties and forties are at risk. Coronary heart disease affects one in ten women over the age of 18 and one in four women over the age of 65.
- **Myth: Chest pain is the most telling sign of a heart attack.** Not always—especially where women are concerned. A study in 2007 funded by the National Heart, Lung, and Blood Institute (NHLBI) found that 30 to 37 percent of women did not have chest discomfort during a heart attack. Women are more likely than men to experience a wider range of vague or subtle symptoms, such as pain in the middle of the upper back, neck, or jaw; indigestion; fatigue; or dizziness.
- **Myth: Hormone therapy (HT) will protect you from heart disease.** Women who get HT experience a small but significant increase in risk for heart attack.
- **Myth: Whether you develop heart disease is largely beyond your control.** Not true. Making lifestyle changes can radically reduce your risk of getting heart disease—even if you have a family history of the disease. More than 80 percent of heart attacks and other cardiac trauma can be avoided if women follow a five-step plan that includes 1) eating healthy foods; 2) getting at least 150 minutes of exercise per week; 3) maintaining a healthy weight; 4) controlling stress; and 5) not smoking. These five steps may sound simple. But unfortunately, only about 3 percent of women are following all five of them. To reduce your chances of getting heart disease, it's important to understand your risks and make a plan to lower them with the help of the guidelines in this chapter and advice from your doctor.

WARNING SIGNS AND SYMPTOMS OF HEART TROUBLE

Early treatment of heart trouble can literally mean the difference between life and death. It's essential for women to recognize the early warning signs of heart disease that are characteristic of their gender. For men, the first sign of heart disease is often a heart attack. For women, warning signs of the disease may be more subtle—vague digestive discomfort or shortness of breath or fatigue while engaging in routine activities such as changing bed linens or other household tasks that have been effortless in the past. One study showed that 95 percent of women who'd had heart attacks experienced symptoms such as fatigue and difficulty sleeping up to a month before their attack.

When we were writing *Strong Women, Strong Hearts*, we interviewed many women who had experienced a heart attack. They told us stories about having just this feeling—of being unusually fatigued for weeks. But when they finally decided to go to the emergency room, a shocking number of them were told that they were probably just stressed-out or had indigestion, and they were sent home. One of the women, Delilah, ended up back at the emergency room a month later with a massive heart attack. Miraculously, she survived.

I can't emphasize this enough: If you are experiencing diffuse symptoms such as feeling unusually tired or fatigued with the simplest of tasks, don't assume that it is just because you didn't get a good night's sleep. Be aware of the full range of symptoms of heart disease, and if you experience any of them, "think heart," and seek emergency medical treatment.

The American Heart Association notes these heart attack warning signs:

- Uncomfortable pressure, squeezing, fullness, or pain in the center of the chest that lasts more than a few minutes or goes away and comes back
- Pain or discomfort in one or both arms, back, neck, jaw, or stomach
- Shortness of breath
- Breaking out in a cold sweat, nausea, or lightheadedness

Women may experience these more subtle symptoms of heart disease:

- Nausea or vomiting
- Indigestion
- Loss of appetite
- Weakness or fatigue
- Cough
- Dizziness
- Palpitations

AM I AT RISK FOR HEART DISEASE?

Every woman should know her risk for developing heart disease so that she can shape a suitable strategy for preventing it. Even women with low risk can benefit from understanding the nature of their own risk, to keep it from creeping up.

Some risk factors for heart disease are beyond your control:

- **Age** (65 and older)
- **Family history** of early heart disease in a first-degree relative such as a parent or sibling—under age 65 in a female relative and under age 55 in a male relative

Other risk factors include conditions and lifestyle choices that you can control:

- **High blood pressure**
- **Abnormal cholesterol**—high LDL cholesterol ("bad" cholesterol) and/or low HDL cholesterol. Even thin people can have high cholesterol and should have their levels checked regularly.
- **High levels of triglycerides**
- **Diabetes.** Some 75 percent of people with diabetes die from some form of heart or blood vessel disease. However, carefully monitoring and controlling diabetes can reduce the risk.
- **Smoking.** Smoking promotes atherosclerosis, damages the lining of the arteries and veins, and raises blood pressure.
- **Overweight and obesity.** Being overweight or obese can raise both blood pressure and blood cholesterol. Having excess body fat, especially in the waist area, is linked to higher LDL cholesterol and triglyceride levels and to lower HDL cholesterol, high blood pressure, and diabetes—all risk factors for heart disease. A waist measurement of more than 35 inches in women increases disease risk. Fortunately, reducing your weight by just 10 pounds can lower your blood pressure and your cholesterol and triglyceride levels.
- **Diet.** Foods high in saturated fats (and, to some extent, cholesterol) elevate blood cholesterol levels, which may accelerate atherosclerosis. Foods high in salt or sodium can raise blood pressure. Refined sugars and highly processed foods are usually higher in calories, which can promote weight gain.
- **Physical inactivity.** A sedentary lifestyle contributes to other risk factors, such as overweight, high blood pressure, low HDL, and diabetes.

- **Stress, anger, and isolation.** Research suggests that stress, whether experienced in the form of depression, anxiety, anger, or another emotion, affects the health of your heart and blood vessels. People who are depressed, for instance, are more likely to develop heart disease. According to one study, women who reported suppressing their anger had higher rates of heart attack than women who didn't. So, too, studies suggest that people with limited social interactions have a two- to threefold greater risk for developing heart disease.
- **Alcohol use.** Overuse can boost blood pressure and triglycerides.

Evidence from recent heart disease research suggests that there are possible additional risk factors:

- **High-sensitivity C-reactive protein (CRP) score.** C-reactive protein is a protein that increases during inflammation. A high score suggests that arteries may be inflamed, a risk factor for heart disease. If you're at low risk for heart disease, there's no need to test for CRP. However, if you're at moderate risk (i.e., you have a 10 to 20 percent chance of suffering a cardiovascular event within the decade—see page 202), you should consult your doctor about getting tested for CRP, because it may help predict a cardiovascular event and warrant further evaluation and therapy. If you're at high risk for heart disease, the test is not necessary, because you should be undergoing aggressive treatment regardless of your CRP level.
- **Elevated blood levels of homocysteine,** an amino acid in blood. Some evidence suggests that homocysteine may promote the development of atherosclerosis and blood clots, but a causal link has not been confirmed. Research at Tufts suggests that homocysteine levels can be reduced by consuming adequate amounts of three B vitamins: folate, B_6, and B_{12}. However, I do not advise using B vitamin supplements to reduce the risk of heart disease. Homocysteine levels in the US population have declined over the past decade because our grain supply is now fortified with folate. Eating a diet rich in fruits, vegetables, and grains is key to maintaining adequate B-vitamin levels.

UNDERSTANDING YOUR HEART AND BLOOD NUMBERS

This section will help you understand the numbers that matter most to your heart and blood vessels, including cholesterol, triglycerides, and blood pressure. Using these numbers, you can determine your own risk for heart disease with the help of the 10-Year Risk Assessment on page 202.

THE SKINNY ON CHOLESTEROL AND TRIGLYCERIDES

Cholesterol is a fatlike, waxy substance produced naturally by the liver to make cell membranes and certain hormones and to fulfill other important functions in the body. Despite what most people think, we make most of our cholesterol in our liver (as much as the body needs) and get very little cholesterol from food.

If there is too much cholesterol in your body, the surplus is deposited in arteries, which can lead to atherosclerosis and heart disease. An elevated level of blood cholesterol is called hypercholesterolemia. About half of all American adults have high blood cholesterol. But the condition does not cause symptoms, so many people are unaware of it. According to a nationwide survey released in 2007 by the Society for Women's Health Research, only 32 percent of women know their cholesterol numbers. Of those women who had recently had a cholesterol test, just over half could recall their numbers.

In caring for your heart, it's vital to know your cholesterol figures, and if they need adjusting, to adopt therapeutic lifestyle changes to lessen your risk of heart disease. Women age 20 and older should have their cholesterol measured at least once every 5 years. The blood test, known as a lipoprotein profile, provides information about:

- **Total cholesterol**
- **Low-density lipoprotein (LDL),** known as "bad" cholesterol, which contributes to heart disease
- **High-density lipoprotein (HDL),** or "good" cholesterol, which offers protection against heart disease
- **Triglycerides,** a form of fat in blood that can also raise the risk of heart disease

Cholesterol is measured in milligrams (mg) of cholesterol per deciliter (dL) of blood.

A **total cholesterol** level of:

- **Less than 200 mg/dL is desirable.** If you have no other risk factors for heart disease, this level means that you have a relatively low risk of developing heart disease. To keep your cholesterol at a healthy level, it's important to maintain heart-healthy habits.

- **200 to 239 mg/dL is borderline high.** If your cholesterol numbers fall between 200 and 239, your doctor should evaluate your LDL and HDL levels and work with you to create a treatment and prevention program that includes lifestyle changes and perhaps medication.
- **240 mg/dL and above is high.** People with a high cholesterol level have double the risk of coronary heart disease as people with cholesterol at the desirable level. Your doctor will order further tests to get a full profile of your lipids and help you create a plan for treating your high cholesterol through lifestyle changes and possibly medications.

An **LDL cholesterol** level of:

- Less than 100 mg/dL is optimal
- 100 to 129 mg/dL is near optimal
- 130 to 159 mg/dL is borderline high
- 160 to 189 mg/dL is high
- 190 mg/dL and above is dangerously high

For **HDL cholesterol,** the higher the number, the better. A level less than 40 mg/dL is considered a major risk factor for heart disease. Levels of 60 mg/dL and higher can help lower your risk.

There are a few factors affecting cholesterol level that are not under your control, among them:

- **Gender.** Estrogen tends to elevate HDL ("good") cholesterol, which may help explain why premenopausal women have a lower incidence of heart disease than men do (until women hit menopause). However, even young women generally have higher triglyceride levels than men do.
- **Age.** As we get older, our levels of cholesterol and triglycerides tend to rise. Before menopause, women are usually protected from high LDL levels because of estrogen's boosting effect on HDL levels. But postmenopausal women—even those with a heart-healthy diet and regular exercise—often experience higher LDL cholesterol levels.
- **Heredity.** Genes partly determine how much cholesterol your liver makes; high cholesterol sometimes runs in families.

Fortunately, cholesterol levels are generally very responsive to lifestyle measures, especially diet, as well as medications. See "Key Actions for Heart Health" on page 204 for guidance on lowering cholesterol through heart-healthy measures.

TRIGLYCERIDES

Triglycerides are a kind of fat found in foods and body fat cells; they are the type of fat in circulation in your blood. Like cholesterol levels, triglyceride levels are affected by both genetics and the foods you eat. Whether high levels of triglycerides are directly associated with risk of coronary artery disease is still a matter of debate. In most cases, high triglyceride levels are linked with low HDL cholesterol, so it's difficult to tease apart the effects of high triglycerides alone. But the best way to lower high triglyceride levels is by improving your diet, especially cutting back on refined carbohydrates, controlling your weight, and engaging in physical activity.

Your doctor can measure your triglyceride levels with a simple blood test. (This is a fasting test, so check with your doctor about food restrictions preceding the test.) The guidelines for triglycerides are:

- Less than 150 mg/dL is normal
- 150 to 199 mg/dL is borderline high
- 200 to 499 mg/dL is high
- 500 mg/dL or above is very high

BLOOD PRESSURE

Blood pressure is the force of circulating blood against the walls of the arteries. It's normal for blood pressure to rise when you're active and to decrease when you're sleeping. But if it stays elevated, a condition known as hypertension, it can increase your risk of heart disease, stroke, congestive heart failure, kidney disease, and blindness.

About one in four women in the United States has hypertension. But because the condition has no symptoms, as many as a third of those with the condition don't know they have it. As women age, they develop hypertension at a higher rate than men do, and more women over the age of 60 have the condition than men of the same age do. Even women with normal blood pressure at age 50 face a 90 percent chance of developing hypertension later in life. Women also have a higher risk if they are pregnant, are obese, have a family history of high blood pressure, or have reached menopause. African American women are at elevated risk.

Blood pressure is measured via a quick and easy procedure that involves a gauge, a stethoscope (or electronic sensor), and a blood pressure cuff. To get an accurate measurement, you should do the following before the test:

- Avoid drinking coffee or smoking cigarettes for a half hour.
- Go to the bathroom.
- Sit and relax for 5 minutes.

A blood pressure reading is measured in millimeters of mercury (mmHg) and consists of two numbers—systolic pressure "over" diastolic pressure. Systolic pressure refers to the pressure at the peak of each heartbeat, when blood is pushed out to the body. Diastolic pressure refers to pressure when the heart relaxes between beats and blood pressure is at its lowest. Systolic pressure is always higher than diastolic pressure and gives the most accurate diagnosis of hypertension.

The following are the guidelines for blood pressure:

- **Less than 120/80 mmHG is considered normal.**
- **120 to 139/80 to 89 mmHG is considered pre-hypertension,** which means that you don't yet have high blood pressure, but are likely to develop it in the future if you don't adjust your lifestyle.
- **Greater than 140/90 mmHG is classified as hypertension.** If you have diabetes or chronic kidney disease, your blood pressure is considered high if it is greater than 130/80 mmHG.

10-YEAR RISK ASSESSMENT

Once you know your numbers, you can assess your risk for having a heart attack in the next 10 years. The National Institutes of Health developed a tool for assessing risk by following thousands of individuals over a period of 10 years and determining which factors, such as cholesterol and blood pressure, predicted risk of heart attack. To calculate your risk you will need to know your total cholesterol, HDL ("good") cholesterol, and blood pressure. I encourage you to go to the Web site nhlbi.nih.gov and answer the five questions in the 10-year risk assessment tool. You'll see that each answer you supply is assigned a certain number of points. Total up the points for all of your five answers, then match the sum with the chart at the end to determine your risk.

Your score on this chart indicates your need for heart disease prevention efforts. As the chart makes clear, if your point total falls below 20, your risk of suffering from heart disease or any of its complications is low, less than 10 percent. If your point total runs between 20 and 22, your risk is moderate, between 10 and 20 percent, which means that you should consider making some lifestyle changes to reduce your risk. A score of 23 or higher means that your risk is high, greater than 20 percent. (Note: Your risk is automatically considered greater than 20 percent if you already have heart disease or diabetes, no matter what your score on these five questions.) If you fall into the high-risk category, you need to take aggressive action to lower your chances of heart trouble—perhaps by losing weight, eating more healthfully, and exercising appropriately. In addition, you should consult with your health care provider about taking preventive medications.

LOWERING YOUR RISK

There is no medical condition that is nearly as responsive to lifestyle changes as cardiovascular disease. Yes, there's a genetic component. But if you're truly fit, active, eating well, and not smoking, your chances of getting cardiovascular disease are radically reduced.

We have heart disease in my family. My grandfather died of a heart attack when he was in his early fifties. I never met him. When my dad entered his forties, he appeared to be heading toward the same fate. He had high blood pressure, smoked, drank too much, and didn't exercise enough. He was also about 30 pounds overweight. But then one day shortly after he turned 48, he had an epiphany. He realized that he was approaching the age at which his father had died. He decided to stop smoking and drinking. He got fit by training for a marathon. He lost 40 pounds.

We recently celebrated my dad's 80th birthday with more than a dozen family members. I toasted him for the gift of life he gave our family, for taking care of himself so that he would be around for me, for my brothers, and for his grandchildren.

It takes many years for heart disease to develop. A 2007 National Heart, Lung, and Blood Institute (NHLBI) study suggests that even adolescents and young adults show some of the warning signs for developing heart disease. Having a high body mass index (BMI) or higher than optimal blood pressure or LDL ("bad") cholesterol between ages 18 and 30 can mean a two to three times greater risk of developing heart disease.

Regrettably, more and more adolescents and young adults are developing these signs because of poor diet and lack of physical activity. You can significantly lower your chances of heart disease by adopting the measures described below.

KEY ACTIONS FOR HEART HEALTH

There are a number of key actions you can take to minimize your risk of heart disease. Consider the list below and evaluate which actions are important for you. For most of us, lifestyle measures, such as eating well, being physically active, maintaining a healthy body weight, and not smoking, are key. For some women, medications may also be necessary.

Control your blood cholesterol. LDL ("bad") cholesterol should be maintained at less than 100 mg/dL and HDL ("good") cholesterol, at over 50 mg/dL. If LDL levels remain in excess of 160 despite lifestyle changes, doctors may recommend therapy with statin, a cholesterol-lowering drug. (See the box Salt: How Much Is Too Much? on page 206.)

Control your blood pressure. Optimal blood pressure of 120/80 mmHg should be maintained. If blood pressure remains elevated despite lifestyle changes, doctors may recommend medication to help lower blood pressure.

Control diabetes. Maintain fasting blood glucose levels below 100 mg/dL and hemoglobin A1C below 7.

Stop smoking. If you smoke, quitting will almost immediately help lower your risk.

Use alcohol moderately. Research shows that a little alcohol reduces heart disease risk. If you enjoy alcohol, limit your intake to one glass of beer, wine, or spirits a day.

Reduce stress and increase positive social interactions. Finding ways to ease stress and depression (such as deep breathing, meditation, tai chi, yoga, or worship) and to enrich your positive social interactions can help lower blood pressure, heart rate, and even high levels of LDL ("bad") cholesterol. (See Chapter 25 for more strategies.)

Maintain a healthy weight and waist measurement. Keep your BMI in the ideal body weight range of 18 to 24 and keep your waist measurement below 35 inches.

Exercise. I firmly believe that there is nothing more important for heart health than being fit. Research shows that aerobic activity not only makes your cardiovascular system stronger and more efficient, but it also dramatically reduces your risk of heart disease. One study of some 122,000 women revealed that those who walk briskly at least 3 hours a week reduce their risk of heart disease by 35 percent.

On the flip side: Women who are sedentary—even if they have healthy blood cholesterol levels and blood pressure levels and don't smoke—have six times the risk of dying from heart disease as do active women with the same heart-health numbers. The fitter you are, the lower your risk. And here's what may be the most important message from this research: The effects of aerobic exercise are immediate. It's what you do today that counts. Both aerobic activities (e.g., walking, running, swimming, biking, raking leaves) and strength-training exercises are important for the conditioning of your whole cardiovascular system. Being physically active not only promotes weight control and better circulation, but it also lowers blood pressure and blood glucose and improves HDL cholesterol levels. (See Chapter 27 for specifics on exercise programs.)

Eat a healthy diet. Eating well has a major impact on reducing your risk of heart disease. The effects are probably a consequence of lowering cholesterol and blood pressure and controlling blood glucose and inflammation. My recommendations for heart-healthy eating incorporate the most important research findings to date:

- Eat an abundance of fruits and vegetables (five or more servings per day).
- Total fat does not matter: It can be high or low; what matters is keeping saturated and trans fats at no more than 7 percent of calories. Saturated fat comes primarily from animals (full-fat milk, red meat, pork, lamb, chicken with skin, etc.).
- Focus on consuming more plant-based proteins such as legumes, beans, seeds, soy, low-fat dairy, and nuts, and fewer animal-based proteins. A recent study followed half a million people and found that those who ate the most red meat and processed meat had the highest mortality rates from heart disease (and also cancer). Numerous other studies have shown similar results.
- Eat more fish. Women who consume at least three servings of fish per week have reduced heart disease, and if they have heart disease, the progression of the disease is slower. Be mindful about how your fish is prepared, however, and try to eat fish that has been broiled, baked, or grilled. Deep-fried fish doesn't count!
- Minimize processed and refined foods. Focus on eating real foods with minimal packaging.
- Keep salt intake to less than 2,300 mg per day (ideally, 1,500 mg per day). The average American typically gets 6,000 mg per day. Most salt comes from processed foods of all types. Select foods low in salt; use spices, onions, and garlic instead of salt to add flavor to your meals. (See the box Salt: How Much Is Too Much? on page 206.)

In describing heart-healthy foods in *Strong Women, Strong Hearts*, I use the **H.E.A.R.T.** acronym:

Heap on vegetables and fruits.
Emphasize the right fats.
Accentuate whole grains.
Revere low-fat and fat-free dairy.
Target heart-healthy proteins.

A very similar approach to this pattern of eating is the DASH (Dietary Approaches to Stop Hypertension) diet. (See the box Healthy Eating Plans on pages 366–367.)

The grocery stores are now full of packaged foods that claim to be heart healthy. This is the result of research on how individual components of food such as fatty

SALT: HOW MUCH IS TOO MUCH?

The body needs salt, but very little. It uses the mineral to maintain fluid balance, conduct nerve impulses, and contract and relax muscles. The kidneys normally do a good job of regulating salt in the body. However, when salt levels get too high, the kidneys can't keep up, and the result is hypertension.

Most experts recommend that daily salt intake for healthy adults should not exceed 2,300 mg. Unfortunately, the average American diet contains between three and ten times that. The greatest contributor to excessive salt intake is processed foods. It's estimated that 77 percent of Americans' salt intake comes from processed and prepared foods; 12 percent from natural sources; 6 percent from salt added while eating; and 5 percent from salt added to foods while cooking. Most natural or whole foods do not contain a lot of salt, but during the processing and packaging of foods, salt is added in large quantities. Until recently, soups have been particularly high in salt; now many manufacturers offer reduced- or low-sodium options. But most cheeses, lunch meats, cured meats, and chips and other snack foods still contain a lot of salt. The best strategy for lowering your salt intake is to avoid processed foods. If they're not a big part of your diet, it's fine to add a dash of salt to your meals.

acids, proteins, carbohydrates, fiber, vitamins, and minerals influence blood cholesterol and risk for heart disease and how much salt and other nutrients affect blood
pressure. The research has led to claims suggesting that products containing oats,
soy protein, or walnuts are heart healthy. The problem with this reductionist
approach is that we don't eat foods in isolation; we eat meals, snacks, beverages, etc.,
which combine nutrients. What worries me is this: As soon as a new research finding
about a specific nutrient is reported, food manufacturers reformulate various packaged foods to reflect the new research and advertise them as the latest "healthy" fare.
This just perpetuates our consumption of processed, packaged foods. For example,
think about the oat cereals that are touted as heart healthy. Simply adding a processed oat cereal to your breakfast and not making any other change to your diet will
not positively affect your heart health. (Moreover, most of those cereals are loaded
with sugar.)

MEDICATIONS FOR CHOLESTEROL

If therapeutic lifestyle changes are insufficient to lower your cholesterol levels, you
should consult with your doctor about combining these with use of cholesterol-
reducing drugs. Among the available drugs are statins, bile acid sequestrants, nico-
tinic acid, and fibric acids. There are currently five FDA-approved statin drugs:
atorvastatin, fluvastatin, pravastatin, rosuvastatin, and simvastatin. Statins all work
similarly in that they block the action of a specific enzyme in the liver that is responsible for making LDL cholesterol. They are safe for most people. (See the box The
Subject of Statins on page 208.) Bile acid sequestrants also reduce LDL levels. Nico-
tonic acid reduces both LDL and triglycerides and raises HDL levels. Fibric acids
work mainly by reducing high triglyceride levels and raising HDL levels. Consult
with your health care provider about which medication or combination of medications may be best for you.

MEDICATIONS FOR HIGH BLOOD PRESSURE

If lifestyle changes do not lower your blood pressure to the normal range, you may need
to supplement these with medications. Ask your health care provider for guidance on
selecting the right medication(s) for you. The main types of drugs are diuretics, ACE
inhibitors, angiotensin antagonists, beta-blockers, calcium channel blockers, alpha-
blockers and alpha-beta-blockers, nervous system inhibitors, and vasodilators.

THE SUBJECT OF STATINS

If I have normal cholesterol, should I take cholesterol-lowering drugs?

New research suggests that even healthy people with normal cholesterol levels benefit from using cholesterol-lowering statin drugs to prevent cardiovascular disease. A study of 17,000 men and women, published in 2008 in *The New England Journal of Medicine,* showed that taking statin drugs reduced the risk of heart attack, stroke, and cardiovascular disease by 47 percent. The study subjects had low levels of LDL cholesterol, but high levels of high-sensitivity C-reactive protein (or CRP), an inflammatory marker associated with elevated risk of heart disease. The subjects were divided into two groups and given either 20 mg of a cholesterol-lowering statin drug called rosuvastatin (brand name Crestor) or a placebo. After just 2 years, the study was halted because it was clear that the cardiovascular benefits were considerable for subjects on drug treatment compared with subjects on placebo. In the Crestor group, LDL cholesterol was reduced by 50 percent; levels of CRP dropped by 37 percent; and risk of heart attack, stroke, and death from heart disease was cut nearly in half. The total risk of death was reduced by 20 percent.

Although these are remarkable findings, I think we should interpret them with caution. Because the trial was only 2 years in duration, the long-term risks of taking these drugs are not known. However, the study does show that lowering your LDL and your CRP—whether with the help of drugs or through lifestyle measures such as diet and exercise—radically reduces your risk of cardiovascular disease.

OTHER HEART PROBLEMS

HEART FAILURE

Heart failure occurs when your heart fails to pump enough blood to meet your body's needs. As a result, the body's tissues receive insufficient oxygen. In addition, blood may back up in the veins, collecting in the lungs, abdomen, lower legs and ankles, and the liver, causing symptoms such as shortness of breath, fatigue, and fluid retention. Congestive heart failure (CHF) is a term used to describe heart failure that includes fluid buildup. The terms are often used interchangeably.

Heart failure may result from other conditions that weaken or damage the heart, such as longstanding coronary artery disease or high blood pressure, as well as cardiomyopathy (disease of the heart muscle), faulty heart valves, previous heart attacks, or arrhythmia. It may develop suddenly or slowly and can be a chronic, long-term condition. More women than men have the disease and women are more likely than men to die from it.

Are You at Risk?

Those at highest risk for CHF are women with hypertension, coronary artery disease, and diabetes. Other risk factors include:

- Previous heart attacks
- Irregular heartbeats
- Sleep apnea
- Congenital heart defects
- Viral infection
- Overuse of alcohol
- Kidney conditions

Warning Signs and Symptoms

General symptoms include breathlessness, irregular heartbeat, fatigue, weakness, reduced ability to exercise, and swelling. However, which symptoms occur depends on which side of the heart is failing. If the left side of the heart is affected, blood backs up into the lungs, causing them to fill up with fluid. This condition, called pulmonary edema, is often marked primarily by shortness of breath. If the right side of the heart fails, blood congests the abdomen, liver, and legs, resulting in bloating, liver malfunction, and swelling of the lower legs and ankles. If both sides fail, swelling occurs in many body tissues, along with breathlessness, fatigue, and weakness.

Prevention

The best way to prevent heart failure is to eliminate risk factors for heart disease by making lifestyle changes, such as:

- Not smoking
- Limiting intake of sodium, fats, and cholesterol
- Limiting intake of alcohol
- Maintaining a healthy weight
- Exercising
- Limiting stress
- Sleeping soundly

Treatment

For most patients, treatment involves a combination of rest, a diet of restricted salt intake, and medications such as beta-blockers and calcium channel blockers, as well as devices to assist the heart in keeping a proper beat. In some cases, surgery is required.

Exercise can also benefit patients. One of the classic symptoms of CHF is fatigue and very low levels of fitness. My colleagues at Tufts have done several studies on CHF. One, on the effects of strength training on women with the condition, found that strength training helps patients maintain their muscle strength over time and boosts their tolerance for exercise. This is exciting research, because this "treatment" has none of the negative side effects that accompany some medications. Trials on the effects of walking have also shown benefit.

VALVULAR HEART DISEASE

Valvular heart disease may involve any of the four valves in the heart, which keep blood flowing in the proper direction. Damaged valves may arise from narrowing (stenosis), leaking (regurgitation), or improper closing (prolapse), all of which can lead to a stretching, enlarging, and weakening of the heart's chambers. Aortic stenosis is a narrowing of the valve that links the heart and the aorta. Aortic regurgitation, an insufficient seal in the aortic valve, allows blood to leak back into the left ventricle. Both conditions make the heart pump harder to move blood through the body. Mitral valve prolapse occurs when the mitral valve, which links the upper and lower chambers of the left side of the heart, prolapses, or balloons out. This may allow blood to flow back into the upper chamber, increasing the risk for endocarditis, an infection and inflammation of the membrane lining the inside of the heart. Some 6 percent of women are diagnosed with the disorder, and it is more common among young women than older women.

Some valve disorders are congenital; others arise from rheumatic fever, infection, some medications, or cancer radiation treatments. Symptoms include fatigue or weakness, chest pain, fainting, dizziness, shortness of breath or difficulty breathing, palpitations, a decreasing ability to exercise at a normal level, and in severe cases, coughing up blood.

ARRHYTHMIAS

Arrhythmias are irregular rhythms of the heart that occur as a result of a malfunction in the electrical impulses that coordinate heartbeat, causing the heart to beat too fast, too slowly, or abnormally. Arrhythmias range in severity from harmless—the occasional skipped or irregular heartbeat—to life threatening. Tachycardia is an exceptionally rapid heartbeat, more than 100 beats per minute. Bradycardia is a slower than normal heartbeat, fewer than 60 beats per minute. If you experience palpitations or abnormal heartbeats not easily explained by exercise, excessive caffeine, or emotional upset, you should consult a physician.

STROKE

A stroke is sometimes referred to as a "brain attack." It occurs when bloodflow to the brain is halted because of a narrowed or blocked carotid artery, a condition called carotid artery stenosis. Every 45 seconds, someone in this country suffers a stroke. Every year, twice as many women die of stroke than of breast cancer. These attacks cause more chronic disabilities than any other disease. The odds of having a stroke more than double each decade after age 55. Although the risk of having a stroke is the same for men and women, more women die from it. For African Americans, stroke is twice as common as for Caucasians.

There are two kinds of stroke. Ischemic stroke, the more common variety, occurs when bloodflow to the brain is interrupted by a blood clot that blocks a carotid artery. Hemorrhagic stroke is caused by a rupture in a blood vessel, which leaks blood into the brain. Both can cause the death of brain cells in the affected areas. Damage to the brain from a stroke can involve the whole body, resulting in mild to serious disabilities, such as paralysis, speech impairment, and dementia.

If you have a stroke, every minute counts! Treatments are available that can greatly reduce the risk of long-term brain injury, but only if the patient arrives at an urgent care

---

LOOKING FOR SIGNS OF STROKE

If you suspect someone is having a stroke, act **FAST** to determine whether she shows telling symptoms:

FACE: Ask her to smile. Does one side of her face move like the other or does it appear to droop?

ARMS: Ask her to raise both arms and hold them straight out for 10 seconds. Does one arm drift downward?

SPEECH: Ask her to repeat a simple statement. Does she have difficulty? Are her words slurred?

TIME: If she displays any of these symptoms, dial 911! Remember that every minute counts.

facility within 60 minutes of the onset of symptoms. It's critical to know the warning signs and act promptly by calling 911. This may be the most important thing that you can do for yourself or a loved one experiencing a stroke.

Any of the following symptoms can be a sign of stroke:

- Numbness or weakness of the face, arm, or leg, usually on one side of the body
- Confusion, difficulty speaking or comprehending speech
- Trouble seeing in one or both eyes
- Difficulty walking, dizziness or loss of balance

- Crushing headache with no apparent cause
- Face or limb pain
- Chest pain
- Palpitations
- Shortness of breath
- Hiccups
- Nausea
- General weakness

Are You at Risk?

Among the risk factors for stroke are:

- A family history of stroke
- High blood pressure
- High cholesterol
- Smoking
- Diabetes
- Being overweight
- Being sedentary
- Taking birth control pills

- Being pregnant
- Using hormone therapy
- Having a waist size larger than 35.2 inches and a triglyceride level higher than 128 mg/dL
- Having migraine headaches, which can increase a woman's risk of stroke three to six times

Prevention

The most common risk factors for stroke are the same as those for heart disease—high blood pressure, diabetes, high cholesterol, and obesity. To prevent stroke:

- Work to lower your blood pressure if you have hypertension.
- Quit smoking.
- If you have diabetes, learn to manage it well.
- If you are overweight, try to lose weight.
- Eat well, following a heart-healthy diet as described earlier in this chapter.

VASCULAR DISEASES

Your body's network of arteries, veins, and capillaries is known as your vascular system. Vascular disorders are relatively common and range from mild conditions, such as varicose veins, to life-threatening aneurysms, or weakened areas in blood vessels that bulge like balloons and may rupture, causing internal bleeding.

Some vascular problems occur when bloodflow in the vessels is impeded because of blood clots that do not dissolve on their own. The tendency of blood cells to form clots is triggered by sluggish bloodflow from long periods of sitting still (say, during an overseas airplane trip) or lying down (during bed rest), and by an increase in clotting factors that may arise during pregnancy, after an operation or injury, from infection, or from medications such as birth control pills.

Other vascular disorders result when excessive pressure in the arteries makes the arterial walls thick and stiff—the condition known as arteriosclerosis, or hardening of the arteries. The most common form of arteriosclerosis is atherosclerosis, when plaque builds up inside the arteries, weakening or clogging them.

The best way to prevent vascular disorders is to follow the heart-healthy measures described on pages 204–206.

Common disorders of the arteries include the following:

- **Peripheral vascular disease (PVD) or peripheral arterial disease (PAD)** occurs when arteries that carry blood to the limbs (usually the legs) become narrow or clogged. The condition can cause "claudication," pain in the legs during exercise. It can lead to severe limitations on activity or even limb amputation. I have become very familiar with PAD over the past couple of years, because my dad, now in his eighties, has significant PAD in his right leg. It became so painful that he needed to have bypass surgery on the leg. Fortunately, he is now recovering and back walking on the golf course. Treatment for mild forms of PVD involves exercise, healthy diet, and quitting smoking.
- **Carotid artery disease** arises when the arteries in the neck become clogged, reducing blood supply to the brain. The condition can lead to stroke. It can be treated with a combination of lifestyle changes, medications, and in some cases, surgery.
- **Pulmonary edema** occurs when increased blood pressure in the vessels of your lungs forces fluid into the small elastic air sacs that normally take in oxygen and release carbon dioxide. This prevents them from absorbing oxygen. Although the condition can be life threatening, prompt treatment and proper therapy can lead to a positive outcome.

- **Pulmonary embolism** occurs when an artery in the lung is blocked by one or more blood clots that may have come from a different part of the body. Symptoms include shortness of breath, sharp chest pain, rapid pulse, sweating, and cough with bloody sputum.

- **Aortic aneurysm.** Aneurysms (bulges or weakness in a blood vessel) may occur in arteries anywhere in the body, but the most common sites are the abdominal aorta—the main artery of the heart—and the arteries at the base of the brain. If these bulges grow large enough, they can rupture, causing life-threatening bleeding.

- **Reynaud's disease.** In Reynaud's disease, arteries that supply blood to the extremities of the body, such as fingers, toes, or nose, temporarily narrow in response to cold exposure or emotional stress, limiting circulation. This may cause extremities to get numb and turn white or blue. The condition is more of a bother than a disability. It is more common among women than men and in those living in colder climates. If you have this condition, it's important to try to keep your body, hands, and feet warm with the right clothing so that they don't get chilled.

Common disorders of the veins include the following:

- **Thrombophlebitis** occurs when a blood clot, or thrombus, causes inflammation in your veins. The condition typically arises in the veins of the legs and is most often caused by prolonged sitting or lying down. If the affected vein is deep within a muscle, the condition is called deep vein thrombosis.

- **Deep vein thrombosis (DVT)** occurs when a clot suddenly forms in the deep veins of the legs. Symptoms may include pain, sudden swelling, reddish blue discoloration, enlargement of superficial veins, and skin warmth. If the condition goes untreated, DVT can cause tissue death or gangrene, which may require amputation.

- **Varicose veins** arise when the valves that control bloodflow in and out of the veins malfunction, and gravity causes blood to pool in the veins. When this occurs in the legs, superficial veins enlarge and bulge, becoming visible as gnarled dark blue vessels just beneath the skin. Smaller varicose veins are known as spider veins. Contributing causes include obesity, pregnancy, tight clothing, standing for long periods of time, and genetics. The condition most often affects women between the ages of 30 and 70. For the majority, varicose veins are primarily a cosmetic concern. However, the condition may also cause pain and discomfort and can lead to more serious circulatory disorders, such as venous stasis disease—when pooling of blood in the lower leg veins causes tissue damage. (See Chapter 6 for more information on varicose veins.)

16

Lungs and Respiration

You may not think of them this way, but your lungs are your body's primary point of contact with the world outside your body. You breathe in and out about 15 to 25 times per minute. Each time you breathe in, you draw into your lungs air from the outside world—about 6 to 10 quarts of air every minute—bringing life-giving oxygen to the tissues of your body and expelling carbon dioxide, their main waste product. This process, called gas exchange, takes place in the lungs, the central organs of the respiratory system.

The process works like this: Air enters though the nose or mouth and passes down the trachea or windpipe, where it is warmed and humidified. From the trachea, the air enters the lungs through large airways called bronchi, like the large major limbs of an upside-down tree. These airways divide into finer and finer branches, or bronchioles, until they reach the alveoli—tiny air sacs where most of the gas exchange takes place. Your lungs hold about 300 million of these air sacs, which are surrounded by the fine network of blood vessels called capillaries. Oxygen and carbon dioxide pass between the alveoli and the capillaries by way of a very thin membrane separating the two.

Because the air we breathe contains potentially harmful substances, from bacteria to pollutants, the inner lining of the respiratory tract possesses an array of defenses aimed at removing or destroying germs and toxic molecules. Mucus lining the respiratory tract traps foreign substances, and specialized cells with hairlike cilia sweep them out and upward so they can be coughed out of the airway or swallowed.

You don't have to think about breathing because the act is controlled by your autonomic nervous system. The rate at which you breathe is controlled by the respiratory centers in your brain stem, or medulla, which automatically sends signals to your diaphragm and other muscles in your chest. These muscles contract and relax at regular intervals, allowing your lungs to expand and fill with air, and then relax and empty. Sometimes the respiratory centers send extra nerve impulses to the diaphragm; the result is unwanted contractions, or hiccups.

WHEN YOUR LUNGS STRUGGLE

Several conditions and diseases of the lungs can make breathing difficult or interfere with the lungs' ability to exchange oxygen and carbon dioxide. The culprit in these disorders is often tobacco smoke, including both active smoking and exposure to passive smoke. Other factors include environmental pollutants, poor ventilation systems, and infections with bacteria, viruses, and fungi. Among the more common disorders or conditions that affect lung function are asthma, chronic obstructive pulmonary disease (chronic bronchitis and emphysema), and pleurisy.

ASTHMA

Asthma is a chronic, but treatable, condition affecting the bronchial tubes, the main airways that transport air in and out of the lungs. Although boys are more likely than girls to have asthma in early childhood, adult women are more likely than men to be diagnosed with the condition. It is likely that a combination of genetics and environmental factors play a role in the development of the disease.

Asthma tends to run in families and to be closely linked with allergies.

In people with asthma, the lining of the bronchial tubes becomes swollen, inflamed, and highly sensitive to irritations or allergens. The disease is characterized by periods of stability, with sporadic episodes or attacks of varying frequency, duration, and severity. During an asthma attack, the muscles squeeze the bronchi, narrowing them and allowing less air to flow through to lung tissue. Often, the cells in the lungs make thick mucus that accumulates in the airways, causing reactions from mild wheezing and coughing to severely restricted or labored breathing, which can be life-threatening.

Triggers of asthma attacks include:

- Allergens, such as animal dander (from skin, hair, or feathers), dust mites, cockroaches, pollen, and mold
- Irritants, such as cigarette smoke, air pollution, cold air, or strong odors from painting, cooking, or scented products
- Medicines, such as aspirin and beta-blockers
- Viral or bacterial respiratory infections
- Sulfites in food or beverages
- Gastroesophageal reflux disease (GERD), a condition in which stomach acid backs up into your esophagus and causes heartburn
- Stress
- Strong emotions
- Physical exertion
- Cold air

Fortunately, most people with asthma can lead active, healthy lives by avoiding triggers and taking medication.

SYMPTOMS

Among the common symptoms of asthma are:

- Wheezing
- Coughing that worsens at night or early in the morning
- Pain or constriction in the chest
- Shortness of breath
- Rapid or noisy breathing

If you are experiencing any of these symptoms, see your doctor. Asthma can be very serious; if you have it, you should learn what things trigger your symptoms and how to avoid them. Your doctor may also prescribe medication to keep your asthma under control. If you are prescribed medication, make sure that you have it with you at all times so that you are prepared to prevent an attack.

PREVENTION

Although there is no known way to prevent asthma, you can control the symptoms to maintain a normal, active life. Follow these guidelines:

- Work closely with a doctor to develop a self-management plan.
- Avoid triggers, such as allergens and other airway irritants. If animal dander is an allergen for you, keep pets out of the house. If pollen is an issue, stay indoors when the pollen count is high. If you're allergic to dust mites, wash your linens and pillows once a week in hot water. If sulfites affect you, avoid foods that contain them, such as dried fruit and wine. Do not allow smoking in your home. If exercise triggers asthma symptoms, talk to your doctor about controlling these exercise-induced symptoms, because it's important to maintain regular physical activity.
- Monitor asthma to respond quickly to signs of an attack. Among the most useful tools is a handheld device called a peak flow meter, which you can use at home to monitor your lung function. The peak flow meter can help warn you of an impending asthma attack even before you're aware of symptoms.
- Take medications as directed.

TREATMENT

How asthma is treated depends on the severity of the disease. Doctors classify asthma severity by how frequently you experience episodes of symptoms:

- **Mild intermittent**—episodes twice a week or less; symptoms at night twice a month or less; between episodes, lung function is normal
- **Mild persistent**—symptoms more than twice a week but no more than once per day; symptoms at night more than twice a month
- **Moderate persistent**—symptoms every day and nighttime symptoms more than once a week
- **Severe persistent**—symptoms throughout the day on most days; frequent nighttime symptoms; physical activity is limited

There are two types of medicines commonly used for asthma:

Quick-relief medicines are used by most asthma sufferers and taken at the first sign of symptoms to provide immediate relief. These include bronchodilators such as inhaled beta-agonists that relax the muscles surrounding your airways.

Long-term control medicines, such as inhaled corticosteroids, leukotriene modifiers, cromolyn, and theophylline, are taken daily to prevent symptoms and attacks. These medicines are used for controlling asthma of all levels of severity.

Many people with asthma benefit from the use of both a quick-relief and a long-term control medicine.

CHRONIC OBSTRUCTIVE PULMONARY DISEASE (COPD)

COPD is a serious lung disease that affects some 24 million Americans. It is the fourth leading cause of death in this country. It typically affects people over the age of 45 who smoke or have smoked in the past or people who have spent many years exposed to lung irritants, such as air pollution or chemical fumes, vapors, and dust. In COPD, the lining of the bronchial tubes becomes inflamed, causing a cough and excess mucus production. In addition, the air sacs, or alveoli, in the lungs lose their shape and become stiff, preventing the critical exchange of oxygen and carbon dioxide. Symptoms include chronic "smoker's cough," shortness of breath (especially with exercise), and wheezing. The disease is treated with daily medications, antibiotics, and oxygen. The best way to prevent COPD is to quit smoking.

PLEURISY

Pleurisy, or pleuritis, results from inflammation of the pleura, the two-layered membrane surrounding the lungs and chest cavity. The ordinarily smooth linings become rough and rub together with each breath. The condition can produce sharp pain during breathing or coughing. Pleurisy may develop as a complication of infections such as flu, pneumonia, tuberculosis, or autoimmune diseases such as lupus and rheumatoid arthritis. It can also result from chest trauma, certain cancers, and asbestos-related disease. Treatment involves addressing the underlying condition and taking pain relievers.

roductive Choices Fertility and Preg
enopause Sexual Abuse and Sexual A
n Teeth Hair and Nails Body Weigh
tabolism Blood Sugar Eating and Exc
scles Bones JointsHeart and Blood I
d Respiration Common Infectious Di
toimmune Disease Cancer Vision He
ell, Taste, and Touch Mental Health
nce Abuse Making Change Managing
d Sleeping Well Shifting Your Food En
nt Getting Active Screenings and H
intenance Reproduction Sexuality an
l Health Reproductive Choices Fertilit
egnancy Menopause Sexual Abuse an
l Assault Skin Teeth Hair and Nails
eight and Metabolism Blood Sugar F
d Excreting Muscles Bones JointsHear
od Lungs and Respiration Common
us Diseases Autoimmune Disease C

PART VI

In Our Defense

We have an ingenious system of self-defense. It's a good thing, too, because the body faces constant challenges from without and within. We live in a matrix of microbes, bacteria, viruses, parasites, and fungi. The vast majority of these organisms are harmless, and many are helpful. But some could cause serious or fatal infections were it not for the intervention of our immune system. This network of cells and chemicals protects us in myriad ways. Cut your finger or contract an infection, and your white blood cells arrive at a moment's notice at the site of injury, whether it be in the epithelial lining of your nose or a knife slice in your thumb. Catch a cold or flu, and the body mounts a complex, coordinated defense against the viral culprit.

Threats to our health may also arise from within, in the form of cells that grow out of control, causing cancer. Most scientists hold that the immune system also protects against cancer, patrolling the body for cancerous cells and nipping them in the bud.

Your immune system is an odd phenomenon. It's not an organ or a body system like any other. You can't transplant it; you can't see the whole thing at once, even with the best imaging technology. It's less like an organ and more like a diffuse intelligence-gathering and communications system made of a network of tissues, organs, and trillions of little sleuthing cells and molecules roaming the blood and lymph.

Twenty-four hours a day, the white blood cells known as lymphocytes patrol your body, looking for intruders. Their mission is to seek out and destroy any invaders they deem a threat. Made in the bone marrow (millions each second, all through life), they inhabit the liver, spleen, lymphoid organs, blood, and tissues. They carry on their surfaces special receptors uniquely fashioned to spot a particular interloper—whether in the form of the bug itself or a little piece of it, as in a vaccine. So diverse are these receptors and fine-tuned in their powers of detection that they can recognize and respond to virtually any molecule in the universe—while (usually) not attacking the molecules and cells of the body itself.

When lymphocytes meet a microbe that matches their receptor, they divide furiously, creating a cloned colony of tens of thousands of cells that release antibodies and other powerful chemicals to fight the infection. What you feel as swollen glands is the burgeoning population of lymphocytes in lymph organs strategically placed in parts of the body where invading microbes are often encountered—say, in your throat. The full flowering of lymphocytes against a specific invader often takes a week.

After the battle, some of the lymphocytes primed against the particular invader remain in the body, ensuring an efficient response to future infection—so rapid and effective that we're often never even aware we've once again met the bug. The encounter is engraved forever in the memory of the body.

The strength of our immune system can also turn against us. Inflammation, the body's natural response to injury or infection, may play a role in atherosclerosis, the buildup of fatty deposits in the lining of the blood vessels that can lead to heart disease. Allergy is inflammation gone haywire, an overzealous response to something that doesn't ordinarily trouble the body. With autoimmune disease, the body's immune cells attack and destroy its own cells and tissues. For reasons not fully understood, autoimmune diseases are far more common in women than in men.

Over the past decade or so, I've thought a lot about how to boost immunity, and in this part of the book, I share the 10 **S.M.A.R.T.** ways to keep your immune system strong.

1. Eat well, exercise, and maintain a healthy body weight.
2. Wash your hands often and thoroughly.
3. Practice basic food hygiene.
4. Practice safe sex.
5. Avoid insect bites.
6. Avoid or minimize exposure to environmental contaminants.
7. Do not smoke.
8. Get recommended immunizations and screenings.
9. Minimize negative stress.
10. Get the sleep you need to feel rested.

17

Common Infectious Diseases

Infectious agents such as bacteria, viruses, parasites, and fungi can enter the body through skin contact or sexual contact, through airways as airborne microbes, in contaminated food or water, through bites from insect vectors such as ticks or mosquitoes, and various other routes.

Some infections, such as measles, HIV, and malaria, are systemic, affecting the whole body. Others, such as the common cold or tuberculosis, are local, involving only one organ or system—though some may cause serious complications if they affect vital organs or spread through the bloodstream. How an infection resolves depends on the virulence and number of agents involved in the infection, and also how your immune system responds.

Fortunately, we've come a long way in our ability to prevent and treat common infectious diseases. Preventive measures include vaccines against such diseases as diphtheria, tetanus, polio, measles, and influenza. Hand washing and sanitary handling of food and water are also valuable preventive strategies.

Antibiotics can be highly effective in the fight against bacterial infections but not viral infections. If you are prescribed antibiotics for a bacterial infection, make sure you follow instructions carefully and complete the full course of treatment. The overuse or misuse of these antimicrobial agents results in many strains of bacteria that are antibiotic-resistant. (See the box Get Smart: Know When to Use Antibiotics on pages 228–229.)

THE ALL-TOO-COMMON COMMON COLD

Most of us get about two to four colds a year. Children get as many as 12 a year. The all-too-familiar symptoms—scratchy throat, runny nose, sneezing—usually last only a week or two. Still, colds account for more doctor visits and missed days of work and school than any other illness. Women, especially those age 20 to 30, get more colds than men do. This may be because of their close contact with children, who pick up colds at day-care centers and schools.

Although folklore suggests that you can catch a cold from getting chilled or over-heated, the real cause of the common cold is viral infection. More than 200 different viruses are to blame for the common cold; among the more frequent culprits are rhino-viruses (from the Greek word *rhin*, meaning "nose"). When a cold virus infects a cell, it hijacks its machinery to make more viruses. The new viruses burst from the host cell to infect other cells. Soon the cold sufferer is experiencing congestion, cough, and a runny nose that spreads the virus to other people.

You can get infected with a cold virus by touching surfaces contaminated with the virus such as hands, door handles, computer keys, or stair rails and then putting fingers to eyes or nose or by inhaling air carrying drops of mucus full of cold viruses. Sleep deprivation, prolonged psychological stress, and allergic diseases affecting your nose and throat can increase your chances of infection.

SYMPTOMS

Symptoms of the common cold most often begin 2 or 3 days after infection and usually last for a week, though they can persist for up to 14 days. They include:

- Congestion
- Runny nose
- Swelling of sinuses
- Sneezing

- Sore throat
- Cough
- Headache

PREVENTION

The best way to avoid a cold is to avoid people with colds. Wash your hands thoroughly and often with soap and water (for at least 15 seconds) and tell your family members to do the same.

Also, avoid touching your nose and eyes. In addition, it may help to:

- Avoid sharing glasses, dishes, silverware, or towels.
- Clean surfaces such as kitchen and bathroom countertops and telephones with sanitizing wipes or a disinfectant to kill viruses that can survive there for hours. There is no advantage to using antibacterial products, because viruses cause colds.
- Minimize stress, which can make you more susceptible to colds.
- Exercise regularly and eat well.

TREATMENT

There is still no cure for the common cold, but there are a few things you can do to ease symptoms:

- At the first sign of a cold, some experts suggest that you take a first-generation antihistamine (such as Benadryl or Chlor-Trimeton) and a nonsteroidal anti-inflammatory drug (NSAID), such as ibuprofen, every 12 hours until symptoms clear (from 3 to 7 days).
- Get bed rest.
- To loosen congestion and prevent dehydration, drink plenty of fluids, such as water, juice, and broth.
- To relieve a sore throat, gargle with warm salt water: Use ½ teaspoon of salt in an 8-ounce glass of water.
- Use saline nasal spray to fight congestion.
- Use products with petroleum jelly to soothe a chafed nose.

Over-the-counter cold remedies such as decongestants can offer adults some relief for symptoms but will not shorten the duration of your cold. Cough suppressants do not treat the cause of your cough and their use is discouraged by the American College of Chest Physicians. Do not treat children younger than 6 with over-the-counter cold and cough medications, because safe dosing recommendations have not yet been established.

Although some people find that aspirin also relieves symptoms, the American Academy of Pediatrics advises against administering aspirin to children and teenagers with viral infections because of the risk of Reye's syndrome, a rare but serious illness. Moreover, research shows that aspirin increases the amount of virus in nasal secretions, possibly increasing the risk of transmitting the infection to others. Ibuprofen and acetaminophen are good alternatives.

Antibiotics are *not* effective against viruses, so do not try to use them to treat a cold. They should be used only when bacterial complications develop.

WHEN TO SEEK MEDICAL ADVICE

Occasionally, colds lead to bacterial infections of the sinus or middle ear, requiring medical treatment. If you develop any of the following symptoms, seek help from a health care provider:

- Fever of 102°F or higher, which may be accompanied by achiness, fatigue, sweating, or chills
- Significantly swollen glands
- Severe sinus pain
- Cough that produces colored phlegm
- Symptoms that worsen or persist for longer than 2 weeks

TO AVOID INFECTING OTHERS

Research suggests that people are most likely to transmit cold viruses in the second to fourth day of infection, when the numbers of viral particles in nasal secretions are peaking. Be kind—stay home from work and avoid public places during this time if you can. Wash your hands with soap and water frequently and avoid touching your nose or contaminating surfaces with nasal secretions. Cover your mouth and nose with a tissue when you cough or sneeze (and be sure to discard used tissues) or use your upper sleeve if necessary.

COLD "REMEDIES"

We can't help but see the massive amount of advertising all around us during the cold season, touting vitamin and herbal remedies for preventing a cold or reducing its symptoms. There is scant evidence that any of these remedies helps prevent colds. If you decide to try a commercial cold preventive or remedy, consult your doctor first, because some of these may have adverse reactions with some medications. Some of the most popular supplements used to avoid a cold are:

- **Echinacea.** There is little evidence of any benefit from taking the herbal supplement echinacea. Some studies show that *Echinacea purpurea* may help relieve symptoms slightly if taken in the early stages. However, it will not prevent colds.

One study by the National Center for Complementary and Alternative Medicine of the National Institutes of Health found that echinacea is not effective for children age 2 to 11.

- **Zinc.** Again, there is no clear evidence that zinc is effective in treating the common cold.
- **Vitamin C.** To date there is no evidence that vitamin C prevents colds. However, it does have a slight drying effect on nasal secretions.

FLU

Also known as influenza, the flu refers to a respiratory infection caused by influenza viruses. It typically strikes during the flu season, from November to March, and is not related to the intestinal ailment sometimes described as "stomach flu." There are many types of flu, including the type of influenza virus known as swine flu. Ordinarily, swine flu causes illness in pigs, but occasionally humans may catch the virus. The outbreak of swine flu in 2009 was caused by a new strain of influenza virus known as H1N1—a genetic blend of swine, avian, and human influenza viruses. Experts strongly recommend vaccination for H1N1 and other flus.

Between 5 and 20 percent of Americans get the flu each flu season. Outbreaks tend to occur in the late fall and winter. Although anyone is susceptible, some people are especially vulnerable, including young children, adults older than 50, and people with immune systems compromised by medications or HIV infection, or with chronic illnesses such as diabetes or heart disease. Most people recover from the illness within a week, sometimes with a lingering cough or fatigue that lasts a little longer. But every year as many as 200,000 people are hospitalized with the illness and 36,000 die of complications.

You can contract flu by inhaling airborne virus particles that travel in droplets released when an infected individual sneezes or coughs. Likewise, you can also pick up the virus from phones, stair rails, door handles, and computer keyboards, and then infect yourself by touching your mouth, nose, or eyes.

You may be at increased risk for flu if you:

- Live or work in a nursing home or other health care facility
- Are pregnant during flu season
- Have regular close contact with young children

GET SMART: KNOW WHEN TO USE ANTIBIOTICS

You're feeling lousy. Your nose is running. Your throat is sore. Your head is pounding. You probably have a cold or flu virus. It would be nice to have a magic pill to make your bug vanish. But the last thing you need is antibiotics.

Antibiotics are powerful drugs that fight infections caused by bacteria, such as strep throat, tuberculosis, and some kinds of pneumonia. They are *not* effective against viral infections, such as colds or flu. Taking antibiotics when they're not needed can be harmful to you and to others.

The misuse of antibiotics for infections that aren't caused by bacteria has given rise to the serious problem of antibiotic resistance—the ability of bacteria to resist the effects of an antibiotic drug. Antibiotic resistance occurs when bacteria evolve in ways that allow them to survive the effects of drugs designed to kill them. A person with a resistant bacterial infection can pass that resistant infection to another person, spreading the hard-to-treat illness.

Almost three-quarters of bacteria that cause infections in hospitals and other health care settings are resistant to at least one of the drugs most commonly used to treat them. Among the most common is methicillin-resistant *Staphylococcus aureus* (or MRSA) infection, also known as "staph." This strain

Once you've had the flu, your body develops antibodies to the particular virus that caused that flu strain. But flu viruses are constantly evolving, so the antibodies can't protect you from new strains.

SYMPTOMS

In its early phases, the flu may appear as coldlike symptoms—congestion, runny nose, sneezing, and sore throat—but it often comes on suddenly and forcefully. Among its other common symptoms are:

- Body aches, especially in the back, arms, and legs
- Chills and sweats
- Fever greater than 101°F
- Headache
- Fatigue and weakness
- Dry cough
- Loss of appetite

of bacteria is resistant to the broad-spectrum antibiotics usually used to treat it and is sometimes fatal.

The key to controlling the spread of resistance is the smart and proper use of antibiotics. Follow these three simple guidelines:

1. Understand that antibiotics are used to fight bacterial infections; don't ask for them if you have a viral illness.
2. Recognize that even some bacterial infections, such as mild ear infections, don't necessarily benefit from antibiotic use.
3. Never take an antibiotic without a prescription. Do not save antibiotics for the next time you get sick and do not take antibiotics prescribed for someone else.
4. Follow the doctor's instructions precisely. To kill all of the harmful bacteria, you need to complete the full course of antibiotics. Do not skip doses. Do not stop taking the medication when you start to feel better. Doing so can allow resistant bacteria to develop.

KEEPING UP WITH THE PREVENTION

By far the best defense against flu is an annual flu vaccine. The vaccines change every year, so you must get a new one each flu season. (See the box Keeping Up with the Flu: The Ever-Evolving Vaccine on page 232.) Because your immune system takes time to react to the flu vaccine, it's best to check with your doctor about the usual start of the flu season in your area and ask to be vaccinated 6 to 8 weeks before this time. Shots are available at your doctor's office, in local clinics, and at supermarkets and drugstores. Protection lasts for up to a year.

In 2003, the FDA approved a nasal spray flu vaccine called FluMist, which is offered by some health care providers. However, a 2006 study found that FluMist was only about 30 to 60 percent effective in preventing flu in adults, compared with 70 to 90 percent for the shot.

Although a flu vaccine can't offer 100 percent protection (especially for older adults), it does reduce your chance of infection and also prevents serious flu-related complications. Health experts recommend vaccinations for:

- Children age 6 months up to their 19th birthday
- Pregnant women
- People 50 years of age and older
- People of any age with certain chronic medical conditions
- People who live in nursing homes and other long-term care facilities
- People who live with or care for those at high risk for complications from flu, including:
  - Health care workers
  - Household contacts of persons at high risk for complications from the flu
  - Household contacts and out-of-home caregivers of children younger than 6 months of age (these children are too young to be vaccinated)

The following simple self-care measures may also help prevent flu:

- Wash your hands frequently with soap and water.
- Keep your immune system strong by eating a healthy diet, getting plenty of sleep, and exercising.
- If you can, avoid air travel in the late fall. When people stopped flying after 9/11, the flu season started later and the illness spread more slowly.

TREATMENT

Most cases of flu can be treated by getting bed rest and drinking plenty of fluids, especially water, juice, and warm broths. Try to drink enough so that your urine stays clear or pale yellow.

If you are at risk for complications, however, or want medicine to treat the illness, you should see your health care provider as early in your illness as possible. Antiviral drugs such as oseltamivir (Tamiflu) or zanamivir (Relenza) are available by prescription. If taken within the first 2 days after your symptoms begin, these drugs can shorten the duration of your illness by a couple of days and help prevent complications. Oseltamivir can also significantly reduce the chances of contracting the flu if there is an outbreak in your family or community.

However, both oseltamivir and zanamivir can cause side effects such as nausea, vomiting, loss of appetite, lightheadedness, and difficulty breathing. Moreover, their overuse or misuse may also lead to the development of drug-resistant strains of flu virus.

WHEN TO SEEK MEDICAL ADVICE

Most cases of flu resolve without intervention. However, in some people, complications may develop, including ear infections, bronchitis, acute sinusitis, and pneumonia. These complications usually emerge after you start feeling better. The most common and most dangerous is pneumococcal pneumonia, a bacterial infection of the lungs. If you have a high fever, shaking chills, a serious cough that produces phlegm, and chest pain with each breath, you may have bacterial pneumonia and need treatment with antibiotics.

PNEUMONIA

Pneumonia is an inflammation of the lungs caused by bacteria, viruses, and sometimes, fungi. The illness ranges in severity from mild (often known as walking pneumonia) to life threatening. Pneumonia contracted during a hospital stay may be particularly deadly. In pneumococcal pneumonia, the most common type, the culprit is a bacterium known as *Streptococcus pneumoniae*, or pneumococcus. In about one out of every three cases of pneumococcal pneumonia, the bacteria move from the lungs into the bloodstream, where they can quickly spread to organs. Other complications of pneumonia include lung abscesses and fluid accumulation and infection of the lining of the lungs, known as pleurisy.

Pneumonia can strike people of any age, but especially at risk are children younger than age 2 and adults 65 and older, as well as people with impaired immune systems, sickle cell anemia, or chronic heart, lung, or liver diseases. Each year, some 60,000 Americans die of the illness.

SYMPTOMS

Symptoms of pneumonia can vary greatly but most commonly include:

- Sudden severe shaking chills
- High fever
- Cough
- Shortness of breath
- Rapid breathing
- Chest pains

These other symptoms may also appear:

- Nausea and vomiting
- Headache
- Fatigue
- Aching muscles

KEEPING UP WITH THE FLU: THE EVER-EVOLVING VACCINE

The viruses that cause flu are cunning microbes, capable of rapid change. Like all viruses, they consist of a strand of genetic material wrapped in a protein coat. As they make copies of themselves, small changes occur. These frequent mutations allow them to continuously alter their appearance, changing the proteins in their outer coats so that our immune systems do not recognize the new disguise. Because the virus evolves in this way, new flu vaccines must be created every year, and experts recommend an annual vaccine. Last year's shot won't protect you against this year's flu.

The process of producing a new flu vaccine begins 9 or 10 months before the start of our flu season. A committee of scientific experts looks at the strains of influenza virus in circulation at the time and tries to predict how they will change and which strains will be most prevalent in the United States in the upcoming winter. Once the committee decides on the likeliest alterations, manufacturers use these recommendations to prepare a vaccine made from inactivated (killed) flu viruses. Because the viruses are inactivated, they cannot cause infection.

Each new vaccine contains three strains of flu virus that are expected to affect people in this country. When there's a close match between the vaccine and the actual flu viruses that are circulating, the vaccine prevents illness in up to 90 percent of healthy adults under the age of 65. (It's somewhat less effective among older people.)

The process sometimes misses unexpected strains. And if the influenza virus changes in a major way from one year to the next, an epidemic or pandemic (world outbreak) can occur. Scientists are working to develop a universal flu vaccine that would confer lifelong immunity.

PREVENTION

To avoid the dangers and complications of this illness, it's best to try to prevent infection in the first place. Because pneumonia sometimes arises as a complication of flu, it's a good idea to get a flu vaccine every year. In addition, vaccines against pneumococcal pneumonia are available for both children and adults. Experts recommend that you get the vaccine if you fall into one of the following risk groups:

- Adults older than age 65
- Smokers
- Those with chronic diseases such as heart disease, sickle cell anemia, alcoholism, lung disease, diabetes, or liver cirrhosis
- Those with immune systems weakened because of HIV or AIDS, cancer, cancer treatment, steroidal treatment, bone marrow or organ transplants, kidney failure, or damaged spleen
- People from an Alaskan Native or other Native American population

As with colds, flu, and other infections, basic self-care techniques may help protect against pneumonia, such as frequent and thorough hand washing with soap and warm water. It's also important to avoid smoking, which damages the natural defenses of your lungs.

TREATMENT

If you suspect you have pneumonia, seek medical care immediately. For bacterial pneumonia, your doctor will likely prescribe antibiotics, which ease symptoms within 12 to 36 hours and address the underlying infection. However, be vigilant about completing your entire course of antibiotics. If you stop medication early, your pneumonia may flare up again. In addition, you may contribute to the growing problem of antibiotic-resistant strains of bacteria.

Your doctor may also suggest using over-the-counter medications to lower your fever, make you more comfortable, and soothe your cough. (However, it's best not to suppress your cough entirely, because it serves to clear your lungs.)

To speed your recovery and reduce chances of complications from the illness, you can take the following measures:

- Drink plenty of fluids, especially water, to prevent dehydration and loosen lung mucus.
- Get rest.
- Take your full course of prescribed medications.
- As your condition improves, follow up with your doctor to make sure you're free of infection.

HEPATITIS

Hepatitis is an inflammation of the liver that affects its ability to function. It may be caused by viruses and other infectious microorganisms; by exposure to alcohol, toxic chemicals, or medications; or by an autoimmune disorder. Symptoms range from mild to severe and include nausea and vomiting, diarrhea, fatigue, loss of appetite, abdominal pain, dark urine, jaundice, headache, muscle aches, and low-grade fever. Usually hepatitis resolves by itself, but in some cases, it may develop into chronic or even fatal liver disorders.

There are three main types of viral hepatitis:

Hepatitis A. The most common and mildest form of the disease, hepatitis A is contracted through contaminated food or water. Healthy people who get this type of hepatitis generally recover within a month or two, but those with anemia, diabetes, heart disease, or other medical problems may suffer complications from the disease. Most cases don't require treatment. The best way to avoid infection is to wash your hands thoroughly and frequently. Vaccines are also available in the form of two shots over the course of several months. If you plan to travel or spend time in a developing country, I strongly urge you to consider getting the hepatitis A vaccination.

Hepatitis B. Spread primarily through sexual intercourse, hepatitis B is a more serious disease than hepatitis A and is responsible for 9 percent of deaths worldwide. Like HIV, it can be contracted through contaminated needles and through body fluids (semen, vaginal secretions, and blood). Most people recover within a few months, but 3 to 5 percent develop chronic hepatitis, which can lead to cirrhosis, and 10 percent become carriers of the virus. You can reduce your risk of acquiring hepatitis B by refraining from use of illegal drugs, by practicing safe sex, and by obtaining a vaccine.

Hepatitis C. The most serious of the three varieties, hepatitis C is most often acquired through sharing contaminated needles for injecting illegal drugs. It frequently leads to chronic infection and chronic hepatitis, or liver disease. It was also present in the supply of blood clotting factors produced before 1987. There is no vaccine available for this infection. The best protection is avoiding unsafe sex and contaminated needles.

For autoimmune hepatitis, see Chapter 18, "Autoimmune Disease."

FOOD-BORNE DISEASES

Every year in this country, 76 million people become ill from food poisoning, or foodborne disease—many of them without ever knowing that their illness was caused by something they ate. At especially high risk for these diseases are infants, pregnant women, the elderly, and those with chronic diseases. The illnesses most often result from the presence of pathogenic bacteria in food. All food carries bacteria, but usually in small numbers. When foods are improperly prepared or handled, the bacteria may multiply and cause illness in those who consume them. Some of these dangerous microbes do not change the smell, taste, or appearance of food. Although bacteria are the most common causes of food-borne illness, viruses, parasites, toxins, and harmful chemicals may also contaminate food.

Among the more common causes of food-borne illnesses are these organisms:

Campylobacter jejuni, a bacterium found in poultry, is the most common cause of bacterial food-borne disease in this country. Infection most often results from eating undercooked chicken or food that has been contaminated with raw chicken or its juices. Infection results in fever, diarrhea, and abdominal cramps, and most people recover within a week. I've had campylobacter, and it's not pleasant.

Salmonella is a group of bacteria often carried in chicken and eggs. Like campylobacter infection, salmonellosis is typically marked by fever, diarrhea, and abdominal cramps that last a week or so. However, for those in poor health or with weakened immune systems, the bacteria may cause life-threatening infections.

Escherichia coli is found in cow feces and can cause illness if food or water contaminated with microscopic amounts of feces is consumed. The most common source of infection is undercooked ground beef, but it can also contaminate vegetables and other foods. The bacterium produces a powerful toxin that causes severe and bloody diarrhea and painful abdominal cramps that can last for hours, even days. In up to 5 percent of cases, infection results in complications, including kidney failure.

Norovirus, also known as Norwalk-like virus or calicivirus, is a common culprit of viral food-borne illness and causes the illness we often refer to as "stomach flu"—nausea, vomiting, diarrhea, and sometimes, low-grade fever, chills, headache, muscle aches, and fatigue—that may last for a day or two. The virus most often spreads when infected kitchen workers contaminate food.

Other causes of food-borne illness are listeria, bacteria sometimes found in soft cheeses and processed meats, which is of special concern to pregnant women and those with compromised immune systems, and giardia, a water-borne parasite found primarily in backcountry streams and lakes, but occasionally at swimming pools and spas. Listeria may cause fever, nausea, diarrhea, and muscle aches. Giardia infection causes nausea, stomach cramps, bloating, and diarrhea.

SYMPTOMS

Symptoms usually occur 24 to 72 hours after the food has been eaten, but may take as long as weeks to appear. The most common signs and symptoms include:

- Diarrhea
- Nausea and/or vomiting
- Abdominal or stomach pain

Most food-borne illnesses improve within 48 hours; however, 3 percent of cases lead to long-term health problems.

If you think you have food poisoning, rest and drink plenty of fluids to keep hydrated. Do not take antidiarrheal medications, because these may inhibit the removal of bacteria from your system. Seek immediate emergency medical help if you:

- Have severe symptoms, such as bloody diarrhea
- Are pregnant, elderly, or in another high-risk group
- Suspect you may have botulism, a rare and deadly form of food poisoning that results from ingestion of the toxin produced by the bacterium *Clostridium botulinum.* The most common source of this toxin is home-canned foods, especially tomatoes and green beans. Symptoms typically begin 18 to 36 hours after eating the contaminated food and may include double vision, blurred vision, headache, drooping eyelids, slurred speech, difficulty swallowing, or muscle weakness—all symptoms of muscle paralysis caused by the toxin.

PREVENTION

Proper food handling and preparation can prevent many food-borne diseases. The World Health Organization has developed the Five Keys to Safer Food to help prevent food-borne illness:

1. **Keep clean.** Wash your hands before handling food, during food preparation, and before you eat. Wash and sanitize all surfaces and food-preparation equipment. Keep insects, pests, and other animals out of your kitchen and away from food.
2. **Separate raw and cooked.** Keep raw meat, seafood, poultry, and their juices separate from other foods. Use separate equipment and utensils, including knives and cutting boards, to handle these raw foods. When storing food, avoid contact between raw and prepared foods.
3. **Cook thoroughly.** Cook meat, poultry, seafood, and eggs completely. Thorough cooking (to a temperature of 158°F) kills almost all microorganisms. Insert a thermometer at the thickest part of meat and make sure juices of meat and poultry run clear, not pink. Bring soups and stews to a boil and let simmer at boiling point for at least a minute.
4. **Keep foods at safe temperatures.** Promptly refrigerate (preferably below 41°F) all cooked and perishable food. Do not leave cooked food out at room temperature for more than 2 hours. Do not thaw frozen food at room temperature—thaw in the refrigerator instead. Do not store leftovers in the refrigerator for more than 3 days, and do not reheat them more than once.
5. **Use safe water and raw materials.** Use safe, clean water for drinking and cooking. Select fresh, wholesome foods, and wash all raw produce thoroughly. Select foods processed safely (such as pasteurized milk), and do not use foods past their expiration date.

Recent outbreaks of illness from contaminated peanuts, spinach, and beef have gained a lot of media attention. Although I believe that our food supply is basically safe, I do worry about the potential for widespread problems. As the peanut story revealed, a problem with contamination at one food processor can lead to the contamination of a wide array of food products—indeed, thousands. It is not uncommon for the parts of a single processed beef cow to end up in food products in almost every state. This is one reason I am a big believer in supporting local food systems. There is less chance of a large outbreak if people draw their foods from smaller, local sources.

18

Autoimmune Disease

Some 80 different illnesses are considered autoimmune diseases, in which the immune system attacks the very cells and organs it is supposed to protect—the liver, thyroid, skin, connective tissues, gastrointestinal tract, and other tissues and organ systems. Autoimmune diseases range from mild to severe and cause a range of symptoms. An individual may have more than one autoimmune disease—even as many as four or five—with a wide array of symptoms.

I have personal experience with autoimmune disease. In the spring of 2000, when I was just 40, I was on a book tour for my *Strong Women, Strong Bones* book. I was in New York, appearing on the *Today Show* and doing newspaper and magazine interviews, when I developed a splitting headache. Tylenol didn't seem to help. I also noticed that I was dragging during my runs. Because my book tours are so grueling—2 weeks on the road, traveling from New York to California and back again—I'm usually very diligent about taking care of myself: getting enough sleep, eating well, and exercising. As the 2 weeks wore on, my runs were getting slower and slower, and yet my heart rate was high. I began to lose weight, a total of 10 pounds in 2 weeks. By the time I reached Minneapolis on my way home, my brain seemed fuzzy, and I wasn't thinking straight. I felt really ill.

When I got home, I consulted with my colleagues at Tufts and submitted to a battery of tests. It turned out that I had silent thyroiditis, an uncommon autoimmune disease that attacks the thyroid, the little butterfly-shaped gland located in the front of the neck that manages metabolism—a condition I share with Oprah Winfrey. The disease was causing my thyroid to swing between hyperactivity (producing too much thyroid hormone) and hypoactivity (producing too little) over a period of several weeks. A decade later, my thyroid has burned out and I take thyroid hormones to replace the ones my body can no longer produce on its own.

For reasons that remain mysterious, roughly three-quarters of all cases of autoimmune disease occur in women, most often during childbearing years. Women have stronger immune responses than men do, which may grant us greater protection from many types of infection but also make us more susceptible to autoimmune disease. Hormones such as estrogen may play a role, too. When estrogen levels are elevated during the early phases of a woman's menstrual cycle, symptoms worsen.

Genetics is another factor: Autoimmune disorders seem to cluster in families as different illnesses. Researchers speculate that people who are genetically susceptible to autoimmune disorders may develop the diseases in response to triggers such as bacteria, viruses, toxins, and certain drugs. Pregnancy can also trigger autoimmune diseases.

As a group, these diseases are the third most common major illness in the United States and the fourth largest cause of disability among American women.

Unfortunately, as of today we know of no way to prevent autoimmune diseases. But it's important to be able to spot the symptoms if you have them so that you can seek prompt treatment.

AUTOIMMUNE SKIN DISEASES

Among the most common skin disorders is psoriasis, an autoimmune disease that results from a malfunction in the life cycle of skin cells. The normal process that produces new skin cells takes roughly a month. But in psoriasis, the process speeds up, resulting in a buildup of thick scales. Some 7.5 million Americans have the condition. It is not contagious. There is a genetic component, and flare-ups are often caused by triggers such as emotional stress, skin injury, reactions to drugs, and certain infections. Treatments include both over-the-counter and prescription topical products, drugs, and light therapy. Another common autoimmune skin disease is vitiligo. This is a condition that causes depigmentation of the skin so that skin coloring appears patchy. One of the most famous people with vitiligo was Michael Jackson, who was diagnosed with this condition in the late 1980s. Usually the extremities are affected. The cause is thought to be a combination of autoimmune and genetic factors. Treatment usually involves makeup to conceal the patches, steroids, or phototherapy.

AUTOIMMUNE ENDOCRINE DISORDERS

GRAVES' DISEASE

Among the most common of autoimmune disorders, Graves' disease arises when immune cells attack the thyroid, resulting in an overproduction of the thyroid hormone thyroxine. The disease strikes women five to seven times more often than men. If you have signs or symptoms of Graves' disease, see your doctor right away. Untreated Graves' disease can lead to heart problems, osteoporosis, and other complications. Symptoms include: weight loss despite normal diet; increased appetite, heart rate, and blood pressure; palpitations; tremors, nervousness, and sweating; anxiety and irritability; trouble sleeping; fatigue; enlargement of thyroid gland causing swelling of neck (goiter); frequent bowel movements; and protruding eyes, known as Graves' ophthalmopathy. If you're experiencing rapid or irregular heartbeat or palpitations, go to an emergency room. This is what I should have done when I first felt ill.

Drug therapy with antithyroid medications is used to decrease the production of thyroxine or block its actions. In some cases, removal or reduction of the thyroid gland by surgery or radioiodine is necessary. To reduce symptoms of Graves' ophthalmopathy, it helps to wear sunglasses, use lubricating eyedrops, apply cold compresses to your eyes, and elevate the head of your bed during sleeping.

HASHIMOTO'S DISEASE

In Hashimoto's thyroiditis, immune cells attack and destroy the thyroid gland. The condition becomes more common with age and occurs in women 10 times more often than in men. Women start developing hypothyroidism in their forties, and the prevalence increases with age to nearly 10 to 15 percent of the population after age 70.

Symptoms vary greatly depending on the severity of the disease. They include: mental and physical slowing; heightened sensitivity to cold; hoarse voice; weight gain despite normal food intake; pale, dry, or coarse skin; puffiness in face; elevated blood cholesterol; muscle aches and stiffness, especially in hips and shoulders; enlargement of thyroid gland (goiter); irregular or absent menstrual periods; and constipation. Treatment for this disorder is thyroid hormone replacement therapy.

TYPE 1 DIABETES

This form of diabetes arises when the immune system attacks the cells of the pancreas, resulting in too little insulin production. Although its onset is most common in childhood or early adulthood, it can occur at any age. Many type 1 diabetics live a normal or close to normal life span. Symptoms include: thirst, increased urination, weight loss, fatigue, nausea and vomiting, and frequent infections.

Treatment consists of monitoring diet and insulin given by injection to control blood glucose. Most type 1 diabetics carry a pump that helps monitor and administer their insulin. I'm very hopeful that the promising research under way around the world will give us a cure for type 1 diabetes within the next decade.

CONNECTIVE TISSUE AUTOIMMUNE DISEASES

SYSTEMIC LUPUS ERYTHEMATOSUS (SLE)

SLE is an inflammation of the connective tissues, which can affect every organ system in your body. It is made worse by exposure to sunlight. The disease is some nine times more common in women than in men and three times more common in black women than in white women. It primarily affects women of childbearing age and tends to decrease in intensity after menopause. For these reasons, scientists suspect sex hormones may affect the course of the disease. If you develop a persistent fever, aching, or fatigue or if you have an unexplained rash, see a doctor right away.

SLE differs widely from case to case. It may develop suddenly or gradually, remain mild or grow severe, be temporary or permanent. It's common for people with SLE to experience flare-ups in their symptoms. The most common symptom is joint inflammation similar to that in rheumatoid arthritis. Other symptoms include: a classic "butterfly" rash on the nose and cheeks; Reynaud's phenomenon—extreme sensitivity to cold in the hands and feet; fever; weight loss; hair loss; mouth and nose sores; fatigue and malaise; and seizures and symptoms of mental illness.

Treatment involves the use of oral steroids for systemic symptoms, anti-inflammatory drugs to control arthritis symptoms, and corticosteroid cream for skin lesions. Anti malaria medications may also be useful in treating symptoms. Experts recommend that those with SLE wear protective clothing and sunscreen whenever they go outdoors.

RHEUMATOID ARTHRITIS

Rheumatoid arthritis is a disorder in which the immune system attacks and inflames the lining of the joints. It can occur at any age but tends to first appear between the ages of 30 and 50. It may also affect the body systemically, damaging the eyes, heart, and lungs. Long-term effects include permanent joint damage, chronic pain, and disability. Symptoms include:

swelling, stiffness, or inflammation of the joints; deformation of the joints from nodules; fatigue; and pain. More information on this disorder can be found in Chapter 14, "Joints."

SCLERODERMA, OR SYSTEMIC SCLEROSIS

In scleroderma, immune-cell activity produces scar tissue in the skin, organs, and small blood vessels. It is especially common in women during childbearing years and strikes black women more often than white women. Symptoms include: Reynaud's phenomenon—extreme sensitivity to cold in the hands and feet, swelling and puffiness of fingers or hands, skin thickening, skin ulcers on fingers, joint stiffness in hands, pain, sore throat, and diarrhea.

The drug D-penicillamine is often prescribed to decrease skin thickening. Other drugs are used to treat symptoms involving blood vessels and organs such as the intestines and kidneys.

SJÖGREN'S SYNDROME

Sjögren's syndrome is a chronic, slowly progressing inability to make saliva and tears. Nine out of 10 cases of occur in women. Symptoms include: dry eyes and mouth, swollen neck glands, difficulty swallowing or talking, tongue ulcers, unusual tastes or smells, thirst, and dental decay.

Treatment involves keeping the mouth and eyes moist by drinking plenty of fluids and using eyedrops, and practicing good oral hygiene and eye care.

NEUROMUSCULAR AUTOIMMUNE DISEASES

MULTIPLE SCLEROSIS (MS)

In multiple sclerosis, the immune system mistakenly attacks the central nervous system—specifically, the fatty substance called myelin that sheathes the nerve fibers in the brain and spinal cord—causing problems that range from numbness and weakness to impaired vision and lack of coordination. The disease strikes women twice as often as men, and most often appears between the ages of 20 and 40. Although the condition has a genetic component, it appears to be triggered by environmental factors such as exposure to certain bacteria and viruses, including the Epstein-Barr virus. Symptoms include: numbness or weakness, most often on one side or one half of the body at a time; tingling, pain, or paralysis in one or more limbs; tremor; lack of coordination or unsteady gait; impaired vision, eye pain, or rapid involuntary eye movement; fatigue; and dizziness.

Treatment includes the drug baclofen to suppress muscle spasticity, corticosteroids to reduce inflammation, medications to combat fatigue, and interferons—genetically engineered versions of natural proteins—to help fight viral infections and regulate the immune system.

MYASTHENIA GRAVIS

This chronic disorder arises when your immune system makes antibodies that block or destroy the action of the chemical acetylcholine, which transmits nerve impulses to your muscles, causing gradual muscle weakness. Fatigue, stress, illness, extreme heat, some medications, and the botulinum toxin can make the condition worse. If you experience any of the following symptoms, see your doctor: muscle weakness in face; drooping eyelids; double vision; difficulty breathing, chewing, swallowing, and talking; or fluctuating weakness in arms and legs.

Several drugs can help improve muscle strength, among them pyridostigmine and neostigmine. Corticosteroids and other medications may also be prescribed to suppress the immune system. For patients younger than 60, surgical removal of the thymus gland can bring relief, though recent research has cast some doubt on its benefits. Physical therapy can also be useful to adjust to handling normal physical tasks.

GUILLAIN-BARRÉ SYNDROME

This rare disorder, in which the immune system attacks the body's nerves, most often occurs after a viral infection of the respiratory or digestive tract and can cause serious nerve damage. If you suspect you have the syndrome, seek medical help immediately. Early treatment is essential; without it, the disease may cause paralysis. Symptoms include: tingling or numbness in the fingers and toes that may spread throughout the body; muscle weakness; trouble with eye or facial movement, speaking, chewing, or swallowing; muscle weakness; slow heart rate or low blood pressure; severe lower back pain; difficulty with bladder control; and difficulty breathing.

In the first few weeks after a severe attack, two treatments may speed recovery: The first is a process called plasmapheresis—also known as plasma exchange—which removes plasma and nerve-damaging antibodies from the blood. The second is treatment with intravenous immunoglobulin from blood donors, which can block the damaging antibodies. Before recovery begins, rehabilitation therapy, in which caregivers manually move your arms and legs, can help maintain muscle strength and flexibility. Whirlpool baths may help relieve pain.

AUTOIMMUNE GASTROINTESTINAL AND LIVER DISEASE

INFLAMMATORY BOWEL DISEASE

Some one million Americans have the most common forms of inflammatory bowel disease (IBD)—ulcerative colitis or Crohn's disease. Both diseases are extremely serious, even life-threatening. They cause inflammation of the lining of the digestive tract, sometimes leading to ulceration or bleeding. Symptoms include severe abdominal pain, diarrhea, even weight loss and malnutrition. Ulcerative colitis is IBD of the large intestine (or colon). Crohn's disease can occur in any part of the gastrointestinal tract, from the mouth to the anus, and may spread deep into affected bowel tissues. There is no cure for IBD, but medications can keep the condition in check. If you think you have IBD, see a doctor immediately. The condition is often misdiagnosed as irritable bowel syndrome, so it's important to educate yourself about the condition and insist on proper diagnosis and treatment.

Symptoms of Crohn's disease include: rectal bleeding, persistent diarrhea, abdominal pain, fever, fatigue, and reduced appetite and weight loss.

Symptoms of ulcerative colitis include: bloody diarrhea, abdominal pain, urgent bowel movements, joint pain, and skin lesions

Treatment includes medications such as steroids and immunomodulators, and/or surgery to repair the colon. Although aggressive treatment is critical, these changes in diet and lifestyle may help ease symptoms:

- Reduce or eliminate intake of dairy products. If lactose intolerance is an issue for you, reducing or eliminating dairy products may help alleviate gas, diarrhea, and abdominal discomfort.
- Limit fiber. Although high-fiber foods are the staple of a healthy diet for most, sufferers of inflammatory bowel disease often have difficulty digesting them. Broccoli, cauliflower, apples, and carrots are often a particular problem. Cooking fruits and vegetables may make digestion easier.
- Reduce meal sizes. Eat five or six small meals instead of three larger ones.

- Drink plenty of fluids, especially water, but avoid alcoholic, caffeinated, and carbonated drinks.
- Avoid certain foods. Some foods, such as spicy cuisine, vegetables in the cabbage family, beans, citrus fruits, and popcorn, may make symptoms worse, so try to eliminate them from your diet.

AUTOIMMUNE HEPATITIS

In autoimmune hepatitis, the immune system attacks the body's liver cells. The disease most often strikes women between the ages of 15 and 40. Symptoms range in severity. The most common symptom is fatigue. Other symptoms include: enlarged liver, jaundice, itching or skin rashes, joint pain, abdominal discomfort, nausea and vomiting, loss of appetite, dark urine, and pale or gray-colored stools.

The disease is treated with daily doses of medicines designed to suppress an overactive immune system, including a corticosteroid called prednisone, and azathioprine. In 70 percent of people, the disease goes into remission within 2 years of the start of treatment.

19

Cancer

More than a million people get cancer every year. Nearly a third of all women in the United States will develop the disease in their lifetime. These are scary statistics. The good news today, however, is that most people survive cancer. Moreover, we've learned that we can reduce our risk of developing many kinds of cancer by modifying our lifestyle—not smoking, for instance, or being more physically active.

Hippocrates, the Greek physician of antiquity, coined the term *cancer* (from the Greek *karcinos*, for "crab"), perhaps to describe the pinching pain caused by the disease or the irregular, crablike appearance of tumors in the body. Now the term encompasses more than a hundred forms of disease, all characterized by the uncontrolled, malignant growth of cells.

Normal cells grow, divide, and die in due time. They live and interact in complex, interdependent societies where individual cells listen to the cells around them and police one another's behavior. But cancer cells violate this scheme, following their own program of inappropriate growth. They do so because of damage to their DNA from viruses, chemicals, ultraviolet rays, and other so-called carcinogens and local environments supportive of their bad behavior.

Our DNA is constantly damaged by factors from within and without, but most of the time the problems are repaired. With cancer, damaged DNA is not fixed. Sometimes people inherit damaged genes, and along with them, the propensity for cancer. More often, though, the damage occurs as a result of exposure to something in the environment, such as cigarette smoke or too much sun.

Although the underlying process of cancer appears to be universal, the various types of the disease can behave very differently. Some cancers, such as breast cancer, form tumors; others, such as leukemia, affect the blood. Sometimes cancer cells travel from the original site to other parts of the body, where they grow and invade normal tissue, a process called metastasis.

Cancer often produces general symptoms such as fever, fatigue, pain, and skin changes. However, specific symptoms vary depending on where the cancer is located, its size, and how much it presses on or affects surrounding organs, blood vessels, or nerves. Some cancers, such as pancreatic cancer, are "silent," causing few symptoms until the cancer has grown quite large. Others, such as certain kinds of brain tumors, produce symptoms early in their development.

Common symptoms that may indicate specific cancers include:

- Persistent cough (lung) or hoarseness (larynx or thyroid)
- Lump or thickening of tissue (breast, lymph nodes)
- Changes in bowel or bladder function (colon or bladder)
- Indigestion or trouble swallowing (esophagus, stomach, pharynx)
- Unusual bleeding or discharge in sputum (lung), in stool (colon or rectal), or in urine (bladder or kidney), or from vagina (cervix or endometrium)
- Sores that won't heal or changes in a mole or wart (skin)

Most Common Cancers in Women

CANCER	Incidence per year per 100,000 people	Mortality per 100,000 people
All cancers	408.5	157.8
Lung	50.2	40.9
Breast	123.8	24.5
Colorectal	42.8	15.4
Lymphoma	18.9	6.1
Skin	17.2	2.1
Cervical	2.5	2.5

Source: National Cancer Institute 2000–2006

Risk factors for cancer include age, sex, family medical history, exposure to cancer-causing factors in the environment, obesity, and lifestyle choices, such as tobacco and alcohol use. Although risk factors vary with each type of cancer, controllable lifestyle factors, such as diet, physical activity, tobacco use, and exposure to infectious agents and radiation, cause about three-quarters of all cancers.

There are many different types of cancer; here we address the kinds most common in women and those for which we can diminish our risk through lifestyle measures. If you need more information on cancer in general or on a specific kind of cancer, consult the Resources section.

ENVIRONMENTAL TOXINS AND YOUR HEALTH

A few years ago, I hosted a Strong Women Summit in upstate New York. We wanted a keynote speaker who would really inspire women, so we invited Erin Brockovich. To our great excitement, she accepted. I had seen the movie about her, but hearing her tell her story in person was gripping. Her account of the residents of Hinkley, California, and the health effects they suffered by being exposed to chromium 6 from groundwater contamination generated by a nearby gas company was heartbreaking.

Erin Brockovich's work, along with the publicity generated by the movie, brought to light the terrible health effects of powerful environmental carcinogens such as chromium 6. There is no doubt that other environmental contaminants put us at risk for cancer. We know that secondhand smoke elevates our risk of lung cancer and other lung diseases. Compounds that have been linked to increased cancer risk include pesticides, bisphenols (chemicals used to make plastics and in the resin that lines cans), polyaromatic hydrocarbons (from fuel combustion), dioxins, alkyphenols (used in some cleaning products), heavy metals, parabens (antimicrobials used in personal care products), and some food additives that are used to enhance growth in cattle and sheep. In addition, there are estrogen-like synthetic chemicals in our environment (so-called xenoestrogens) that may increase our risk of cancer. Some of these chemicals have also been tenuously linked to early puberty, infertility, low-birth-weight babies, miscarriages, and birth defects.

BREAST CANCER

Breast cancer is a cancer that starts in the tissues of the breast as a result of the abnormal growth of breast cells. Although it is second to lung cancer in cause of cancer deaths among American women, it is the disease women fear most. Roughly one in every eight women will develop breast cancer in her lifetime. However, the rate of new postmenopausal breast cancer cases in the United States has fallen sharply in recent years, which is related to a national decline in the use of hormone therapy. Moreover, death rates from cancer are decreasing in this country, perhaps due to more widespread screening and more effective treatment.

So what to do? You can't avoid all environmental contaminants, but there are a few things you can do to reduce your exposure to everyday toxins:

- Ask about the history of a property before you buy.
- Have your tap water tested and use a simple water filter on all faucets, including shower and bath.
- Buy and eat foods that are local, organic, minimally processed, and free of food additives.
- Do not microwave your food in plastic containers; always use glass or ceramic.
- Use natural home cleaning products and dust and vacuum weekly.
- Avoid home products with artificial fragrances, such as air fresheners, fabric softeners, and dryer sheets.
- Use natural kinds of cosmetics, toiletries, and grooming products. Avoid any that include paraben or phthalate (often referred to as "fragrance" or as diethylhexyl or dibutyl). If there are no ingredients listed, check the list of personal care products at the Web site Cosmeticsdatabase.com.
- If you choose to have your clothes dry-cleaned, do so at a dry cleaner that does not use perchloroethylene (perc).
- Try to avoid car and truck fumes.
- Stay away from secondhand smoke.

Scientists have recently come to understand that there are several types of breast cancer, which vary in how aggressive they are. Some are limited to the tumor site and never metastasize or spread; others have the potential to wreak havoc in the body if they're not caught early; still others are highly aggressive and can spread and cause problems in the body even if they're detected early, when they're still very small.

There are two main types:

- **Ductal carcinoma,** the most common type, starts in the ducts that transport milk from breast to nipple.
- **Lobular carcinoma** begins in the lobules, the parts of the breast that produce milk, at the ends of the ducts like leaves on a tree.

In addition, there are at several subtypes based on tumor characteristics:

- **Hormone sensitivity.** Some breast cancers are sensitive to estrogen and/or progesterone (called estrogen receptor, or ER, positive); others are not (called estrogen receptor, or ER, negative). Women with ER-positive tumors are often treated with hormone-modulating treatments such as tamoxifen or aromatase inhibitors.
- **Epidermal growth factor overexpression.** A percentage of women have a subtype of breast cancer in which breast cells possess too many copies of an oncogene known as HER2, which normally helps cells grow, divide, and repair themselves. An overabundance of this oncogene in a cell pushes it to grow quickly, much like pushing down on a car accelerator. Women with HER2-positive cancers are treated with a targeted therapy that blocks this message.
- **Triple negative.** Tumors that are not sensitive to hormones and do not overexpress HER2 are termed triple-negative, or basal, tumors. Although there are no targeted therapies for this group, chemotherapy is very effective.

ARE YOU AT RISK?

As with many diseases, there are some risk factors for breast cancer that you can't control, such as your gender, age, and family history. Others you can do something about, including exercise, diet, and weight control. It's important to remember that having a certain risk factor or even a combination of risk factors does not mean that you will develop cancer. It just means that you are at increased risk for the disease.

Here are some risk factors beyond your control:

- **Gender.** Being female is the single largest risk factor. Women are 100 times more likely to get breast cancer than men are.
- **Age.** Your risk of developing breast cancer rises as you get older. Some 80 percent of breast cancers occur in women over the age of 50. Before the age of 40, your risk is 0.5 percent (1 in 233); from ages 40 to 49, it's 1.5 percent (1 in 68); from 50 to 59, it's 2.7 percent (1 in 37); from 60 to 69, it's 4 percent (1 in 26); by age 85, it's about 12 or 13 percent (1 in 8).
- **Family history of cancer.** You are at increased risk if you have a first-degree relative (e.g., mother, sister, or daughter) with breast, ovarian, uterine, or colon cancer. Having a mother or sister with breast cancer, for example, doubles a woman's risk. If you are concerned about your family history, you may wish to seek genetic counseling to determine your risk.
- **Genetics.** Only 5 to 10 percent of breast cancer is hereditary, due to the inheritance of defective genes. The major mutations are in the BRCA1 and BRCA2 genes (BR for breast, CA for cancer), which normally make proteins that protect cells from cancerous growth. Women of Ashkenazi Jewish descent are at especially high risk of carrying these types of mutations. Women with defects in these genes have a 40 to 80 percent chance of developing breast cancer over their lifetime, depending on the specific abnormality and the nature of your own body. Much rarer are other inherited mutations that increase risk, including those in the p53 tumor suppressor gene, the ataxia-telangiectasia gene, and the cell cycle checkpoint kinase-2 (Chk-2) gene.
- **Personal history.** If you have had cancer in one breast, you have a 10 to 15 percent chance of getting a new cancer in that breast again or in the other breast.
- **Menstrual cycle.** The growth of breast cells—both normal cells and cancerous cells—is stimulated by the presence of estrogen and progesterone. Extended exposure of breast tissue to cycles of estrogen and progesterone is a risk factor. Women who start their periods before the age of 12 and go through menopause after the age of 55, or menstruate for more than 40 years, have a greater risk for breast cancer.
- **Breast density.** One of the most significant risk factors is breast density—the presence of more glandular tissue than fat—as measured on a mammogram. Similar to genetics, there is nothing that you can do to change the density of your breasts.
- **Precancerous changes.** A breast biopsy can detect precancerous changes, which can lead to breast cancer over time.

- **Pregnancy.** Although some may consider this a modifiable risk factor, for most it is not. If you have never been pregnant, or if your first full-term pregnancy occurs after the age of 30, you have a greater risk. Being pregnant more than once or becoming pregnant before age 30 reduces your risk.
- **Radiation.** Women who received radiation treatment to the chest as children or young adults are more likely to develop breast cancer. The risk is greatest if radiation was given during breast development.

The National Cancer Institute provides an online tool, the Breast Cancer Risk Assessment Tool, to help you determine your overall risk. See Cancer.gov/bcrisktool.

SYMPTOMS

Early-stage breast cancer usually causes no symptoms. As the cancer grows, symptoms may include a lump in your breast or armpit that is firm, with uneven edges or a change in the size, shape, or feel of your breast or nipple, such as a change in texture, redness, or dimpling.

PREVENTION

Although there is no sure way to avoid getting breast cancer, there are some things you can do to reduce your risk:

- **Minimize the use of hormone therapy.** If needed, use the smallest dose for the shortest period of time. It is clear that exposure to estrogen contributes to breast cancer risk, but for most women the additional risk is very small. If you have had treatment for menopausal symptoms with combined estrogen and progestin for more than 2 years, you may be at greater risk. This risk disappears within 2 years of stopping the drugs. In postmenopausal women who have had a hysterectomy, estrogen alone has been found to increase breast cancer risk after 10 years of use.
- **Maintain a healthy weight.** Although the relationship between overweight and breast cancer is still controversial, there is evidence that excess weight raises the risk of breast cancer in postmenopausal women, probably by increasing the production of estrogen in the body. (Extra fat cells make extra estrogen that causes more cells to divide.) This is especially true if you put on the extra pounds after menopause. Excess body fat on the upper half of your body also increases risk. Try to maintain a BMI in the ideal range between 18 and 25.

- **Stay physically active.** A program of regular cardiovascular exercise (at least 150 minutes per week) has been shown to reduce your risk of developing breast cancer and to increase your survival rate if you have the disease.
- **Don't smoke.** Smoking has been linked with a small rise in risk for breast cancer.
- **Limit use of alcohol.** Drinking more than a glass or two of alcohol each day elevates your risk by about 20 percent. Alcohol limits your liver's ability to regulate blood levels of estrogen.
- **Avoid unnecessary radiation.** Before you have an x-ray, ask the health care provider if it is absolutely necessary and how the results will influence your care.
- **Eat a healthy diet.** Although there has been no conclusive link found between a specific food and breast cancer, research has shown that an overall wholesome pattern of eating (plenty of vegetables, fruits, and whole grains) does reduce risk. These foods have natural cancer-fighting properties.

If you are at very high risk for breast cancer, you may want to consider these preventive measures:

- **Chemoprevention.** Studies suggest that the drug tamoxifen, used for women age 35 and older who are at high risk of developing breast cancer, can reduce ER-positive breast cancer risk by a third to a half. Raloxifene, a medication also used for osteoporosis, has been shown to reduce the likelihood of developing ER-positive breast cancer in high-risk postmenopausal women.
- **Preventive surgery.** In women with a very high risk of breast cancer because of personal or family history, preventive surgery can reduce risk. Prophylactic mastectomy involves removing one or both breasts and reduces the risk of breast cancer by half. Prophylactic oophorectomy involves surgically removing the ovaries before menopause and reduces the risk of breast cancer by 70 percent.

DETECTION AND SCREENING

Screening is looking for cancers that are already there. Detection can sometimes prevent them from becoming more aggressive. Not all cancers detected by mammograms are necessarily aggressive. One recent study showed that 25 percent of cancers found on mammograms will disappear if left alone. This likely reflects the fact that different types of cancers are more or less aggressive than others. Also, the nature of the stroma (tissue or neighborhood where the mutated cells are located) strongly influences whether the cancer will be dormant or active. For the new guidelines on screening for breast cancer, see the box New Guidelines for Breast Mammography below.

- **Know your breasts.** Although the evidence is mixed on whether doing a formal breast self-exam every month makes a difference in cancer detection, it is clear that knowing your own breasts and how they change during the

NEW GUIDELINES FOR BREAST MAMMOGRAPHY

In fall of 2009, the US Preventive Services Task Force, a federal advisory panel of experts, issued new guidelines on breast cancer screening that overturned the long-held recommendation that every woman should have an annual mammogram starting at age 40. The new guidelines—that women age 50 to 74 have mammograms every 2 years—arise from the unanimous consensus of six research groups from independent academic institutions. The recommendations reflect our new understanding of breast cancer biology and the benefits and harm of annual screening. They are intended to reduce unnecessary tests and treatment. Research shows that screening every other year offers almost the same benefit of screening yearly, with about half the number of false positives (which can result in unnecessary biopsies and overtreatment).

I have been watching these data closely over the past few years and have expected that the guidelines would change. As my colleague Dr. Susan Love explains, there are many different kinds of breast cancer. Some types grow slowly and go away by themselves; others grow quickly and spread aggressively. "We need to stop finding the cancers that will never do anything, and stop over-treating women who have them," says Dr. Love. The goal of breast cancer screening should be to find the cancers that may kill, and treat them with appropriate interventions.

The new guidelines hold for women who have no unusual cancer risks such as smoking or a family history of breast cancer. For women without these risk factors, the recommendations are as follows:

- Women age 40 to 49 years should not have routine screening mammography. Screening for women in this age group results in a large number of false positive mammograms, which may lead to unnecessary biopsies and stress. A woman under age 50 should month is very important. Make it a point to be familiar with your own breasts and underarms and check them periodically to see whether you notice changes.

- **Regular clinical breast exams.** Some experts recommend clinical breast exams by a medical professional at least once every 3 years for women ages 20 to 39 and once a year for women over age 40.

decide with her health care provider whether to start regular mammography based on her individual breast cancer risk and her understanding of the benefits and harms of screening.

- Women age 50 to 74 years should have mammography every 2 years. Studies show that biennial mammograms achieve most of the benefits of annual screening, but with less harm. In other words, the results are roughly the same whether you have a mammogram every year or every 2 years. Even for women with aggressive forms of cancer, annual screening is unlikely to make a difference in survival.

- For women age 75 and older, the panel states that there is insufficient evidence to assess the benefits and harms of screening.

It may be surprising to some women that the new guidelines recommend against teaching patients breast self-examination. The reason for this is that the success of breast self-exams at finding cancers at a curable stage has never been supported by clinical studies. And like mammograms in younger women, self-exams may turn up false positives. The guidelines also state that there is not enough information to determine whether clinical breast examination by a professional provides additional benefit beyond mammography. Finally, the guidelines suggest that there is insufficient information to determine whether newer kinds of mammography, such as digital or magnetic resonance imaging, are any better than regular mammography in detecting cancer.

It should be noted that the American Cancer Society has not changed its guidelines in response to the new federal recommendations, and many health care providers also continue to recommend screenings according to the old guidelines.

- **Mammograms.** There is still some controversy over recommendations for mammograms. Experts differ in their advice for frequency of screenings. The new federal guidelines issued in 2009 recommend screenings every 2 years, beginning at age 50, for women at low risk of breast cancer. The American Cancer Society continues to back the old guidelines recommending mammograms every 1 to 2 years, beginning at age 40. MRI screening is recommended for women who carry the BRCA mutation. (See screening recommendations in Chapter 28.) For women with dense breast tissue, experts recommend digital mammography.

TREATMENT

In the past decade, we've made many advances in treating breast cancer. We now have more therapies than ever and a better understanding of how to use them. Treatment for each case varies, depending on the type and stage of the cancer, and whether it is ER positive or HER2 positive or triple negative. Surgery and radiation are used to treat breast cancer locally and prevent it from recurring. Chemotherapy and hormone therapies target cancer cells that may already be elsewhere in the body. Most women receive a combination of these therapies. You will need to consult with your doctor to determine the appropriate treatment for you.

CERVICAL CANCER

Cervical cancer begins in the cells on the surface of the cervix, the lower part of the uterus that opens into the vagina. The surface of the cervix is composed of two types of cells, squamous and columnar. Most cervical cancers arise in squamous cells. The disease develops very slowly. It begins with a precancerous condition called dysplasia, which is detectable by a Pap test and is 100 percent treatable. If these precancerous changes progress, however, they can develop into cervical cancer, which may spread to the bladder, intestines, lungs, and liver.

Although cervical cancer is the third most common type of cancer in women worldwide (after lung and breast), it is much less common in the United States because of preventive screening through Pap tests. Since the 1940s, when Pap tests were introduced, there has been almost an 80 percent reduction in incidence of the disease. Still, more than 11,000 women in this country are diagnosed with the disease each year, and nearly 4,000 die from it. The majority of women diagnosed with cervical cancer have not had regular Pap tests or have not followed up on abnormal results.

Most cases of cervical cancer are caused by various strains of the human papilloma virus (HPV), an infection transmitted through sexual intercourse. If a woman is exposed to HPV, her immune system will normally disarm the virus. However, in some cases, the virus may survive and cause cancer. The availability of a vaccine against the virus holds the best promise of ending this disease. (See the box The Human Papilloma Virus (HPV) Vaccine on page 32.)

ARE YOU AT RISK?

Age is a factor in cervical cancer. Some 50 percent of cases occur in women between the ages of 35 and 55. However, the most significant risk factor is exposure to HPV. Other risk factors include:

- **Early sexual activity** (before age 18). Immature cells are more susceptible to the precancerous changes caused by HPV.
- **Having multiple sexual partners.** Having many sexual partners increases your risk of infection with HPV.
- **Having sexual partners who have multiple partners or engage in high-risk sexual activities.**
- **Compromised immune system.** If your immune system is weakened by a health condition such as HIV/AIDS, and you acquire HPV, you may be more likely to develop cervical cancer.
- **Infections with other sexually transmitted diseases (STDs).** Genital herpes, gonorrhea, syphilis, HIV/AIDS, or chronic chlamydia infections increase your chances of acquiring HPV.
- **Smoking.** Tobacco use appears to increase the risk of precancerous and cancerous changes in the cells of the cervix.

SYMPTOMS

Although early cervical cancer rarely has symptoms, as the cancer progresses, some signs may appear, including:

- Continuous vaginal discharge that is watery, pink, brown, or bloody, or with a foul odor
- Abnormal vaginal bleeding between periods, after intercourse, or after menopause
- Periods that are abnormally heavy and longer than usual
- Pain during intercourse

PREVENTION

To reduce your risk of getting cervical cancer, follow these guidelines:

- **Get vaccinated against HPV.** Gardasil, the first vaccine designed to prevent a cancer, provides protection from the two forms of HPV responsible for 70 percent of cervical cancer cases. The vaccine is given as a series of three injections over a 6-month period. The second dose is given 2 months after the first dose and followed by a third dose 4 months later. Experts recommend vaccination for girls ages 11 and 12, preferably before they become sexually active. This allows for the highest antibody levels before they're likely to encounter HPV. They also recommend immunization for girls and women ages 13 to 26 who have not yet been vaccinated. (See the box The Human Papilloma Virus (HPV) Vaccine on page 32.)
- **Get regular Pap tests.** The Gardasil vaccine cannot prevent infection from every virus that causes cervical cancer. Therefore, it's recommended that all women get regular Pap tests. During a Pap test, a health care provider takes samples of cells from your cervix and sends them to a laboratory to be examined for abnormalities. Routine Pap tests are the most effective way to detect cervical cancer in the earliest stages, when treatment is most likely to be successful and the disease is rarely life threatening.
  - In 2009, the US Preventive Services Task Forces issued new guidelines for cervical cancer screening. The guidelines suggest an initial Pap test within 3 years after a woman becomes sexually active, but not later than age 21. Then, from ages 21 to 29, experts recommend a Pap test every 1 or 2 years; from ages 30 to 69, experts recommend a Pap test every 2 or 3 years, provided you've had three normal Pap tests in a row and are monogamous. If you're 70 or older and have had three or more consecutive normal tests and no abnormal results in the past 10 years, you may stop having Pap tests.
  - Women at high risk for cervical cancer should consult with their doctors about having more frequent Pap tests.
- **Practice safe sex.** Use condoms to reduce your risk of getting HPV and other sexually transmitted diseases. (See pages 37–38.)
- **Have fewer sexual partners.**
- **Do not smoke.**

TREATMENT

Treatment of cervical cancer depends on the stage of the cancer, the size and shape of the tumor, the age and overall health of the woman, and her desire to maintain fertility in the future.

Early, noninvasive cancer involves removal of the cancerous and precancerous area of cells through:

- **Cone biopsy,** the removal of a cone-shaped piece of cervical tissue
- **Laser surgery,** the use of light to kill cancerous and precancerous cells
- **Loop electrosurgical excision procedure (LEEP),** which uses electricity to remove abnormal tissue
- **Cryotherapy,** which freezes abnormal cells
- **Hysterectomy,** a major surgery to remove the cervix and uterus—but it is rarely performed in cases of early, noninvasive cancer

Later-stage, invasive cancer requires more extensive treatment, including:

- **Hysterectomy,** simple (removing just the cervix and uterus) or radical, which involves removing the uterus and much of the surrounding tissues, including lymph nodes and the upper part of the vagina. In either case, removing the uterus makes future pregnancy impossible.
- **Radiation**
- **Chemotherapy**

COLON CANCER

Colon cancer begins in the large intestine (colon) or the rectum (the last 6 inches of the colon). Most cases begin as small, benign polyps in the colon, which may slowly develop into cancer. This is why it's so important to have a colonoscopy after the age of 50. Doctors can find polyps and snip them out before they become cancerous. Fortunately, the death rate for colon cancer has dropped in the past decade, thanks primarily to increased screening by colonoscopy. However, fewer than half the people who should get screened actually submit to the test; if they did, it would likely reduce the death rate by half.

ARE YOU AT RISK?

Age is a significant risk factor for colorectal cancer. Some 90 percent of people with the disease are over the age of 50. You are also at increased for colorectal cancer if you have:

- **Colorectal polyps.** There are three types of polyps, which vary in their potential to become cancerous. Hyperplastic polyps rarely develop into colorectal cancer; inflammatory polyps, which often follow a bout of ulcerative colitis, sometimes become cancerous; and adenomas, which can become cancerous, are often removed during screening tests.
- **A family history of colorectal cancer or polyps.** If a family member such as a parent or sibling has colorectal cancer, your risk is greater. The association can be due to shared genes or shared lifestyle or exposure to cancer-causing environmental factors.
- **A personal history of colorectal cancer**
- **Inflammatory diseases of the colon,** such as ulcerative colitis or Crohn's disease
- **A diet consisting largely of high-fat,** low-fiber foods, and red meat and processed meat
- **An inactive lifestyle**
- **Obesity**
- **Diabetes**
- **Smoking and/or heavy use of alcohol**

SYMPTOMS

Colorectal cancer is often a silent disease, with no apparent symptoms. However, the following symptoms may occur:

- Blood in stool
- Diarrhea, constipation, or other bowel changes
- Unexplained anemia
- Pain or tenderness in the lower abdomen
- Unexplained weight loss
- Narrow stools

PREVENTION

Experts recommend that nearly all women age 50 and older have a colonoscopy. Doctors use a colonoscope to view the interior of your colon and rectum. If polyps are found, they may be removed immediately or biopsied for further analysis. Although some people are squeamish about getting the tests, the procedure is actually painless. It's the preparation that people often find most unpleasant: fasting on clear liquids and drinking a laxative to clean out your colon. It's important to drink plenty of water to replace lost fluid. Experts emphasize that the discomfort of the tests is a small price to pay to avoid a deadly disease.

After the initial colonoscopy, the American Cancer Society recommends having *one* of the following five tests on a regular basis:

- Colonoscopy every 10 years
- Fecal occult blood test or fecal immunochemical test every year
- Flexible sigmoidoscopy, in which your doctor uses a scope to examine the lower part of the colon, every 5 years
- Stool test with sigmoidoscopy every 5 years
- Test with barium enema and x-rays every 5 years

If you're at high risk for colorectal cancer, you should discuss with your doctor having earlier screening or more frequent screenings.

You can also reduce your risk of the disease by following these guidelines:

- **Eat a variety of healthy, minimally process foods,** with plenty of whole grains and five or more servings per day of fruits and vegetables, which contain fiber, vitamins, minerals, and antioxidants. Try to minimize saturated fats from red meat, dairy products, and coconut and palm oils.
- **Limit your consumption of alcohol to no more than one drink a day.**
- **Maintain a healthy body weight.**
- **Stay physically active.**
- **Consult with your doctor** if you have a high risk of colorectal cancer about taking aspirin or other anti-inflammatory medications to reduce the risk of precancerous polyps or colorectal cancer.

TREATMENT

Treatment most often involves surgery, chemotherapy, and/or radiation, alone or in combination, and depends on the location of the cancer and its stage, or how far it has spread.

ON THE HORIZON

New and improved screening tests for colon cancer are under development. These include an improved stool DNA test, which involves checking a stool sample for signs of DNA mutations, as well as new methods for increasing the accuracy of a technique called virtual colonoscopy, which uses a CT scanner to produce images of the interior of the colon.

ENDOMETRIAL CANCER

This cancer starts in the endometrium, the lining of the uterus. Its cause is not known, but it may be related to increased levels of estrogen, which stimulate the buildup of the uterine lining. Most cases occur in women aged 60 to 70. Because the disease produces recognizable symptoms—vaginal bleeding between menstrual periods or after menopause—it is often detected early and can be successfully treated through hysterectomy 90 percent of the time. In 2007, 39,000 women in this country contracted the disease; 7,400 died from it.

ARE YOU AT RISK?

You have a higher risk of endometrial cancer if you:

- Have a history of endometrial polyps or other growths of the uterine lining
- Have had or are on estrogen replacement therapy
- Have taken tamoxifen for breast cancer
- Have diabetes
- Have never been pregnant
- Started menstruating before age 12
- Are infertile
- Started menopause after age 50
- Are obese
- Have been diagnosed with polycystic ovary syndrome (PCOS) or metabolic syndrome

SYMPTOMS

The following symptoms may occur:

- Abnormal bleeding between normal periods before menopause; vaginal bleeding after menopause
- Exceptionally long, heavy, or frequent episodes of vaginal bleeding during the perimenopausal years
- Thin pink, white, or clear vaginal discharge after menopause
- Pain in the lower abdomen or pelvic cramping
- Pain during intercourse
- Weight loss

PREVENTION

Experts recommend that all women have regular pelvic exams starting with initial sexual activity (or at age 21). Women at higher risk should consult with their doctors about more frequent screening, including endometrial biopsy. Use of oral contraceptives for more than 1 year can reduce the risk of endometrial cancer by more than 40 percent.

TREATMENT

In the early stages of the disease, treatment involves abdominal hysterectomy and sometimes removal of the fallopian tubes and ovaries. For more advanced cases or recurrent disease, surgery combined with radiation therapy or chemotherapy may also be used.

LUNG CANCER

Most women are unaware that lung cancer is the number one cancer killer in the country. More women die each year from lung cancer than from breast cancer. Of the 172,000 or so new cases of lung cancer that occur every year in this country, almost half will affect women.

The air you inhale through your nose and mouth travels down your windpipe and into the lungs through tubes called bronchi. Lung cancer tends to begin in the cells lining these bronchi.

There are two main types of lung cancer:

- **Non-small cell.** Some 80 percent of lung cancers are of this type, including the most common type of lung cancer in women, adenocarcinoma, found in the mucus glands of the lungs.
- **Small cell.** This type accounts for 20 percent of cases.

ARE YOU AT RISK?

Lung cancer most often strikes those between the ages of 55 and 65, but the disease tends to develop in women at a younger age than men, as early as the mid-forties. Cigarette smoking is the leading cause, accounting for 85 to 95 percent of lung cancers. The statistics are grim: Women who smoke increase their risk of death from lung cancer by more than 12 times. The earlier you start smoking and the more cigarettes you smoke each day, the higher your risk of lung cancer. On the other hand, risk declines dramatically when you stop smoking. After a decade of not smoking, risk is reduced by 30 to 50 percent.

If you smoke, now is the time to quit! Easy to say, of course. Quitting smoking can be an extremely difficult task. Addiction to nicotine is as powerful—if not more so—as heroin addiction. Fortunately, there are good behavior modification programs and medications for people who wish to quit smoking permanently.

Lung cancer can also occur in people who have never smoked. Breathing secondhand smoke raises your risk. So does a family history of cancer of the esophagus, head, neck, breast, prostate, or colorectum, or exposure to heavy air pollution, radon, asbestos, and carcinogenic chemicals such as vinyl chloride, coal products, uranium, beryllium, nickel chromates, mustard gas, gasoline, and diesel exhaust.

You are at increased risk for lung cancer if:

- You are or have been a smoker.
- You have a blood relative with lung cancer.
- You have been exposed to secondhand smoke for long periods of time or to carcinogenic chemicals.

SYMPTOMS

Common symptoms include:

- Persistent cough or cough that produces sputum containing blood
- Change in color of sputum or increase in volume

- Shortness of breath or wheezing
- Chest or back pain
- Recurrent pneumonia or bronchitis
- Loss of appetite
- Loss of weight despite normal food intake
- Fatigue or weakness
- Hoarseness
- Headache

PREVENTION

The best way to prevent the occurrence of lung cancer is to never smoke. If you smoke, quit. You should also try to avoid inhaling secondhand smoke from other people's cigarettes, cigars, or pipes. It may also help to eat a diet rich in fruits and vegetables.

DETECTION AND SCREENING

Unfortunately, there is no approved screening test for lung cancer. If you are experiencing any of the symptoms of lung cancer, or if you're at high risk for the disease, you should seek medical help. Your health care provider may perform any of the following tests:

- Physical examination
- Chest examination
- Chest x-ray
- CT scan, the best test for detecting lung cancer
- PET scan or MRI of the chest
- Sputum cytology test
- Blood work
- Biopsy

TREATMENT

Treatment for lung cancer depends on the stage of the disease. Early-stage lung cancer is most often treated with surgery to remove the affected area. Chemotherapy is used to treat larger tumors and when there's a chance that the cancer has spread. It can be used alone or in combination with radiation, which is also used to treat cancer that has spread to bones of the ribs or spine. There are now targeted therapies for lung cancers that overexpress an epidermal growth factor; these are showing very good results.

OVARIAN CANCER

Ovarian cancer occurs when normal cells in the ovaries—the female reproductive organs that produce eggs—begin to grow uncontrollably, producing tumors. Each year, about 22,000 American women develop the disease; roughly 15,000 die from it. Its cause is unknown. If it is detected early and can be treated when it remains in the ovary, the 5-year survival rate is about 94 percent. But it is hard to catch in its early phases, because it rarely causes symptoms. Most cases (between 50 and 80 percent) are not detected until the cancer has spread into tissues and organs beyond the ovaries, and the 5-year survival rate drops to 30 percent. Recently, cancer organizations have emphasized the need to be aware of a list of persistent symptoms that might indicate the presence of the disease in its earliest stages: bloating, abdominal or pelvic pain, difficulty eating or feeling full quickly, urgent or frequent urination, and constipation.

ARE YOU AT RISK?

Factors that affect risk for developing ovarian cancer include:

- **Genetic inheritance.** An important risk factor is inheriting a mutation in the breast cancer genes BRCA1 and BRCA2. Women of Ashkenazi Jewish descent are at particularly high risk of carrying these mutated genes.
- **A family history of breast or ovarian cancer.** Having a close relative—mother, daughter, or sister—with ovarian or breast cancer increases your risk of developing ovarian cancer, but not to the same degree as possessing an inherited genetic defect does.
- **Age.** More than 60 percent of deaths from ovarian cancer occur in women older than 54. A quarter of ovarian cancer deaths occur in women between 35 and 54.
- **Childbearing status.** The more children a woman has had, and the earlier in life she has given birth, the lower her risk of ovarian cancer.
- **Oral contraceptives.** The Pill may offer some protection.
- **Infertility.** Women who have had difficulty conceiving may be at increased risk. The risk seems to be greatest among women with unexplained infertility and women with infertility who never conceive. However, the link is still unclear, and research continues.
- **Obesity in early adulthood.** If a woman is obese at age 18, she has a slightly greater risk of developing ovarian cancer before menopause.

SYMPTOMS

The need for early detection of ovarian cancer is clear. It's important to be aware of persistent symptoms of generalized discomfort in the abdominal or pelvic area. The most common symptoms of ovarian cancer are often nonspecific—abdominal or pelvic discomfort or pain, bloating, urinary urgency, loss of appetite, or a premature sensation of fullness during eating. They resemble those of other disorders, such as digestive conditions or bladder disorders. However, in these other conditions, symptoms come and go; with ovarian cancer, they persist and may worsen. Other symptoms, albeit rare, include:

- Persistent gas, indigestion, or nausea
- Unexplained changes in bowel habits, including diarrhea or constipation
- Unexplained weight loss or gain or increased abdominal girth
- Pain during intercourse
- A persistent lack of energy
- Low back pain

PREVENTION

Research is ongoing to find a good screening test for ovarian cancer analogous to mammography for breast cancer or a Pap test for cervical cancer. For women with mutations in the BRCA1 and BRCA2 genes, prophylactic surgery to remove the ovaries can dramatically reduce risk.

TREATMENT

The preferred treatment for ovarian cancer is surgery, with chemotherapy used afterward to treat any remaining disease.

SKIN CANCER

Skin cancer is the irregular growth of skin cells. It is the most common form of cancer in this country, with more than a million cases diagnosed each year. In the past 3 decades, the number of women under age 40 diagnosed with basal cell carcinoma has more than doubled. The rates for squamous cell carcinoma and melanoma for women have also increased. The most common cause of skin cancer is overexposure to the sun, but it can occur in areas of the body not exposed to light. Early detection is the key to successful treatment. If you notice any abnormal changes in your skin, see your health care provider immediately. There are three main types of skin cancer:

- **Basal cell carcinoma.** The most common form of skin cancer, this type usually appears as a small waxy bump on the face, ears, or neck or a flat brown discolored area on the back or chest and is relatively easy to treat.
- **Squamous cell carcinoma.** This type shows up as a scaly flat lesion on the face, ears, neck, arms, or hands or as a red nodule on the face, lips, ears, neck, arms, or hands. If detected early, it can be treated easily.
- **Melanoma.** The deadliest kind of skin cancer, melanoma can show up in normal skin or in moles and may take many different forms, including large brown, speckled areas; firm, shiny bumps; or lesions with irregular borders. In women, melanomas most often appear on the legs rather than the torso. One in every 61 women will develop melanoma in her lifetime.

ARE YOU AT RISK?

Among the risk factors for skin cancer are:

- Too much unprotected sun exposure, including severe sunburns in childhood
- Fair skin and light hair and eyes
- Frequent sunburns
- Many moles
- Living in a sunny place or at a high altitude
- Family history of skin cancer

PREVENTION

The Skin Cancer Foundation recommends the following guidelines for preventing the disease:

- Wear sunscreen with an SPF of 15 or above all year round. Apply 1 ounce (2 tablespoons) of sunscreen to your entire body 30 minutes before going outside. Reapply every 2 hours.

- Seek the shade, especially between 10 a.m. and 4 p.m.
- Do not burn.
- Avoid tanning and UV tanning booths.
- Cover up with clothing, including a broad-brimmed hat and UV-blocking sunglasses.
- Examine your skin head to toe every month.
- See your physician every year for a professional skin exam.

DETECTION AND SCREENING

The American Cancer Society urges people to follow the **ABCD** rule when checking their skin for melanoma:

- **A** for Asymmetry: One half of a mole or mark looks different from the other half.
- **B** for Border: Edges are irregular—ragged, notched, or blurred.
- **C** for Color: Color is uneven, with different shades of brown or black or other colors, such as red, white, or even blue.
- **D** for Diameter: The mole or mark is larger than 1 inch in diameter or is growing.

TREATMENT

Treatment for cancerous and precancerous skin lesions varies according to the location and severity of the condition. The abnormal cells may be surgically excised, frozen off, or destroyed with topical medications.

roductive Choices Fertility and Pregn
enopause Sexual Abuse and Sexual A
in Teeth Hair and Nails Body Weigh
etabolism Blood Sugar Eating and Exc
scles Bones JointsHeart and Blood
d Respiration Common Infectious Dis
toimmune Disease Cancer Vision He
ell, Taste, and Touch Mental Health
ce Abuse Making Change Managing
d Sleeping Well Shifting Your Food En
ent Getting Active Screenings and H
intenance Reproduction Sexuality and
l Health Reproductive Choices Fertilit
egnancy Menopause Sexual Abuse and
l Assault Skin Teeth Hair and Nails
eight and Metabolism Blood Sugar E
d Excreting Muscles Bones Joints Hear
ood Lungs and Respiration Common
us Diseases Autoimmune Disease C

PART VII

Sensing:
Staying in Touch with the World

Our sensory view of the world—how we take in information through our intricate and efficient sensory organs—has a great impact on our well-being. Vision, hearing, taste, smell, and touch all affect our ability to communicate, to enjoy activities and social interactions, and to register crucial changes in our environment. Think of the tune of an aria or the whine of a siren; think of the fresh, earthy scent of new-fallen rain or the acrid odor of smoke; envision the snowcapped mountains that you love to climb.

Although each of our senses may receive input from our surroundings in a different form (light waves, sound vibrations, chemical stimuli), all five senses work by converting this input into electrical impulses that travel along sensory nerves to the brain, which analyzes and interprets the stimuli as meaningful perceptions.

As we age, our senses become less acute. For the brain to perceive a sensation, it requires a minimum amount of stimulation, known as a threshold. Aging often raises this threshold, so we need more sensory input to register a sensation. Fortunately, we can stave off or accommodate some of these changes by making minor adjustments in lifestyle; for other changes, help is available in the form of glasses, hearing aids, and other medical treatments.

Because of my family history, I think often about eye health and try to stay on top of the latest research. My mother has macular degeneration, a deterioration of the macular area of the retina, which can cause the loss of vision. My father's eyesight is affected by mild cataracts. At Tufts, my colleagues are working on promising new research about the effects of nutrition on the aging eye. It turns out that what we eat has a profound influence on our eye health. The antioxidants found in colorful fruits and vegetables, for instance, can help delay progression of early macular degeneration. Antioxidants also delay changes that are associated with cataracts and boost eye health. On the other hand, diets high in white bread, white rice, high-fructose corn syrup, and other easily metabolized carbohydrates such as those found in highly refined, sugary foods can contribute to macular degeneration. Here's another great reason to eat your fruits and vegetables and cut out foods such as sweetened drinks and doughnuts.

Hearing is also a family issue for me. Multiple ear infections in childhood left my father-in-law deaf from the time he was a teenager. His hearing loss profoundly affected his life. I worry about my husband in this respect. He is a professional violinist, so an acute sense of hearing is vital; unfortunately, he has experienced hearing loss in his left ear because of regular exposure to music at a high volume from his own instrument.

Even if it does not affect our profession, the fading of any sense diminishes quality of life. My close friend Corey has lost his sense of taste. He once savored a good meal; now everything tastes the same. I think about the sensual pleasure I get from a wonderful meal and can't imagine not being able to sense the delicious variety of flavors.

Your senses are precious and deserve to be treated with care. I always wear good-quality sunglasses and a hat to protect my eyes when I go outside. I'm keenly sensitive to noise, so I avoid loud concerts and plug my ears if I'm exposed to a shrill siren or blasting jackhammer. I also work hard to avoid smoky environments, because smoke "burns" all senses.

These **S.M.A.R.T.** suggestions will help you preserve the acuity of your senses and the health of your sensory organs:

1. Protect your eyes from bright sunlight by wearing good sunglasses and a hat.
2. Eat a diet low in refined sugars.
3. Eat plenty of green leafy vegetables.
4. Avoid smoky environments.
5. Avoid loud noises that can damage your ears, or wear protective earplugs.
6. Treat eye and ear infections promptly and appropriately.
7. Protect yourself from exposure to temperature extremes.

20

Vision

The sense that gives us access to the images around us—from the smile lines in our own face to a sunrise over the Grand Canyon—involves both the complex structure of the eye and a large part of the brain. Our eyes work with the vision cortex in the brain to tell us the color of an object; its size, shape, and texture; and its nearness and direction and speed of movement. They register depth and adapt to changes in our environment so that we can perceive our surroundings in bright or dim light.

I find how the eye works complex and fascinating. Vision begins when light reflected from an object enters the eye through the dome-shaped transparent cornea, which focuses the light before it passes through the hole of the pupil. The size of the pupil is adjusted to accommodate the level of light by the surrounding muscles of the iris, which may narrow the pupil to less than $\frac{1}{5}$ inch in diameter in bright light, or dilate it to $\frac{1}{3}$ inch in low light or dark.

Just behind the pupil lies the lens, a clear disk about the size and shape of an M&M, which works like a camera lens to further focus the light with the help of a tiny ring of muscles that surround it. These muscles change the lens shape, making it thicker to accommodate light from near objects and thinner for far ones. Together the cornea and lens finely focus the light rays so they form a clear, inverted image on the retina, a sheet of neurons and light-sensitive photoreceptors lining the back of the eye. The retina is a mosaic of hundreds of millions of visual receptors, known as rods and cones, which convert the light into electrical signals. Rods are sensitive to dim light and detect shades of gray; cones work in bright light and are responsible for seeing in color and detecting detail. Within the retina is a small, specialized area called the macula, where photoreceptors are most dense. This area helps us see fine details. Signals generated by the retina's photoreceptors are carried by the optic nerve—a bundle of millions of nerve fibers—to the visual cortex of the brain, which interprets them as visual images.

WHAT IS GOOD VISION AND HOW IS IT MEASURED?

Visual acuity, or the sharpness of your eyesight, is most commonly measured by a standardized test called the Snellen eye chart. This familiar chart has a series of letters, beginning with large letters at the top, followed by rows of letters of diminishing size. The test is performed on each eye, one at a time, with the chart normally held 20 feet away.

Visual acuity is expressed as a fraction, such as 20/20 or 20/40. The top number indicates your distance from the chart, and the bottom number refers to the distance at which a person with normal vision could accurately read the same line that you read. The fraction 20/40, for instance, means that the line you read accurately at 20 feet could be read by a person with normal eyesight at a distance of 40 feet. Contrary to popular belief, 20/20 is not perfect vision, but rather a reference standard. Normal vision is usually one or two lines better (20/15 or 20/10).

A chart held 14 inches from your face is used to test the acuity of near vision.

CARING FOR YOUR EYES
AND PRESERVING YOUR VISION

Following these simple guidelines can help you preserve your vision as you age:

1. **Get a complete eye exam** every 1 or 2 years after the age of 40. Don't wait until your vision weakens for your first exam. Find out whether you are at risk for any eye diseases. If you have a family history of eye disease or other risk factors, you should have more frequent exams. Regular eye exams are the keystone of maintaining visual health!
2. **Have routine physical exams** to check for high blood pressure and diabetes, which can cause eye disease.
3. **Eat a healthy diet.** Nutrition can make a big difference in preserving your vision and staving off age-related eye diseases such as macular degeneration and cataracts. We've all been told to eat carrots to keep our eyes healthy. It's true that carrots contain beta-carotene, which can be converted into vitamin A, a

vitamin essential for our eyes. But many other fruits and vegetables are also important for eye health. These include dark green leafy vegetables that contain antioxidants and vitamins C and E, which may help preserve vision, in addition to being beneficial for overall health.

To keep your eyes at their best, avoid highly refined, sugary foods. (See the box Eating for Eye Health: Avoiding the Sugar Spike below.) Eat foods low in saturated fats to prevent the buildup of cholesterol and waste products, which can block the transfer of vitamin A and its derivatives from reaching the rod cells in the retina. Eat fish and other foods rich in omega-3 fatty acids to protect eyes against retinopathy (a deterioration of the retina), age-related macular degeneration (AMD), and other age-related eye diseases. If you have signs of AMD, you should consider talking to your eye care specialist about taking

EATING FOR EYE HEALTH: AVOIDING THE SUGAR SPIKE

My colleague Dr. Allen Taylor, chief of the Laboratory for Nutrition and Vision Research at Tufts University, suggests that eating fewer simple carbohydrates—foods high on the so-called glycemic index (GI)—may help slow the eye tissue damage that occurs in age-related macular degeneration (AMD) and cataracts.

Using data from long-term studies, Allen's research looked at people's diets in relation to their incidence of cataracts and AMD. He found that people who consumed diets with a high GI had a significantly higher risk of developing AMD and cataracts. They also developed these diseases at a younger age. "The intake of simple sugars sets up the body for damage when the sugar is oxidized," Allen explains. In people who ate lower-GI diets, with more complex carbohydrates, the disease progressed more slowly. Allen suggests that 20 percent of the cases of advanced AMD might have been prevented if those individuals had consumed a low-glycemic diet.

Allen recommends making an immediate change in your diet. "I'm not talking about drastic change," he explains. "You can go from a high- to a low-glycemic diet by simply replacing the five slices of white bread you eat every day with five slices of whole wheat and cutting down on sugar-sweetened beverages. That would shift your GI to a healthier range."

vitamin preparations based on the results of the 10-year National Eye Institute's Age-Related Eye Disease Study (AREDS).

4. **Don't smoke.** People who smoke have a markedly higher risk of developing AMD and cataracts.

5. **Whatever your age, protect your eyes from UV rays** by wearing sunglasses and a wide-brimmed hat when you are out in the sun for long periods of time. Your sunglasses should protect your eyes from both UVA and UVB rays. Buy your sunglasses from a reputable company and look for a label that specifies 99 to 100 percent UV protection. The lenses should be dark enough to reduce glare but not distort colors. A broad-brimmed hat can offer protection from sunlight that may enter from above and from the sides of sunglasses.

6. **Maintain a healthy body weight.** There is more and more evidence that obesity puts people at an increased risk for AMD and cataracts as they grow older.

7. **Watch for warning signs.** See your eye doctor immediately if you notice:

   - Abrupt changes in vision
   - Sudden eye pain, swelling, or redness
   - Sudden burst of eye floaters or flashes of light
   - Double vision
   - Appearance of a dark curtain moving over a portion of your visual field
   - Gradual or sudden narrowing of peripheral vision
   - Gradual loss of central vision
   - Cloudy or blurred vision
   - Blind spots
   - Sensation of scratchiness or irritation

COMMON VISION PROBLEMS

REFRACTIVE ERROR

Among the most common vision problems is refractive error, when the eye cannot properly focus an image. Examples are:

- **Nearsightedness (myopia):** Nearsightedness occurs when light from objects beyond close range converges in front of the retina rather than on it, blurring distant vision. It affects about one in five people and is often first noticed in childhood. It may worsen in adolescence and after the age of 40.

- **Farsightedness (hyperopia):** Farsightedness occurs when light from objects closer than a certain distance converges just behind the retina, making it difficult to focus on anything up close—though far-off objects can be seen clearly. It may be caused by congenital factors or, after the age of 40, by a loss of elasticity in the lens called presbyopia.
- **Astigmatism:** Astigmatism occurs when a misshapen cornea disrupts focus of near and distant vision.

Correcting Refractive Error

Fortunately, refractive errors are usually easy to correct with eyeglasses, contacts, or refractive surgery. If you suspect you have a refractive error, the condition can be diagnosed by an optometrist; if there's a chance that you have a more serious eye problem, you should see an ophthalmologist, a doctor trained in diagnosing and treating eye disorders.

Eyeglasses

Prescriptions for eyeglasses are ordered by an optometrist or ophthalmologist and can be filled by an optician. They are measured in diopters; the higher the diopter, the stronger the prescription. The measurement starts at zero (called "plano") for 20/10 or 20/15 vision, and increases by negative quarter diopters, -0.25 (a quarter diopter) or -0.50 (half a diopter).

Contact lenses

Contact lenses fit over the cornea of the eye and help refocus light on the retina. They must be fitted by an optometrist or ophthalmologist. Contact lenses provide greater convenience and durability than eyeglasses, as well as a wider field of vision. (They also can't fall off your head and break, although they do occasionally pop out.) However, they carry a risk of corneal infection, because they reduce the amount of oxygen reaching your cornea. They are not recommended for people with impaired coordination or the condition known as dry eye (see page 279).

Three basic types of contact lenses are available—soft, hard (or gas permeable), and hybrid:

- **Soft lenses.** These are thin and flexible, easily conforming to the curve of your eye. They are used to correct nearsightedness and farsightedness and are generally more comfortable than hard lenses. However, they tend to be fragile and, depending on type, can be costly to replace. Soft lenses come in three forms: daily wear, extended wear, and disposable.

- **Hard lenses (or gas permeable).** These lenses can be used to correct astigmatism and other visual problems as well as nearsightedness and farsightedness. They allow a freer flow of oxygen and carbon dioxide between the lens and the cornea, diminishing the risk of corneal irritation and infection. Hard lenses require a longer period of adjustment than soft lenses do, but they're relatively easy to care for and more durable than soft lenses, requiring replacement only every 2 or 3 years.
- **Hybrid.** A new kind of lens first marketed in 2006 blends the positive features of both soft and hard lenses. A gas-permeable center provides better visual acuity and a surrounding soft outer ring offers greater comfort.

Refractive Surgery

Millions of Americans have opted for refractive surgery to correct their routine vision problems. Most of the time the results are good. But occasionally the surgery actually impairs vision. If you opt for refractive surgery, be a smart consumer and make sure the center you visit is accredited and run by an experienced, knowledgeable staff of doctors. Your eyes are some of the most valuable real estate in your body. Take care of them and get the best possible medical advice on the right treatment.

LASIK surgery is a wonderful option for some people. Before you go this route, you should know the risks, make sure that you are a good candidate for the procedure, and plan to have the surgery performed at a top-notch medical center. Several surgical techniques can be used to treat refraction errors, including:

- **LASIK** (laser-assisted in-situ keratomileusis) eye surgery is used to correct nearsightedness, farsightedness, or astigmatism. With the help of a laser, an eye surgeon removes a small amount of tissue from your cornea to flatten the curve or make it steeper so that light rays focus more precisely on your retina.
- **LASEK** (laser epithelial keratomileusis) is similar to LASIK except that it involves peeling back a thin surface layer of the cornea to apply the laser on parts of the cornea that need reshaping. Once this is done, the flap is replaced.
- **Photorefractive keratectomy (PRK)** is used to treat low to moderate nearsightedness or farsightedness. In this procedure, an eye surgeon removes a thin surface layer of the cornea and then uses a laser to flatten the cornea or make it more steeply curved.
- **Radial keratotomy** is a form of microsurgery with a scalpel used to correct nearsightedness and certain kinds of astigmatism. A surgeon makes spokelike incisions in the cornea to flatten it.

- **Corneal transplant** is sometimes used to treat conditions that distort the cornea or diminish its transparency, such as clouding, swelling, or scarring of the cornea from infection or injury. In a cornea transplant, a surgeon replaces a portion of your cornea with one from a donor.

OTHER COMMON EYE PROBLEMS

- **Benign essential blepharospasm (BEB).** In BEB, involuntary muscle contractions cause spasms and twitching of the eyelid muscles. BEB is especially common in middle-aged and elderly women. The condition often begins gradually with increased frequency of eye blinking linked with eye irritation and is thought to be due to abnormal functioning of the basal ganglia, a part of the brain involved in coordinating movements. The treatment of choice is botulinum toxin injections, which relax the muscles and stop the spasms.
- **Conjunctivitis.** Conjunctivitis is an inflammation or infection of the conjunctiva, the tissue that lines the inside of the eyelid. It may be caused by a virus, a bacteria, irritating substances, allergens, or sexually transmitted diseases. A common kind of conjunctivitis called pinkeye is a contagious infection in which the eyes become pink and watery. It's usually treated with antibiotic eyedrops. Although conjunctivitis is harmless to your sight, it's highly contagious for up to 2 weeks, so it's a good idea to seek diagnosis and treatment early.
- **Retinal detachment.** Retinal detachment is when the retina is lifted or pulled from its normal position. If not promptly treated, it can cause blindness. Symptoms include the sudden appearance of many "floaters" (little spots, specks, or strings that float about in your field of vision), sudden flashes of light, or the appearance of a dark curtain moving over your field of vision. If you experience any of these symptoms, you should see an eye care doctor immediately. Surgery is the only effective therapy.
- **Sty.** A sty is an infection of an eyelash follicle. It is best treated by applying warm compresses and sometimes, with antibiotics.
- **Dry eyes.** The problem of dry eyes is most often age-related. The lacrimal glands in our eye sockets produce a layer of tears, mucus, and oil that protects the delicate orb of the eyeball. As we age, our eyes make fewer tears, causing burning, stinging, and other discomfort. Women age 50 or older are twice as likely as men to suffer from dry eyes, perhaps because of a decline in chemical signals that help maintain tear film. Treatment consists of the use of artificial tears or prescription dry-eye medications.

HOW DO OUR EYES CHANGE WITH AGE?

As we age, many of us experience problems with our vision. If you're over 40, maybe you have to hold this book a bit farther from your eyes to follow the text or use reading glasses to decipher the small print. Maybe you find that you need brighter light to read. Or perhaps when you're driving, you have to squint to read road signs or have difficulty seeing in the dark. All of these changes are normal effects of aging.

Beginning in our forties, many of us develop presbyopia—decreased visual acuity—and reduced sensitivity to light. As we move into our fifties, the problem may become more noticeable, requiring more frequent changes in eyeglass or contact lens prescriptions or different eyeglasses for different uses.

In our later years, diminished strength in the tiny muscles that control pupil size makes our pupils slower to respond to changes in lighting. People in their sixties typically have difficulty adjusting their eyes from dim light to bright sunlight and have weaker night vision. In addition, with aging we lose nearly a third of the rod cells in our retinas, those crucial to sensing shades of light and dark, and the ones that remain don't work as well, exacerbating poor night vision. Likewise, loss of sensitivity in our retinal cone cells as we age can cause colors to look washed-out or less bright.

More serious age-related eye problems include:

- **Age-related macular degeneration (AMD).** As I mentioned at the start of this part, macular degeneration is the deterioration or scarring of the macular area of the retina, the small area that produces the sharpest vision. In this country, the condition is the most common cause of vision loss among the elderly, affecting about one in three people age 75 and older. The cause of macular degeneration is unknown in most cases, but it tends to run in families. Atherosclerosis may contribute to the development of AMD, possibly by affecting bloodflow to the eye. New research suggests that smoking nearly doubles the risk for AMD. Likewise, diets high in refined, sugary foods also contribute to the disorder. (See the box Eating for Eye Health on page 275.) On the other hand, eating fish frequently (especially salmon and other fish rich in omega-3 fatty acids) may decrease the chances of developing the disorder. Although the damage caused by AMD can't be reversed, it can be limited if caught early and treated. If you have signs of AMD, you should consider talking to your eye care specialist about taking vitamin preparations based on the results of the 10-year National Eye Institute's Age-Related Eye Disease Study (AREDS).

- **Cataracts.** Cataracts are a clouding of the eye's lenses that may result from chemical changes in the lenses. They may begin as a small opacity that is barely noticeable, but as the cloudiness grows, it can disrupt vision, making it harder to see at night, increasing sensitivity to light and glare, fading colors, and producing double vision. Cataracts occur rarely in young people but are most common in the elderly and are most often treated with surgery. Some 50 percent of all Americans age 75 and over have the disorder. Surgical treatment usually results in complete vision restoration.

- **Diabetic retinopathy.** High blood sugar in the body can damage the blood vessels in the eye, causing them to leak or bleed. This may lead to diabetic retinopathy and vision loss. The National Eye Institute estimates that 40 percent of people over the age of 40 who have been diagnosed with diabetes have some degree of diabetic retinopathy. If the condition is treated promptly, vision loss can be avoided. If you are diabetic, you should have a dilated eye exam at least once a year.

- **Glaucoma.** The group of eye disorders known as glaucoma is characterized by increased fluid pressure within the eye that can damage the optic nerve, causing partial or complete blindness. Although it can occur in young people, it is much more common among older adults. Those at higher risk include people over age 60, African Americans over age 40, and people with a family history of the disease. Other risk factors are diabetes and other medical conditions, as well as use of corticosteroids. Although the condition may be silent, symptoms include sensitivity to light, loss of peripheral vision, difficulty differentiating shades of light and dark, and trouble seeing in low light. If detected early, glaucoma can be treated with medication or surgery. If you experience these symptoms or if changes in your vision are associated with severe eye pain, headache, or nausea, seek medical attention immediately. Treatment involves drug therapy. The best way to avoid the disorder is to get regular screening every 2 years after the age of 40.

21

Hearing

From the fluty notes of a songbird in spring to the boom of your teenager's bass drum, the sounds processed by your ears all involve the same mechanism: Sound waves enter the external ear and are funneled through the external auditory canal to the tympanic membrane, or eardrum, a thin, rigid, and highly sensitive piece of skin only about 10 millimeters in diameter. In response to sound waves of different amplitude and frequency, the tympanic membrane vibrates at different speeds, transmitting the vibrations to the ossicles of your middle ear. (This part of the ear is connected to the throat by way of the Eustachian tube.) The ossicles—a set of tiny bones called the malleus, the incus, and the stapes—amplify the vibrations before passing them along to the inner ear. Here they encounter a fluid-filled spiral passage known as the cochlea, which contains some 16,000 hair cells. These cells have microscopic hairlike projections that respond to the vibrations and send electrical impulses through the cochlear nerve to the brain, which interprets them as birdsong or bass drum.

Your ears also have a second job: to maintain equilibrium. In the semicircular canal of your inner ear are fluid and small hairlike sensors that help the brain monitor the motion of your head and maintain balance. Sensations of vertigo or dizziness may result from inflammation in the inner ear (called acute vestibular neuronitis or labyrinthitis) or Ménière's disease, an excessive buildup of fluid in the semicircular canal.

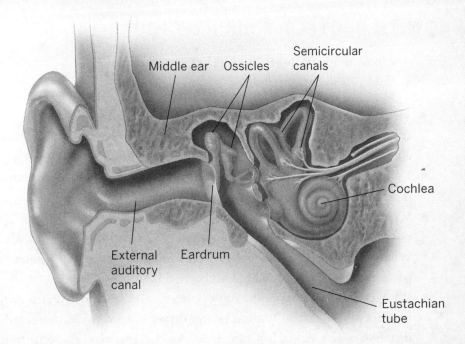

Sound waves enter the ear through the external auditory canal and are converted into vibrations by the inner ear. There they cause cells in the cochlea to create nerve signals, which travel to the brain, where they are interpreted as sound. The semicircular canals send the brain messages about head position to maintain balance. The Eustachian tube acts as a valve to equalize pressure around the eardrum.

HOW HEARING IS TESTED

Hearing specialists measure hearing with a battery of tests, including tone and speech tests, assessments of your middle ear function, and other diagnostic tests. The results of these tests are recorded in an audiogram, which charts your ability to hear sounds of various frequencies (measured in hertz, or Hz) at varying degrees of loudness (measured in decibels, or dBs). Your hearing threshold is the softest level at which a sound is still audible to you. A hearing threshold of between zero and 25 dB is considered normal.

The audiogram helps the hearing specialist determine your hearing ability relative to normal adult hearing levels—and, if you have a hearing loss, where it occurs and its type or classification. Most people hear sounds in the range of 20 to 20,000 Hz, with best sensitivity in the middle range. Ordinary conversation usually occurs at frequencies between 500 and 3,000 Hz.

HOW TO PROTECT YOUR PRECIOUS HEARING

Among the most common causes of hearing loss is exposure to loud noise, which is usually preventable. To protect your hearing:

- Be aware of hazardous noises above 85 decibels in your environment, such as from heavy traffic, trains and subways, concerts, lawn mowers, snow blowers, etc., which can cause damage. (See the box Sound Advice on page 286.)
- Limit your exposure to loud noise when possible. When exposed, wear earplugs, fluid-filled earmuffs, or other hearing-protective devices.
- When using earphones or other stereo headsets, keep the volume low. If someone standing 3 feet from you can hear the music, it's too loud.
- When purchasing toys, appliances, recreational equipment, and power tools, pay attention to the noise rating and choose quiet models.
- When cleaning your ears with a cotton swab, do so gently and never use it on the inside of your ear. If you have wax buildup in your ears, consider using eardrops that soften wax, followed by a warm water douche. This may help keep ears from becoming clogged.
- If you think you may have hearing loss, make an appointment with an otolaryngologist (ear, nose, and throat specialist) and get a hearing test by an audiologist.

COMMON HEARING PROBLEMS

The ability to hear higher frequencies tends to diminish as we get older. But hearing loss is common across all ages. It may be caused by genes, birth defects, side effects from medication, frequent exposure to very loud noise, or untreated ear infections, such as those suffered by my father-in-law before the invention of penicillin. To determine whether you might have hearing loss, ask yourself the following questions:

- Do you have trouble hearing on the phone?
- Do you strain to understand conversation?
- Do you have trouble hearing when there's noise in the background, e.g., at a cocktail party?
- Do you have to turn the TV or radio volume up high to hear?
- Do you often ask people to repeat what they've said?
- Do you find that you misunderstand what people say?

If you answered yes to some of these questions, you may benefit from a hearing evaluation by an audiologist, an otolaryngologist, or an otologist (a physician specializing in hearing disorders).

CAUSES OF COMMON HEARING PROBLEMS

- **Genetic defects.** Hearing loss is often linked with genetic defects. Scientists have identified more than 120 genes that play a role in hearing loss; defects in these genes can interfere with the ear's development and function. Examples of genetically caused syndromes of hearing impairment include Ushers, Waardenburg, and Pendred, which causes a deformation of the inner ear. Certain genes may also make people more prone to hearing loss from noise, drugs, or infections. Close to half of all cases of deafness have a genetic component.

- **Noise-induced hearing loss (NIHL).** NIHL occurs when our ears are exposed to noises that are too loud or loud noises that last a long time. (See the box Sound Advice on page 286.) This harmful noise damages our hair cells, the tiny sensory cells in our inner ear that convert sound energy into electrical signals. Once these cells are damaged, the loss is permanent; the cells will not grow back. NIHL can be caused by a single exposure to one loud sound, such as an explosion (120 to 150 decibels), or by long-term or repeated exposure to loud noises (above 85 decibels), such as the sound generated by a jackhammer. People of any age can develop NIHL. Some 22 million Americans may already have suffered permanent hearing loss because of routine excessive noise exposure.

- **Infection.** Otitis media, an infection or inflammation of the middle ear, is primarily a disease of infants and young children, but it can also affect adults. The inflammation often begins when a viral or bacterial infection that caused a sore throat or cold spreads to the middle ear. Otitis media can cause temporary hearing problems, which can become more serious if the infection is left untreated.

- **Tinnitus.** Tinnitus, or ringing in the ears, affects some 12 million Americans. It can be intermittent or continuous, a low roar or a high-pitched squeal, annoying or debilitating. It has numerous causes, including different kinds of hearing loss, overexposure to loud noise, medicines, allergies, tumors, and Ménière's disease, a relatively common disorder associated with a sense of spinning. There is no cure for tinnitus, but some treatments may give relief, including hearing aids, electronic devices that mask the ringing or roaring, and some medicines and drug therapies.

HEARING CORRECTIONS

How hearing loss is treated depends on its cause and severity. Sometimes the treatment is as simple as removal of earwax blockage. If the loss is the result of damage to the inner ear, a hearing aid may be helpful. For severe hearing loss, a cochlear implant is often a good option. You can discuss with your hearing specialist which device is best for you.

- **Hearing aids.** A hearing aid is an external device that amplifies sound and directs it toward your ear canal. Although it won't restore all of your hearing, it

SOUND ADVICE
Know Your Noises and Protect Your Ears

It's important to pay attention to noise levels in your environment and know which noises can damage your ears. When you're exposed to loud noises for any length of time, protect your ears with earplugs.

Decibel Level

150   Firecracker
140   Jet engine
120   Ambulance siren
110   Rock concert
Regular exposure of more than 1 minute to any noise above 110 decibels can cause permanent hearing loss.
100   Snowmobile, Jet Ski, chain saw, drill
More than 15 minutes of unprotected exposure to any noise above 100 decibels may cause hearing loss.
95   Motorcycle
90   Power lawnmower, truck traffic, subway
85   Heavy traffic, alarm clock
Prolonged exposure to any noise above 80 decibels may cause hearing loss.
60   Normal conversation, dishwasher
40   Refrigerator humming
30   Whisper

can make it easier to cope with hearing loss. Unfortunately, up to 60 percent of people who need hearing aids or would benefit from them go without—perhaps because they're not aware of their hearing problem or because they don't want to wear a clunky device.

If you think you need a hearing aid, make an appointment with a hearing specialist who can help find and adjust the best device for you. Recent technological advances have led to the development of small, sophisticated hearing aids. The new models come in a vast array of shapes, sizes, styles, and prices to address individual needs and desires. Some fit in your outer ear or inside your ear canal, where they are barely noticeable; others sit behind your ear and feed amplified sound to your ear canal through a small tube. All include a microphone to gather sounds, an amplifier to make sounds louder, and an earpiece to transmit the sounds to your ear canal. There are two basic types:

○ **Analogue** hearing aids transmit sounds to the ear in real time.

○ **Digital** hearing aids convert sounds into bits and manipulate them before amplifying the signal. They can be tailored to the user's need with the help of a minicomputer. Some models include advanced directional microphones that can help people who have difficulty hearing in noisy surroundings.

• **Cochlear implants.** For people who are deaf or profoundly hearing impaired and unable to use a hearing aid, one option is a cochlear implant, a device surgically implanted in the ear that takes over the function of the damaged cochlea. Cochlear implants have been a technological miracle for thousands of children and adults who have profound hearing loss. The devices improve hearing ability and facilitate lipreading. The newer models include a microphone to pick up sounds, which travel via a thin cable to a computerized speech processor worn behind the ear or on a belt. The speech processor then sends the signals to a surgically implanted electronic chip that stimulates the hearing nerve. In this way, the signals bypass the damaged area of the hearing system and are recognized as sounds by the brain.

SIGN LANGUAGE

Most people with hearing loss can achieve normal communication with a hearing aid and lipreading. However, for those who are deaf or profoundly hearing impaired, sign language—a complex language that uses signs made with the hands, facial expressions, and body posture—can be essential. Different regions use different forms of sign language. American Sign Language (ASL) is said to be the fourth most commonly used language in this country. (For more information, go to nidcd.nih.gov and type in the key words "American Sign Language.")

WHAT HAPPENS TO OUR HEARING AS WE GET OLDER?

As we age, many of us experience a gradual loss of hearing known as presbycusis, especially if we have been exposed to a lot of noise over our lifetime. One in three people between the ages of 65 and 75 has presbycusis and as many as half of all people 75 and older have it. The hearing loss usually affects the ability to hear high-pitched sounds such as birdsong or the ring of a telephone. People with the disorder often have difficulty hearing and understanding speech.

Presbycusis may arise from changes in the middle or inner ear or along the auditory nerves leading to the brain. It is exacerbated by the cumulative damage to the cochlea from the effects of chronic exposure to loud noise such as traffic, music, and noisy equipment. Medical conditions such as heart disease, high blood pressure, and other circulatory disorders that alter the blood supply to the ear can also contribute to the problem.

To avoid hearing loss from damaging noise, minimize your exposure to lawn mowers, leaf blowers, snowmobiles, loud appliances, and other machinery by using earplugs or fluid-filled earmuffs.

To cope with your hearing loss, it may help to:

- Reduce or eliminate background noise in your environment or pick a quiet place to converse.
- Be direct with others about your need for them to speak clearly.
- Face your conversation partner.
- Consider training in speech-reading—using visual clues to better understand spoken speech.
- Explore the use of hearing aids or assistive listening aids such as built-in telephone amplification devices and radio- and TV-listening systems.

22

Smell, Taste, and Touch

We're generally most aware of our senses of vision and hearing and get the regular checkups we need for eyes and ears. But our other senses—smell, taste, and touch—are just as vital, protecting us from harm and allowing us to fully experience the world. They deserve equal attention and care.

SMELL

Your sense of smell gives you the ability to perceive the aroma of baking bread and the fragrance of a gardenia. It enhances the flavor of food; in fact, 75 percent of what you think of as flavor is actually food odors released into your mouth when you eat. Part of a marvelous chemical sensing system, smell also allows you to detect danger in the form of spoiled food, the smoke of a fire, or the pungent fume of a gas leak. Its loss can be devastating, destroying your enjoyment of food and other aromatic pleasures of life. It can even be dangerous, robbing you of a vital way to gain information about the safety of your environment.

Loss of smell can also signal more serious underlying conditions or diseases, such as Alzheimer's, Parkinson's, multiple sclerosis, malnutrition, and diabetes.

Normal smell occurs when tiny molecules released by the substances around us (coffee, fresh basil, sea breeze) stimulate sensory cells known as olfactory cells in a small patch of tissue high up in the nose, the olfactory epithelium. The cells there respond to the molecules by sending messages along the olfactory nerves to our brain, which interpret the messages as specific odors.

HOW SMELL IS TESTED

Special tests designed to determine the ability to smell include "scratch and sniff" tests, which determine how well you can identify various common odors; tests that measure your odor threshold—the smallest amount of odor you can detect; and tests that ask you to compare the scents of various chemicals. Nasal examinations with a nasal endoscope, x-rays, and CAT scans can also help determine whether there is a problem anywhere in your nasal passages.

HOW TO PRESERVE YOUR SENSE OF SMELL

To maintain a good sense of smell:

- Don't smoke.
- Wash your hands often, especially during the cold season, to protect yourself from upper respiratory infections.
- Get a flu vaccine every year.
- If you have allergies, avoid allergens such as ragweed and pet dander.
- Wear a seat belt and, when riding a bike, wear a helmet to avoid head injuries.

COMMON PROBLEMS WITH SMELL

By some estimates, more than 200,000 people visit a physician each year for smell-related problems. Hyposmia, the reduced ability to detect odor, is a common result of upper respiratory infections such as the common cold, or of nasal congestion from chronic sinus disease. It usually diminishes or disappears when the infection goes away. Anosmia is the complete inability to detect odor. It is sometimes caused by head trauma, and rarely, by a genetic defect.

Other causes of smell-related problems include:

- Exposure to toxic chemicals such as insecticides or solvents
- Radiation
- Allergies
- Dental problems
- Certain medications such as antibiotics and antifungals and drugs to lower cholesterol and blood pressure
- Nasal polyps, small growths in the nose or sinuses that can block smell molecules from reaching the olfactory patch in your nose

- Smoking, which impairs the ability to distinguish odors
- Thyroid abnormalities
- Vitamin deficiencies

If you think you're having trouble with smell, see your doctor. Smell disorders are often curable. Because some medications may be the source of the problem, adjusting dosage or changing medications may alter the impact on smell. If polyps or other nasal obstructions are the issue, surgery can help restore airflow. Sometimes loss of smell signals a more serious health problem, such as a disease of the nervous system. Early diagnosis may lead to effective treatment of an underlying condition.

HOW THE SENSE OF SMELL CHANGES WITH AGE

Like vision and hearing, our sense of smell may decline as we grow older, especially after age 60. Some 30 percent of Americans between the ages of 70 and 80 and some 60 percent of those over 80 have a problem with their sense of smell. This may be the result of degeneration of the nerves that control smell. Although you can't avoid the age-related problems with smell, you can help prevent their development by following the measures to preserve smell outlined above.

TASTE

Who could argue against the importance of taste? This vital sense allows us to enjoy everything from the rich flavor of chocolate to the juicy tang of a fresh orange.

However, taste serves a purpose beyond allowing us to enjoy the pleasures of food. It helps us detect the bitterness that sometimes signals poisonous substances. It also helps us regulate our diets. If our sense of taste is impaired or distorted, we may eat too little or too much, putting us at risk for chronic disease. Or we may consume too much salt or sugar—a particular problem for people with diabetes or high blood pressure.

Although taste is a discrete sense, with its own receptors, it is intimately entwined with other senses. What we think of as flavor—the sensation that tells us whether we're eating a peach or an apple—is the result of a complex combination of perceptions, including taste, temperature, texture, and, especially, odor.

Taste itself is limited to detecting five basic sensations: sweet, salty, sour, bitter, and umami, or savory, the taste of glutamate, a building block of proteins found in bacon, chicken broth, and certain cheeses. Tastes are detected by taste buds embedded in the tongue, mouth, and throat. Those on the tongue are found in the little bumps, or papillae (from the Latin for "pimples"). When we're born, our tongues possess 5,000 taste buds. Each taste bud consists of up to 100 sensory cells that respond to the different categories of taste. The sensation of taste occurs when tiny molecules released by the food we eat stimulates our taste cells in our taste buds. The signal then travels along taste nerves to taste centers in the brain stem responsible for basic responses to food, and also to higher brain areas in the cerebral cortex for conscious perception of taste.

Not everyone's ability to taste is the same. When it comes to tasting particular bitter compounds, 25 percent of Americans are "nontasters," unable to detect the compounds; 25 percent are "supertasters," especially sensitive to the bitterness; and the rest are medium tasters, somewhere in between. This is important because the ability to detect bitterness in foods often affects our food choices. Supertasters may avoid broccoli, Brussels sprouts, and other vegetables because the bitter taste is too intense.

As with smell, loss of taste can signal serious underlying conditions or diseases, including diabetes, malnutrition, and diseases of the nervous system such as multiple sclerosis.

HOW TASTE IS TESTED

Your doctor can determine your ability to taste with the help of several tests. Some are designed to measure your taste threshold, the lowest concentration of a chemical that you can detect. Others measure your ability to compare tastes of different chemicals and detect increasing intensity of the chemicals' concentration.

HOW TO PRESERVE YOUR SENSE OF TASTE

To maintain a good sense of taste:

- Don't smoke.
- Practice good oral hygiene. Tell your dentist if you notice any problems with your sense of taste.

If you've lost some of your ability to taste, try adding flavor by preparing foods with aromatic herbs, hot spices, sharp cheese, olive oil, or toasted nuts.

COMMON PROBLEMS WITH TASTE

True problems with taste, which result from an interruption in the transfer of taste sensations to the brain, are very rare. The most common taste-related troubles include hypogeusia, or the reduced ability to taste—usually a temporary disorder; disgeusia, a persistent bad taste in the mouth, often bitter or salty, which most often affects older people; and ageusia, the inability to detect one or more of the five taste categories, most often caused by head trauma, radiation therapy, and surgical procedures. Frequent sources of taste problems are:

- **Medications.** Certain medications, such as antibiotics, drugs to lower cholesterol or blood pressure, antidepressants, and antianxiety drugs, can create a bad taste in your mouth or cause you to lose taste. Some combinations of medications may reduce saliva, causing dry mouth and taste problems.
- **Dental problems.** These include gum disease, inflammation, dentures, and mouth infections.
- **Head injuries.** Injuries to the base of the skull can damage facial nerves involved in smell, which affects taste.
- **Infections.** In particular, middle ear infections and upper respiratory infections such as colds and flu may temporarily affect taste.
- **Heavy smoking**, especially pipe smoking.

Other causes include vitamin deficiencies, radiation therapy for cancers of the head and neck, and certain diseases, including Bell's palsy and Sjögren's syndrome.

If you think you have a problem with taste, see your doctor. In addition to the taste tests noted above, an x-ray or a CAT scan can reveal trouble with the nerves in your mouth or head. If impaired taste is properly diagnosed, it can often be treated with medication.

HOW THE SENSE OF TASTE CHANGES WITH AGE

After the age of 50 we may lose some taste buds, but in general, our sense of taste remains robust into old age. More often, the age-related decline in our sense of smell accounts for the diminished ability to enjoy flavors. Serious taste problems are not usually the result of normal aging but are caused by medications, injury, or disease.

TOUCH

Touch is the sense we use to explore and evaluate our physical environment, to avoid harm from hot, cold, or damaging substances, and to enjoy stroking the soft fur behind our dogs' ears or the relaxing heat of a warm bath. It's what allows us to feel that mosquito landing on our skin and the hammer dropped on our toe.

Unlike our other senses, which originate in particular locations in the body, our sense of touch is spread all over, residing in millions of microscopic nerve endings, or receptors, tucked into the layers of our skin. Some 20 different kinds of touch receptors respond to movement, pressure, temperature, and pain. When they're stimulated, these receptors flash the signal to the spinal cord, which carries the touch messages to the brain, where they are interpreted.

Touch receptors are not evenly distributed in our skin, which is one reason we're more sensitive to touch on our lips and fingertips than on our backs or thighs. The density of touch receptors in a particular area determines its sensitivity.

Some touch receptors, known as proprioceptors, give the brain vital information about changes in the position of limbs and the condition of internal organs.

HOW TOUCH IS TESTED

Neurologists may test the sense of touch by measuring "two-point discrimination"—the ability to discriminate two points pushing on your skin. Your fingertips can normally distinguish the sensation of two touch stimuli just 2 to 3 millimeters apart; your thighs can distinguish the two points only if they're 42 millimeters apart. If you have cut your finger badly, a test for two-point discrimination will reveal whether a nerve has been severed.

Other tests to evaluate your tactile sense involve the neurologist lightly touching with a tissue your fingers and toes while your eyes are closed and asking you to identify when you feel the sensation. Your ability to sense pain is tested by having the neurologist touch your fingers and hand alternately with the sharp tip of a safety pin and the blunt end to determine whether you can discern the difference. Your sense of vibration is tested by holding a vibrating tuning fork on the nail bed of your index finger.

HOW TO PRESERVE YOUR SENSE OF TOUCH

To protect yourself against dangers associated with changes in your sense of touch, it may help to follow these tips:

- Inspect your body for injuries, and pay special attention to your feet. If you find a cut or other injury, treat it.
- Adjust the maximum temperature on your water heater to reduce the risk of scalding.
- Dress according to the temperature, taking care to wear warm socks and gloves or mittens in cold weather.

COMMON PROBLEMS WITH TOUCH

Some people experience the sensation of "pins and needles" (known as paresthesia), pain for no apparent reason (dysesthesia), and sensory loss, usually in the hands and feet. Changes in the sense of touch may arise from other health problems, including:

- Poor blood circulation
- Skin or nerve damage caused by trauma
- Nerve damage caused by chronic disease such as diabetes
- Thiamine deficiency
- Neurological disorders
- Spinal cord lesions
- Certain medications

If you suspect you've experienced an alteration in your sense of touch, see your health care provider. You may be referred to a neurologist, a doctor who specializes in diseases of the central nervous system (brain and spinal cord) and peripheral nervous system (nerves to organs and muscles).

HOW THE SENSE OF TOUCH CHANGES WITH AGE

As we age, our sensitivity to touch often diminishes. This may occur because of decreased bloodflow to touch receptors or to the brain and spinal cord, or because aging skin becomes thinner, drier, and less elastic, reducing sensitivity to pressure, vibration, and temperature. Peripheral neuropathy, nerve damage in our fingers, toes, and feet, may also cause loss of touch sensitivity.

Whatever the cause, this loss may put older people at risk for injuries, such as damage to feet and fingers, pressure sores and ulcers, burns, frostbite, heatstroke, and hypothermia. After the age of 50, some people have a diminished sense of pain and reduced proprioception—the sense of where the body is in space—increasing the risk of falls.

roductive Choices Fertility and Preg
enopause Sexual Abuse and Sexual A
in Teeth Hair and Nails Body Weigh
etabolism Blood Sugar Eating and Exc
uscles Bones Joints Heart and Blood
d Respiration Common Infectious Di
utoimmune Disease Cancer Vision He
hell, Taste, and Touch Mental Health
nce Abuse Making Change Managing
d Sleeping Well Shifting Your Food En
ent Getting Active Screenings and H
aintenance Reproduction Sexuality an
l Health Reproductive Choices Fertilit
egnancy Menopause Sexual Abuse an
l Assault Skin Teeth Hair and Nails
eight and Metabolism Blood Sugar
d Excreting Muscles Bones Joints Hear
ood Lungs and Respiration Common
us Diseases Autoimmune Disease C

PART VIII

Headstrong
Minding Your Emotional and Mental Health

Most of us would agree: Good physical health begins with mental well-being—feeling self-confident, calm, and fulfilled. Although more and more health care professionals are beginning to embrace this connection between mind and body, we still have a long way to go. Unfortunately, many of us still do not pay attention to our mental health the way we do our physical health. We're far more apt to seek treatment for a sprained ankle than anxiety. Our teenage girls are more likely to get professional help for acne than for stress or eating disorders. This unconscionable situation may be rooted in the stigma attached to mental health issues. Because of the shame we associate with mental health problems, we fear naming them and instead try to ignore, minimize, or discount mental or emotional difficulties. The problem, of course, is that depression, anxiety, and excessive stress all have a profoundly negative impact on both body and mind. Stress suppresses immunity. Depression is a serious risk factor for chronic diseases such as osteoporosis and heart disease.

As a young adult, I had serious bouts of depression and severe anxiety attacks. I was lucky: I received excellent professional help from a psychiatrist I saw regularly for a couple of years while I was at college. He gave me essential tools for recognizing my emotions, strategies for dealing with them, and the awareness to know when I needed to get help. Dr. Edwards, more than any other health care provider I've ever had, made a profound difference to my well-being. I credit him with my present state as a happy, well-adjusted, and productive woman.

Statistics suggest that most women at some point in their lives will be affected by a mental health issue. The problem affects people of all races and all socioeconomic and educational strata. The sad reality is that most don't get the help they need and instead are at risk for experiencing prolonged periods of distress.

My advice is this: Keep an open mind about seeking assistance from a mental health professional. Pay attention to your state of mind and your mental health concerns—whether it's anxiety, depression, or substance abuse—and address them just as you would a broken bone. Life is too short to lose months or even years to unhappiness. Your mind—and your body—deserve better. Think of your mental health not just as the absence of mental illness but as a positive, productive state of mind that you can strengthen, nourish, and protect.

To foster positive mental health and well-being, follow these **S.M.A.R.T.** strategies:

1. Protect your head; wear seat belts and, when appropriate, helmets for certain sports.
2. Build vigorous activity into your week.
3. Exercise your brain.
4. Maintain social connections.
5. Get the sleep you need to feel rested.
6. Manage stress.
7. Avoid substance abuse.
8. Seek mental health help when you need it.

23

Mental Health

To understand mental health, you need to understand a little about the brain.

Your brain defines you, determines everything you think, feel, understand, remember, sense, and say. All of this essential mental activity is contained within a mass of pinkish gray tissue weighing only about 3 pounds. Given its array of powers, it's no wonder the brain is an energy hog: It requires massive amounts of oxygen and glucose to run smoothly. Although it makes up only 2 percent of your body weight, it uses up about 20 percent of the oxygen and fuel in your body. Like other body parts, it needs special care and maintenance, especially as it ages.

The brain is divided into regions that work together to allow its wizardry of functions. Deep in the center lies a set of core structures responsible for instinctive behaviors vital to our survival. These include the brain stem, which controls such basic, automatic functions as breathing, digestion, blood pressure, heart rate, and alertness. Right above the brain stem is the hypothalamus, a small structure that controls your pituitary gland, which releases hormones and regulates drives such as hunger, thirst, and sex. At the back of the brain is the cerebellum, which helps coordinate your movements, all the walking, eating, and dancing you do in a day. Above these core central structures resides the cerebrum, the bulging hemispheres that fill your skull, making up more than 80 percent of your brain mass. Capping the cerebrum is a slender layer of deeply convoluted "gray matter" known as the cerebral cortex, which produces your thoughts and language, your ability to learn and solve problems. Scientists have mapped areas, or lobes, of the cortex that specialize in specific tasks. The frontal lobe is the seat of many higher cognitive functions, such as reasoning, planning, solving problems, and making decisions; the parietal lobe processes sensory information related to touch, pressure, temperature, and pain. The temporal lobe is concerned with perception and recognition of auditory stimuli and memory, and the occipital lobe processes and interprets visual information.

Our brains are also divided into right and left halves. The right side controls the left half of your body; the left side controls the right half of your body. For most people, the right side is critical for spatial and perceptual faculties; the left side, for speech. The left and right hemispheres are connected by the corpus callosum, a thick band of nerve fibers that allow for communication between the two hemispheres.

The real work of your brain goes on in its 100 billion or so individual nerve cells, or neurons. These cells link with one another at junctions called synapses to form networks that communicate in a flash of electricity and chemistry. Each of the brain's neurons can send and receive signals from millions of other neurons. In this way, messages flash through the brain's elaborate networks of nerves, creating thoughts, sensations, memories, and moods. The signals move through individual neurons as a little electrical charge, or nerve impulse. They pass between neurons by traveling across a synapse in a tiny burst of chemicals called neurotransmitters. Among the dozens of neurotransmitters active in the brain are adrenaline, dopamine, and serotonin. When these neurotransmitters lock on to receptors on adjacent neurons, they may trigger nerve impulses in that neuron. Certain neurological illnesses and mental health disorders may be linked with too much or too little of these neurotransmitters. Alzheimer's, for instance, appears to be associated with low levels of the neurotransmitter acetylcholine, and Parkinson's disease may be linked with insufficient dopamine.

WHAT'S SO SPECIAL ABOUT THE FEMALE BRAIN?

Your brain, just like the rest of your body, differs in subtle ways from a man's. Although male and female brains are alike in many ways, recent research suggests that there are significant sex differences in their construction and chemistry.

Women's brains are smaller than men's by about 15 to 20 percent. However, size is by no means the whole story. Men may have more neurons, but women have more connections between them. We tend to have more elaborate and extensive linkage from cell to cell, especially in the "executive center" of the brain, the frontal region involved in judgment and decision making. We also have more cross talk between the two halves of the brain. And in some regions, we have a higher density of nerve cells. In the center of the cortex specialized for aspects of language and hearing, for example, women have 11 percent more neurons than men do.

Science suggests that an important factor in shaping the male and female brain is the level of exposure to sex hormones that bathe the fetal brain early in development. These hormones play a key role in directing the brain's organization and wiring. Thanks in part to these hormonal differences in early development and to environmental effects, a woman's frontal cortex is generally bulkier than a man's, as are portions of her limbic system, the region of the brain involved in emotional responses. Parts of a woman's hypothalamus—a key player in sexual behavior—are smaller, as are portions of her parietal cortex—important for spatial perception—and her amygdala, involved in fear and processing emotionally arousing information.

These differences go well beyond explaining why women have a bigger vocabulary than men do or are more inclined to ask for directions. They may actually point to important distinctions in how we keep our brains healthy, especially for women who may suffer from conditions such as depression, addiction, and post-traumatic stress disorder (PTSD). For instance, male and female brains have different ways of processing stressful or emotionally arousing events and images into memory—a distinction that may affect how women are treated for PTSD. In addition, it turns out that women metabolize serotonin (a neurotransmitter involved in mediating emotional behavior) differently, which may suggest one reason that we're more susceptible than men are to depression. This difference may also have implications for treatment.

STAYING FIT FROM THE NECK UP: MAINTAINING BRAIN AND MENTAL HEALTH

As we grow older, our brains lose some of their tissue mass and ability to make neurotransmitters; they also may become less agile in certain ways. Many scientists believe that with aging comes deterioration in executive brain functions such as memory, learning, language use, attention, and concentration. *Age-related cognitive decline* is the medical term for this gradual erosion of mental power, and women may be a little less vulnerable to these age-related changes than are men. On the other hand, women are more prone to dementia.

Although there are no guarantees, you can help minimize these changes by making a few brain- and mind-centered lifestyle changes:

- **Protect your head.** To prevent head injuries, always wear seat belts and use a helmet when bicycling. A few years ago, a seat belt and air bags saved my head in a head-on car collision. I can't count the number of times I've been saved by wearing a helmet. When I was young, I suffered two major head traumas while horseback riding; both times my helmet saved my life. Now I have two different helmets, one for each of my favorite sports—rock climbing and bike riding.

- **Know your cholesterol and blood pressure numbers and manage them.** High blood pressure, diabetes, and heart disease can boost your risk of memory loss and dementia. High cholesterol in your forties has been linked with an increased risk of Alzheimer's disease. Take action to keep your numbers—especially your cholesterol, body weight, blood pressure, and blood sugar—at recommended levels.

- **Build vigorous activity into your week.** Research suggests that people who exercise have a reduced risk of Alzheimer's disease and other cognitive disorders compared with people who do not exercise. They also have less overall cognitive decline and better executive brain functioning. Evidence suggests that vigorous aerobic exercise boosts bloodflow to the brain. It also stimulates the production of hormones and a chemical called brain-derived neurotrophic factor (BDNF), important in the birth and growth of brain cells. In my view, if there is one reason to exercise, this is it. Do whatever exercise you like to get your blood pumping: Walk for a half hour, dance, swim, do yoga or tai chi, golf, play tennis, or lift weights.

- **Exercise your mind.** Although many of us are conscientious about exercising our bodies, we need to be equally vigilant about exercising our minds and keeping intellectually stimulated. The old adage is true: Use it or lose it! Mental activity fortifies brain cells and the links between them. Exercise your cognitive functions by reading, writing, playing card games, doing crossword puzzles, learning a foreign language, or mastering a new computer program.

- **Maintain social connections.** Research shows that social activities keep stress levels low, which helps boost the health of brain cells. Keep your social connections by working, volunteering, spending time with neighbors, and engaging in community and civic activities.

- **Get enough sleep.** Sleep plays a large role in maintaining the brain's functions. There is no set amount of sleep that is right for everyone, but if you are tired, your body is trying to tell you that you need more sleep. (See Chapter 25 for tips on getting sufficient rest.)

- **Manage stress.** Chronic stress can actually rewire parts of the brain involved in emotion, memory, and decision making, making us more susceptible to anxiety and depression. (See Chapter 25 for strategies to help deal with negative stress.)
- **Avoid substance abuse.** Don't smoke or use illicit drugs. Limit your alcohol intake. New research shows that people who smoke or drink heavily (more than two drinks per day) develop Alzheimer's disease 2 to 5 years earlier than those who do not smoke or drink heavily.
- **Eat a brain-healthy diet.** A healthful diet rich in whole grains, nuts, seeds, fruits, vegetables, and fish provides you with all of the vitamins and minerals that you need to maintain good mental health as you grow older. We know that the B vitamins (especially folate, B_6, and B_{12}), vitamin E, and omega-3s that come from these foods are important for cognition as we grow old. At this point, there is little evidence that supplements offer any advantage; in fact, they may cause some harm.
- **Get mental health help when you need it.** If you're feeling blue for more than a few weeks or if anxiety is impeding your ability to work, play, or enjoy life, seek out the help of a mental health professional.

HEADACHES

According to the World Health Organization, headaches are extraordinarily common among women all over the world. They occur in us more frequently than they do in men, are more intense, and last longer. Stress and hormones may play a role in this.

I'm lucky that I don't often get headaches. If I do get one, I take an acetaminophen, and it usually goes away. But a number of my close friends and colleagues get migraines, and I know how debilitating they can be. For them, relief has been slow in coming. Fortunately, we're making better progress now in the prevention and treatment of migraines and other serious headaches, and there are a number of effective preventive, self-care, and medical treatments to help you manage them.

If you get headaches regularly, consider keeping a headache diary. (You can view a sample headache diary at headaches.org.) Note what you are doing when your headaches strike and try to identify possible triggers (such as lack of sleep, a specific food or drink, or stress). This diary will help you understand the patterns of occurrence and provide useful information for your health care provider.

ANATOMY OF A HEADACHE

So what causes that throbbing, stabbing, or aching head pain? Not your brain, which lacks pain-sensitive nerve fibers. Rather, it's the vast network of pain-sensitive nerves that run over your scalp and in the muscles of your head and neck, in the blood vessels at the base of your brain, and in the meninges (the membranes covering your brain and spinal cord). These nerves are capped by nociceptors, endings that can be triggered by stress or dilated blood vessels, firing a pain signal that travels to the brain.

There are several common types of headaches:

Tension Headache

This is the most prevalent type of headache, accounting for about 90 percent of all cases. It's more common in women than in men, and especially in people ages 20 to 50. The pain ranges from mild to moderately intense and may feel like a dull ache or a squeezing of the forehead, scalp, or neck. A tension headache can last for just half an hour or a whole week. It may occur rarely or frequently. Among the triggers are stress, poor posture, inadequate sleep, lack of physical activity, anxiety or depression, and hormonal changes.

Despite their prevalence, tension headaches are not well understood. Until recently, scientists believed that the pain was caused by muscle tension or contraction in the face, scalp, and neck resulting from stress or emotion. But new research suggests that tension headaches may be linked to fluctuations in the brain chemicals that help nerves communicate, including serotonin and endorphins. These chemical changes may activate pain networks in the brain and interfere with its ability to suppress pain signals.

Tension headaches are generally treated with analgesics such as aspirin and acetaminophen. Some people benefit from a hot shower, massage, or relaxation therapy.

To help prevent tension headaches, follow these guidelines:

- Stick to regular eating and sleeping schedules.
- Stay physically active.
- Use stress management techniques.
- Maintain good posture to minimize strain.
- Do stretching and strengthening exercises for your neck, shoulders, and back.
- Avoid excessive caffeine (the amount depends on your individual tolerance).

Migraines

Migraine headaches are second only to tension headaches in prevalence among women. Up to 17 percent of women have experienced at least one migraine—a number that is two to three times the rate of migraine occurrence for men. Migraines in women may be hormonally driven. My coauthor, Jenny, began getting migraines when she was 12 years old. Her migraines are preceded by an "aura," a set of symptoms such as scotoma (a small blind spot surrounded by bright light and zigzagging lines that tends to expand), difficulty speaking, and numbness in her limbs. The severe headache that follows is accompanied by nausea, vomiting, intolerance to light and sound, and other symptoms. She's lucky: Her migraines occur only rarely now, and she staves off the worst of them by resting in a dark, quiet room.

Migraines are usually marked by severe pain in the temple or behind the eye on one or both sides of the head that typically lasts from 4 hours to a few days. They may occur several times a week or just once or twice a year.

Many people who get migraines have a family history of the disorder. (Jenny's dad had migraines, too.) The nature of the genetic link is unknown; it may be related to an inherited abnormality in the regulation of blood vessels. Migraines are thought to involve sudden changes in the function of the brain's blood vessels. Recent research points to the possible role of serotonin, a neurotransmitter in the brain that can act to constrict blood vessels, as well as chemicals that cause inflammation and swelling.

There are two main types of migraines, classic and common. People with the classic variety typically experience an aura 10 to 30 minutes before the onset of the headache. As in Jenny's case, this often takes the form of a scotoma and may also include numbness in the hands and arms that extends upward to the face, difficulty with language and speech, and confusion. Those who get the more prevalent "common" migraine do not experience the aura. Both types are characterized by intense, incapacitating head pain that can last for days.

Some evidence suggests various triggers for migraines, including:

- **Hormonal changes.** Fluctuations in estrogen appear to trigger migraines in some women. The headaches often begin in women around the time of puberty and occur just before or after their periods. Sometimes headaches develop or their pattern changes during pregnancy or menopause. If this is the case for you, your headaches may worsen if you're taking contraceptives or hormone therapy.

- **Foods.** Among possible food triggers are red wine, aged cheese, chocolate, milk, nuts, cured or smoked meats containing nitrates, coffee, tea, and monosodium glutamate (MSG), although evidence of food triggers is largely anecdotal and has not been proven.
- **Skipping meals** or fasting
- **Bright or flickering lights** or other strong sensory stimuli, such as intense perfumes or other scents
- **Disruptions in sleep-wake patterns**—either getting too little or too much sleep
- **Intense physical exertion**
- **Fatigue**
- **Stress**
- **Changes in weather,** barometric pressure, season, or altitude
- **Some medications**

If you experience an aura or feel a headache coming on, try to lie down in a dark, quiet, cool room. Put a cold compress over your eyes or on the back of your neck. Some women find they can decrease the frequency and severity of migraines by making lifestyle changes. These include avoiding the triggers listed above, getting regular aerobic exercise (e.g., swimming or brisk walking), eating meals regularly, getting enough sleep (but not oversleeping), and practicing meditation or deep relaxation. If estrogen seems to trigger your migraines, you may want to talk with your doctor about avoiding or reducing the use of birth control pills or hormone therapy.

Although there is no cure for migraines, medications for managing the pain and preventing full-blown attacks have improved dramatically in the past 5 to 10 years. If you get chronic migraines, discuss with your doctor possible medications to prevent attacks or relieve the pain.

Sinus Headaches and Other Headaches Caused by Infections

A sinus headache occurs when the membranes lining your sinuses (the air-filled cavities in the head) become infected as a result of a bad cold or an allergy. As the cavities fill with fluid from the inflamed membranes, they become tender and painful. Treatment includes antibiotics, decongestants, and analgesics. I get a sinus infection and the accompanying headache about once a year, usually when I have a bad head cold and have to fly. If it is a full-blown sinus infection, I take antibiotics, and the infection and headache go away within a day or two. However, I should say that recent research suggests that several types of sinus infection are not bacterial and thus not affected by antibiotics. If you have a sinus headache for more than a few days, see your health care provider for proper care.

Headaches can also occur with the fever that accompanies pneumonia, mumps, measles, the flu, strep throat, and tonsillitis.

Cluster Headaches

These are a relatively rare form of headache marked by episodes of intense, piercing pain on one side of the head, usually around the eye, occurring in clusters at the same time(s) of day for several weeks. The pain typically lasts for an hour or two before dissipating. Other symptoms include nausea, runny nose, agitation, and sensitivity to light, sound, and smell. The headaches typically begin between age 20 and 50 and are strongly linked with cigarette smoking. Medications are available to reduce pain and ward off future attacks.

WHEN TO WORRY

Headaches, even when they're severe, do not usually indicate underlying disease. However, occasionally they signal a serious medical problem, such as an aneurysm, a stroke, or a brain tumor. If you have any of the following symptoms, see your doctor or go to an emergency room:

- Sudden, severe headache
- Headache with stiff neck, fever, rash, seizures, convulsions, weakness, numbness, eye or ear pain, vision trouble, speaking difficulties, confusion, or loss of consciousness
- Serious headache after a blow to the head
- Chronic, progressive headache that is precipitated by coughing, exertion, straining, or a sudden movement
- Onset of new, persistent headache pain
- Headache that disrupts daily life

MENTAL HEALTH, MOODS, AND EMOTIONS

Your thoughts, feelings, moods, and emotions have a powerful influence on your overall physical well-being. The most common mental health issues—depression and anxiety—can deeply affect your health and compromise your quality of life. Likewise, chronic stress and your reaction to it may harm your mind, brain, and other organs. Fortunately, there are some excellent strategies for managing these issues. Ways to identify negative stress and strategies for neutralizing its toxic effects are dealt with in Chapter 25, "Managing Stress and Sleeping Well."

ANXIETY

Everyone has mild, temporary anxiety in the course of normal life: Feeling nervous when you have to speak in public, for instance, or worrying about the health of a spouse or friend is entirely normal. In fact, a little anxiety is a good thing, part of a survival instinct rooted in predicting harm and learning to avoid it. But some people suffer from excessive anxiety.

When I was a teenager, I developed severe anxiety. People have always thought of me as social and outgoing, but I often feel ill at ease in social situations. In fact, I still get physically anxious when I'm going to a large social gathering where I don't know many people. But because of the mental health counseling I received, I learned some basic strategies for dealing with the problem. I've learned to cope with these feelings and to function well despite them.

Specialists define an anxiety disorder as persistent anxiety that lasts 6 months or longer. Different anxiety disorders have different symptoms, but they tend to center on irrational fearfulness, uncertainty, or dread. Most can be successfully treated with psychotherapy, including cognitive-behavioral therapy (therapy aimed at changing thoughts, attitudes, and responses so that feelings will change), and sometimes medication.

- **Generalized anxiety disorder (GAD).** You may have GAD if you worry excessively about a variety of everyday problems for at least 6 months. GAD affects 4 to 7 million people in this country, including twice as many women as men. People with the disorder constantly expect the worst and obsess about money, health issues, or family or work troubles. They often have trouble sleeping and experience headaches, fatigue, edginess, irritability, sweating, and nausea. GAD tends to run in families and is most often treated with medication or psychotherapy.

- **Panic disorder.** This is marked by sudden and repeated attacks of terror that are accompanied by a cluster of severe physical symptoms, including chest pain, pounding heart, shortness of breath, dizziness, and sweating or feeling chilled. The disorder affects about 6 million American adults, and occurs twice as often in women as men. It appears to have a genetic component. Panic disorder can be successfully treated with medication or cognitive psychotherapy to help change thinking patterns.

- **Obsessive-compulsive disorder (OCD).** People with OCD have persistent, upsetting obsessions that create deep anxiety (e.g., a fixation on germs). They use rituals, or compulsions (such as excessive hand washing), to try to control the anxiety. The disorder most often appears in youth or early adulthood. Recent studies suggest that roughly 2 percent of women and men ages 18 to 54 have this disorder. It is often successfully treated with medications and/or a form of cognitive-behavioral therapy that involves desensitizing sufferers to situations that cause them fear or anxiety.

- **Phobias.** These are persistent, irrational fears of objects or situations that pose little or no threat. Common examples include heights, enclosed spaces, water, spiders, flying, and injuries involving blood. People with phobias may know that their fears are irrational but nonetheless are unable to control them, so that they suffer a panic attack, severe anxiety, and disruption of social interactions or daily life. Twice as many women as men are affected by phobias. They tend to first appear in youth and respond well to specific cognitive-behavioral techniques, such as desensitization.

- **Social phobia, or social anxiety disorder.** This disorder is marked by a tendency to feel excessively anxious and self-conscious in normal social situations to the point where ordinary activities become the focus of dread. People with social phobia have an overwhelming fear of being observed and judged by others. Symptoms include trembling, trouble talking, flushing, and profuse sweating.

- **Post traumatic stress disorder (PTSD).** This severe form of anxiety may develop after a traumatic incident such as a natural disaster, bombing, war experience, plane crash, car accident, mugging, rape, torture, intimate partner violence, or child abuse. People with PTSD typically relive the trauma through flashbacks, nightmares, and hallucinations. Symptoms most often begin within a few months of the incident but sometimes occur much later. Women are more likely than men to develop the disorder. It is usually treated effectively with medication and cognitive-behavioral therapy. I had a mild form of PTSD after I was in a horrific head-on car crash several years ago. Although the physical trauma healed quickly, I was fixated on the crash for months and relived it in my mind over and over throughout the day. Fortunately, the trauma eased eventually, and I suffered no long-lasting effects.

VIOLENCE, SEXUAL ABUSE, AND EMOTIONAL HEALTH

According to the World Health Organization, sexual violence, sexual abuse, and intimate partner violence against women is a major public health problem. Each year, women in this country experience about 4.8 million intimate-partner–related physical assaults and rapes. If you're sitting around a table with a group of a dozen women or so, it's very likely that three or more of them have been sexually abused or sexually assaulted at some point in their lives. All women, regardless of marital or social status, race, religion, or age, are at risk for sexual assault. However, young women are especially at risk. Some 67 percent of victims of sexual assault reported to law enforcement agencies were under age 18; about 34 percent of all victims were under age 12.

Apart from the serious physical dangers violence and abuse may inflict, this kind of trauma may have profound negative consequences on emotional health, increasing risk of depression, post-traumatic stress disorder, sleep difficulties, eating disorders, and emotional distress. If you have suffered sexual assault or sexual abuse and you need help, call the National Sexual Assault Hotline at 1-800-656-HOPE (4673). If you have experienced intimate partner violence, call the National Domestic Violence Hotline 1-800-799-SAFE (7233), or 1-800-787-3224 TTY, or visit www.ndvh.org. If you have experienced violent trauma of this kind, seek counseling and support at a counseling center from a knowledgeable person who is experienced in helping victims of sexual assault or intimate partner violence. Try to talk openly about the experience, and expect that healing will take time.

Treatment

If you think you may have one of the disorders listed above, seek immediate evaluation and treatment from a licensed and experienced mental health professional.

DEPRESSION

It's important to distinguish between sadness and depression. Sadness is a normal human response to unfortunate situations. It can be a useful emotion, one that helps us learn from our mistakes. It's usually short-lived and should not be treated with medications but allowed to run its course. Taking medications for normal sadness may dull your motivation to improve an unhealthy situation that's causing you sorrow.

Depression, on the other hand, is characterized by persistent negative feelings of sadness, hopelessness, worthlessness, anxiety, or emptiness that disrupt daily life, interfering with the ability to work, eat properly, sleep, and enjoy life. Women are twice as likely to become depressed as men are. This may have to do with the interaction between our sex hormones and our stress response. Symptoms vary dramatically in kind, severity, and duration, but they may include crying spells, difficulty sleeping, diminished libido, lack of interest in activities you once enjoyed, and irregular eating patterns.

Depressive disorders sometimes run in families, suggesting that there may be a hereditary component. They are likely brought on by a combination of genetic, environmental, and psychological factors and appear to be linked with lower activity of the neurochemicals serotonin and norepinephrine. Medications that affect the levels of these chemicals can be effective in relieving symptoms. Bouts of depression may occur only once in a lifetime or recur several times, and may be triggered by excessive stress, chronic illness, or difficulties in some aspect of life, such as marriage troubles or financial difficulties. Disruption of the body's natural rhythms, known as circadian rhythms, can also cause depressive episodes.

All my life I've had short, transient bouts of depression. These "blue periods" tend to be seasonal, occurring in late September and early October and sometimes in February, too. Over the years, I've come to recognize the pattern of these depressive bouts. I expect them, understand them, and know that they're short-lived, nothing to panic about. When I'm feeling low, I have more conversations with my very understanding husband, to try to identify situational causes of my unhappiness. Often, I have a *eureka!* moment, when I realize that there is something in particular about life that's troubling me, and then I can address it. Sometimes it's a matter of needing a short break from work or family, or getting more regular exercise. If the depression persists, however, I don't hesitate to get professional help.

Depression can heighten risks for other illnesses, including heart disease, osteoporosis, HIV, and asthma, and it may lead to suicidal feelings. It can often be successfully treated with psychotherapy, antidepressant medications, and, as a last resort in extreme cases, electroconvulsive therapy. There is also now solid research that moderate to vigorous exercise can treat and manage moderate to severe depression.

Among the types of depression are:

- **Bipolar disorder.** Once known as manic depression, bipolar disorder is a chronic, often recurring condition marked by a spectrum of moods, ranging from depression to mania. The mood changes may be sudden and dramatic or gradual. The depressive phase of the disorder is marked by feelings of hopelessness, guilt, pessimism, and helplessness; a loss of interest in usually pleasurable activities; insomnia; diminished or increased appetite; fatigue; trouble concentrating; and irritability. The manic phase may include inappropriate elation, a racing mind, trouble sleeping, irritability, and lapses in judgment and/or social behavior. People with the disorder sometimes also have issues with alcohol and drug abuse. The disorder often runs in families and tends to begin in late adolescence, but it is sometimes not diagnosed until later in life. It can be managed with appropriate treatment, which may include medications and/or psychosocial interventions. Patients with bipolar disorder are at an increased risk of suicidal behavior.

- **Seasonal affective disorder (SAD).** Seasonal affective disorder is a type of depression that occurs cyclically with the seasons. It may result from the effect of reduced sunlight on the body's circadian rhythms, including its production of melatonin, a hormone that fosters sleep, or serotonin, a neurotransmitter involved in regulating mood. Symptoms usually appear in the late fall or early winter and lift during the sunnier days of spring and summer. They include significant seasonal changes in mood, including heightened feelings of hopelessness, anxiety, stress, fatigue, loss of interest in activities you normally enjoy, cravings for carbohydrates or other appetite changes, weight gain, and difficulty concentrating. The disorder most often begins in early adulthood and is diagnosed more often in women than men. You may be more at risk for SAD if you live at higher latitudes or if you have a family history of the disease. To ease symptoms, maximize your time in natural light—get outside on sunny days in winter and sit near bright, sunny windows when you're indoors. Exercise outdoors if you can, practice stress reduction techniques, and stay socially connected. You may also want to consider light therapy, or phototherapy—using a box that emanates bright artificial light to mimic natural light. The therapy is thought to affect circadian rhythms and suppress the body's release of melatonin, which helps alleviate symptoms of SAD.

Are You at Risk?

If you are concerned that you may have depression, ask yourself the following questions:

- Do you have persistent sad, anxious, or "empty" feelings?
- Do you have feelings of hopelessness and/or pessimism?
- Do you have feelings of guilt, worthlessness, and/or helplessness?
- Are you irritable or restless?
- Do you have a loss of interest in activities or hobbies that you once found pleasurable, including sex?
- Do you experience greater than normal fatigue and decreased energy?
- Do you have difficulty concentrating, remembering details, and making decisions?
- Do you experience insomnia, early-morning wakefulness, or excessive sleeping?
- Do you overeat or have a loss of appetite?
- Do you have thoughts of suicide or have you made suicide attempts?
- Do you have persistent aches or pains, headaches, cramps, or digestive problems that do not ease even with treatment?

If you answer "almost always" to more than one of these questions, you may be depressed. Talk to your health care provider to determine whether you need help from a mental health specialist. Of course, if you answered "yes" to having thoughts of suicide, you should seek immediate care.

I can't say it strongly enough: If you think you may be suffering from depression, get help now. Most forms of the condition are effectively treated with therapy or medications.

GRIEF AND LOSS

Unlike depression, grief is a form of sadness, a normal, healthy response to the loss of someone or something you hold dear. It may be painful and long-lasting, reappearing in waves throughout life, and it can have serious psychological and physical effects. But unlike depression, it serves an important purpose, helping you move toward a feeling of peace with your loss.

In the past couple of years, my husband has lost both of his parents. We mourned their passing, but also celebrated their full, rich years that extended until the natural end of their life span. It was a different sort of grief our family experienced when my sister-in-law died of cancer in early midlife, leaving behind two young children. The pain was keen, and we felt it both physically and mentally. We knew it was important to experience our grief fully, to let ourselves feel the magnitude of her loss. This is natural and healthy. Although her loss will always be with us, with the help and support of family and friends we eventually moved on with our lives.

Grief becomes unhealthy only when it is sustained, when a grieving person can't "come out of it." Then it's important to seek professional help.

Grief is highly personal and highly individual: No two people grieve alike. However, there are some strategies that help many people cope:

- **Get support from other people.** This is the most important action you can take to facilitate your own healing. Seek the company and comfort of friends and family, support groups, online communities, your church or other organizations to which you belong, and therapists. Ask for help—whether in the form of a conversation, a meal, or just a hug. Surrounding yourself with others who have been—or currently are in—the same situation can be very helpful. Being with those who "get it" provides significant relief.

- **Take care of yourself.** People who are grieving often neglect their own physical needs. Make sure you eat well, get sufficient sleep, exercise regularly, and avoid alcohol and drugs as a means of avoiding or numbing your pain.

- **Find an outlet.** This may take the form of journaling or writing a letter to your loved one, creating a memorial, bonding with a pet, listening to music that you love, or watching favorite movies. You may want to let out your emotions with your therapist or simply wrap up in your favorite blanket and cry on the couch.

EATING DISORDERS

Eating disorders are distressingly common among women; almost all of us have either experienced one ourselves or know someone close to us who has. The information and advice I offer here may be applicable to you or to someone you know and love.

An eating disorder is a severe disturbance in eating behavior—extreme undereating or overeating, vomiting after meals, or obsessive calorie counting—that is rooted in negative, self-critical, and often distorted attitudes about food, body image, and weight. It is a serious mental health problem. People with eating disorders often use food to deal with emotional discomfort or pain: Holding back from eating may help them feel in control of their lives; overeating may temporarily relieve feelings of anxiety, anger, depression, or loneliness. People with eating disorders often lose all perspective on themselves and come to focus on food and weight to the exclusion of all else.

These disorders often start in adolescence and occur along with other conditions, such as depression, substance abuse, obsessive-compulsive disorder, or anxiety disorders. They can cause serious damage to the heart, kidneys, bones, and teeth and may be life threatening.

Studies suggest that eating disorders affect almost 5 percent of all young women in the United States. Women and girls are much more likely than men are to develop an eating disorder, with females accounting for about 85 to 95 percent of cases of anorexia or bulimia and about 65 percent of cases of binge-eating disorder.

Sometimes it's difficult to distinguish between an eating disorder and normal concerns about weight, diet, and body image. However, there are some warning signs specific to eating disorders. These include skipping meals or making excuses to avoid family dinners, having a distorted image of your own body shape or weight, dieting even when you're thin, obsessing about calories and serving size, using laxatives or diet pills to lose weight, or eating in secret.

Eating disorders are complex, and their biological, behavioral, and social causes are not well understood. They may include:

- **Biological causes.** Twin studies indicate that vulnerability to eating disorders may have a genetic component. Other research points to the possibility that neurological or hormonal imbalances play a role. Some evidence suggests that brain chemicals such as serotonin or dopamine may be abnormal in people with eating disorders.

- **Psychological issues.** Researchers have suggested that various psychological factors may make women more susceptible to eating disorders, including low self-esteem, a tendency toward overachievement and perfectionism, anger management or impulse control issues, family conflicts, or a desire to feel "in control" of life. Women who have been through stressful events such as losing a loved one by death or divorce or other difficult emotional or psychological experiences are more prone to developing an eating disorder. Some researchers believe that women with these disorders may be using food to self-medicate pain and distress.

- **Social issues.** The tendency in our society, and especially in the media and entertainment industries, to equate thinness with beauty and success may exacerbate body image issues. I cringe when I watch television or other media channels with my teenage daughters and see poor body-image messages being conveyed!

The main types of eating disorders are:

- **Anorexia nervosa**—an intense and irrational fear of weight gain or being fat and purposely losing weight to the point of starvation. If you're anorexic, food, calories, and concern with body weight and shape become an obsession. To lose weight, an anorexic may severely restrict her food intake, overexercise, or purge her system of undesired calories by vomiting or using laxatives. The disorder almost always causes amenorrhea (cessation of menstruation)—in fact, this can be one of the deciding symptoms of anorexia. Many times the disorder also causes heart arrhythmias. Anorexic women typically have a BMI of 17.5 or less. (If a person does not have a low BMI but displays other symptoms, the problem is generally diagnosed as a different eating disorder.) Up to 10 percent of people with anorexia nervosa die from it. The mortality rate has been estimated at more than 0.5 percent a year, which is roughly 12 times higher than the annual death rate from all causes for females ages 15 to 24.

- **Bulimia nervosa**—involves a secretive cycle of quick, helpless eating of vast quantities of food, followed by feelings of shame, and purging through vomiting, excessive exercise, fasting, diet pills, diuretics, or laxatives. Symptoms may include damaged teeth and gums, menstrual irregularities, bloating, abnormal

bowel function, dehydration, fatigue, and irregular heartbeat. People with bulimia are usually normal weight or a bit overweight.

- **Binge eating**—compulsive, out-of-control eating beyond the point of comfortable fullness. It differs from bulimia in that the bingers do not regularly
purge after they have eaten. However, they may have feelings of shame or
self-loathing and make repetitive efforts to diet. Body weight varies from
normal to severely obese.

Are You at Risk?

Although the causes of eating disorders are not fully understood, there are some factors, situations, and events that can increase the risk of developing one:

- **Gender and age.** More than 90 percent of people with anorexia and bulimia are
female, and 95 percent are between the ages of 12 and 25. Disturbing recent
research shows that anorexia is affecting more and more girls under the age
of 12.
- **Genetics and biology.** Recent research has focused on the role of genetic and
biological factors in the development of eating disorders. Some studies suggest that women with a mother or sister who has had anorexia nervosa are 12
times more likely than others to develop the disorder themselves.
- **Body shape and weight.** Being overweight or obese can also predispose women
to developing an eating disorder when dissatisfaction with body shape and sub-
sequent dieting spin out of control.
- **Occupation or avocation.** Eating disorders are common in women whose jobs
or favorite activity depend on thinness, such as models, dancers, gymnasts, jock-
eys, and figure skaters.
- **Family background and patterns.** If you feel insecure in your family or your
parents or siblings are critical of you and tease you about your appearance, you
are at higher risk of developing an eating disorder.

The following 10 questions are from a more complete questionnaire offered by an eating disorders organization called Something Fishy. These questions will help you discern whether you, or someone you know, may have an eating disorder.

FEELINGS			
Are you a perfectionist, a person who always wants to be in control, or an overachiever? And/or do you think no matter what you do, it is never enough?	YES	NO	MAYBE
Within your family and/or circle of friends, are you considered "the strong one" who everyone comes to with problems and/or you never seem to talk much about your own?	YES	NO	MAYBE
Do you continuously feel that you are overweight even though others have told you that you are not?	YES	NO	MAYBE
Do family members and/or friends often express concern for your weight loss/gain, your appearance, and/or your eating habits?	YES	NO	MAYBE
Are you depressed, suicidal, stressed out, and/or fatigued? Or do you suffer from anxiety or panic attacks, mood swings, rage, and/or insomnia?	YES	NO	MAYBE
BEHAVIORS			
Do you eat, self-starve, or restrict, binge and/or purge, and/or compulsively exercise when you are feeling lonely, badly about yourself or about a situation, or emotional pressures?	YES	NO	MAYBE
When eating do you ever feel out of control or like you will lose control and not be able to stop? And/or do you try to avoid eating because of this fear?	YES	NO	MAYBE
Do you typically feel guilty after a binge, or after any snack or meal? Do you feel as if you have almost instantly gained weight, like you are a failure, and/or like you have sabotaged yourself?	YES	NO	MAYBE
Do you use self-starvation, purging, diet pills, laxatives, diuretics, and/or obsessive exercise as a way to attempt to lose weight?	YES	NO	MAYBE
Do you weigh yourself often and does the number on the scale dictate your mood and/or self-worth for the day? And/or do you find you are continuously trying to get that number lower?	YES	NO	MAYBE

BEHAVIORS			
Are you constantly "on a diet," and/or counting calories and fat grams? And/or do you feel like you've tried every fad diet or quick-weight-loss scheme?	YES	NO	MAYBE
Do you do any of the following: hide and/or steal food, take laxatives and/or diet pills; eat and/or exercise secretively; avoid eating in public or around others; wear clothes that hide your weight; and/or make excuses (such as "I don't feel well") to avoid meals?	YES	NO	MAYBE
Do you spend a lot of time obsessively cooking for others or reading recipes, and/or studying the nutritional information on food (calories, fat grams, etc.)?	YES	NO	MAYBE

If you have answered *yes* or *maybe* to more than two of these questions, or if you suspect that you may have an eating disorder—or if someone you care about displays typical symptoms—I suggest that you go to either of these two Web sites for more information: something-fishy.org or nationaleatingdisorders.org. Both of these sites have good resources for people with eating disorders.

Treatment

If you think that you have an eating disorder, I urge you to see a health care professional. Without treatment, eating disorders get worse and may cause serious physical and emotional damage. A health care provider can diagnose the disorder, treat any medical problems involved, evaluate possible coexisting conditions such as depression or anxiety disorders, and offer treatment.

Eating disorders are treated most successfully when they're treated early. To effectively address both the physical and the psychological aspects of the disorder, treatment often involves a combination of psychotherapy to help with underlying emotional issues, nutritional counseling, group support, and sometimes medication. Most patients can be treated as outpatients, but some need hospital care. The goal of treatment is to address medical needs, encourage a healthy attitude toward food and body image, and offer productive ways of dealing with life's challenges.

SUBSTANCE ABUSE

Substance abuse is the compulsive or excessive use of controlled substances such as alcohol, illegal drugs, or prescription medications to achieve a "high" or to self-medicate—regardless of the harmful and often dangerous physical, psychological, and social consequences. Drugs and alcohol produce a high by triggering the release of dopamine in the brain, the chemical that activates the brain's pleasure centers. Repeated use of these substances, however, desensitizes the dopamine system so that a person needs more drugs or alcohol to achieve the same high feeling—a phenomenon known as tolerance.

Almost every family has been faced with substance abuse issues of one sort or another. My family is no exception, and it has taken a large toll on us over the years.

In the past, more men than women in this country have been substance abusers, but the gender gap is narrowing. The National Center on Addiction and Substance Abuse (CASA) estimates that 15 million American girls and women use illegal drugs, 32 million smoke cigarettes, and 6 million are alcohol abusers or alcoholics. The economic burden is estimated at several hundred billion dollars a year, and the cost to society in terms of damage to individuals and families is enormous.

The most common form of substance abuse for women is abuse of prescription medications such as painkillers, tranquilizers, and diet pills. A report from the National Institute on Drug Abuse (NIDA) suggests that women are almost 50 percent more likely than men to be prescribed an addictive drug such as a painkiller, a sedative, or an antianxiety drug, and that young women become addicted to antianxiety drugs at almost twice the rate of men.

New brain research suggests that women may be especially vulnerable to addiction in part because of the presence of progesterone in our bodies. Progesterone makes the brain's dopamine-producing cells more sensitive to the effects of drugs, which can lead to greater craving for them. This effect is especially potent in the second half of the menstrual cycle.

Other research shows that the female brain is more susceptible to visual cues, such as advertising for alcohol or cigarettes. So women are more driven than men to desire a drug if they observe someone else indulging in it.

Commonly abused substances include:

- Alcohol
- Nicotine
- Narcotic painkilling drugs
- Marijuana
- Club drugs

Various factors may affect your likelihood of abusing a drug or becoming addicted. These include:

- **Genes.** Drug abuse and addiction tend to run in families and likely involve many genes.
- **Experience.** Growing up in a chaotic home environment, especially where substance abuse is present in family, peers, and community, heightens the risk of substance abuse. Research by CASA shows that 69 percent of women in treatment for substance abuse say they were sexually abused as children.
- **Psychological factors.** Drug dependence is more common in people with other psychological issues, such as anxiety, depression, loneliness, post-traumatic stress disorder, or attention-deficit/hyperactivity disorder.

Among the behavioral signs and symptoms of an alcohol or drug problem are:

- A feeling that you need to drink alcohol or use the drug regularly, sometimes more than once a day
- Planning alcohol or drug use in advance
- Repeated failures to stop use of alcohol or drugs
- Having to drink more or use more drugs to get the same high
- Avoiding friends or family in order to use drugs
- Drinking or using other drugs alone
- Driving under the influence of the drug
- Having "blackouts," when you can't remember what you did the night before
- Efforts to maintain a steady supply of the drug, sometimes including actions you would not ordinarily engage in, such as stealing
- A feeling that using the drug helps solve your problems or offers the only way to have fun and relax

If you think you have a substance abuse problem and want help, contact your doctor or a help line or hotline. (See Resources section.) Most substance abusers who try to stop using drugs on their own do not succeed, in part because long-term drug use changes the brain, strengthening the compulsion to use the drug. Drug abuse and addiction is most often treated with a combination of counseling and medication to control cravings and ease withdrawal symptoms. The sooner you seek help, the greater your chances are for long-term recovery.

COGNITIVE DECLINE

Although gradual age-related cognitive decline is considered normal, sudden or major declines in memory or the ability to learn new information are not; they may signal dementia or degenerative brain disorders that affect the ability to function effectively in daily life. These disorders, which usually occur later in life, are of greater concern to women in part because of our longer life spans. They include:

- **Alzheimer's disease.** Alzheimer's is the most common cause of dementia. It is characterized by structural changes in the brain—tangles of filaments within nerve cells and accumulations of so-called beta-amyloid plaques outside them— that interfere with the transmission of nerve signals, eventually leading to the death of brain cells. There are two types:
  - **Early-onset Alzheimer's,** which affects people ages 30 to 60, is rare and appears to run in families. Some families have a mutation in selected genes on certain chromosomes. Mutations in each of these three genes appear to cause more damaging beta-amyloid to be made in the brain. In families with these mutations, if a parent has the disease, the children have about a 50/50 chance of developing it.
  - **Late-onset Alzheimer's** is more common. Ten percent of people over age 65 and half of those over 85 have the disease.

  My grandmother suffered from Alzheimer's disease beginning in her early to mid-seventies. She lived until her late nineties. It was very difficult for our family to witness her decline. Born in the late 1800s, she had been a high-powered businesswoman well before it was considered normal for women to enter business. She was smart and able, a force to be reckoned with. To see her mind disintegrate was a terrible thing. I admit that getting Alzheimer's is the thing I worry about most as I grow older. Right now I definitely have difficulty with short-term memory, but I'm chalking it up to early menopause.

  Women are at higher risk for Alzheimer's and may suffer more damage from the disease. A common early sign is memory loss—difficulty remembering recent events or the names of familiar people or things. Other signs are trouble with normal daily tasks such as paying bills, increased anxiety, and confusion about the location of familiar places. As the disease progresses, it can cause profound confusion and irritability and the loss of language, reasoning, and comprehension. People with Alzheimer's typically live about 8 years after the onset of symptoms. Treatment includes drugs that may boost brain functioning, but there is currently no cure.

- **Vascular dementia.** Vascular dementia, the second most common type of dementia, occurs when bloodflow to the brain is obstructed. Studies show that about a third of people who have cognitive decline and dementia have damage to the small blood vessels that feed the brain—the kind of damage caused by high blood pressure and diabetes. These conditions increase the risk of vascular dementia, as does smoking, high cholesterol, and a history of heart disease. Mini-strokes often cause the disease. Symptoms of vascular dementia can mimic those of Alzheimer's disease, including diminished capacity for memory and cognitive functioning. Medications are available to help boost blood circulation to the brain and reduce the risk of stroke.

CENTRAL NERVOUS SYSTEM DISORDERS

- **Amyotrophic lateral sclerosis (ALS)** is a rare neurodegenerative disease that attacks the body's motor neurons, causing degeneration in the brain and spinal cord. Often called Lou Gehrig's disease after the baseball player who died of it in 1941, ALS causes muscle weakness, disability, and ultimately, death. It most often strikes people between the ages of 40 and 70. Early symptoms include weakness in a hand, a foot, an arm, or a leg; difficult walking; and slurred speech. Some 1 or 2 percent of cases are inherited, the result of a mutation in a particular gene, but the cause of most cases is a mystery. There is no known cure for the disease; some medications may slow the progression of symptoms.
- **Parkinson's disease** is a chronic progressive movement disorder that results from damage to nerve cells in the brain that control movement and coordination. It most often develops after age 60, but it may occur in younger people as well. Symptoms include tremors, muscle stiffness or rigidity, poor balance, slowed movement, impaired speech, and trouble walking. Although the cause is unknown, there may be a genetic component. If you have a close relative with the disease, your risk is increased by about 5 percent. No cure is currently available, but there are several treatment options, including medication and surgery, to manage the problems associated with the disease.

If you have any of the symptoms associated with these diseases, see your doctor right away. Getting an accurate diagnosis is critical to getting prompt and effective treatment.

eproductive Choices Fertility and Preg
enopause Sexual Abuse and Sexual A
kin Teeth Hair and Nails Body Weigh
etabolism Blood Sugar Eating and Exc
uscles Bones JointsHeart and Blood
nd Respiration Common Infectious Di
utoimmune Disease Cancer Vision H
nell, Taste, and Touch Mental Health
ance Abuse Making Change Managing
nd Sleeping Well Shifting Your Food En
ent Getting Active Screenings and
aintenance Reproduction Sexuality an
l Health Reproductive Choices Fertili
regnancy Menopause Sexual Abuse an
l Assault Skin Teeth Hair and Nails
eight and Metabolism Blood Sugar
nd Excreting Muscles Bones JointsHear
ood Lungs and Respiration Common
us Diseases Autoimmune Disease C

PART IX

Flipping the Switch:
An Action Plan for Health

Up to this point, *The Strong Women's Guide to Total Health* has offered information on the spectrum of health issues important to all women. This section is designed to help you make the changes in your lifestyle and behavior necessary to address your individual health concerns and enhance your overall well-being.

If you could alter certain aspects of your life to improve your health, what would they be? Here's my list of things I'd like to do more consistently every day:

1. Be active in some way.
2. Spend more time with my family, especially sharing meals together.
3. Make time to meditate to calm my active mind.
4. Sit less.
5. Write in my journal.

After reading this book, you probably have a pretty good idea of the health behaviors you do consistently and which you need to work on. You probably also now have a good idea where your health concerns lie. Maybe it's overweight. Or stress. Or lack of sufficient physical activity or sleep. Maybe it's poor dental hygiene.

We all lead busy lives, so it's important to prioritize. Some chapters in this section will resonate for you; others won't. To tailor your own better-health plan, pick and choose what pertains to you. If your concern is weight control, then the eating and physical activity chapters will be of greatest interest. If stress is your nemesis, then start with the chapter on managing stress.

As a general rule, these **S.M.A.R.T.** behaviors will boost your well-being in every way:

1. Take a moment during the day to quiet your mind and body through meditation, yoga, or any other calming activity.
2. Get the sleep you need to feel rested.
3. Create a healthy food environment to eat a little less and eat better.
4. Try to be active in some way every day.
5. Break a sweat at least once a week.
6. Be vigilant about getting regular medical checkups and screenings.
7. Be confident in your ability to make needed change in your life.

24

Making Change

Whatever health issue concerns you, large or small, the key to addressing it most likely lies in changing your behavior.

Behavior is not what we think or feel or believe, but what we *do*. A few years ago, I was not getting enough exercise. It had been that way for close to a decade. I was raising three kids and working long hours, and it was hard to squeeze in the time to run or bike or even lift weights. I walked my dog on the weekends and occasionally got a short run in, but I knew that I wasn't nearly as active or fit as I wanted to be, especially given my profession. After all, I've been working in the field of nutrition and physical activity for more than a quarter century. I know the benefits of exercise and tout them virtually every day on the job. But I was not taking the time myself to practice what I preached.

Then came one day in the spring of 2004 when I was conducting a performance review for my staff. After the review was complete, I asked Rebecca, my close colleague, if there was anything she wanted to discuss with me. She hesitated, and then she said, "Yes, there is. But it's not easy for me to say it."

I encouraged her to go on.

"You're a really bad role model," she told me, "especially considering your job here. You get into the office early. You eat at your desk. We never see you exercise. You're the leader here," she explained. "Those of us who work for you don't feel comfortable taking time in the middle of the day to go out for a run or hit the gym. Your behavior doesn't suggest a culture of valuing exercise even though that's the mission of your job."

It was a sobering moment for me. I realized that Rebecca was absolutely right. I *was* a poor role model. I'm the kind of person who needs something big to get me going.

After a few days of thought, I decided to train for the Boston marathon with my university's team. I began slowly, running a couple of miles three times a week and gradually building up to greater distances. I ran in the late morning or at lunchtime and invited my staff to get out and run with me. It was good for them and good for me.

Now, whenever I can, I try to build exercise into my workday and I urge my colleagues to join me. I'm happier being a better role model and being in much better shape, able to do things that I couldn't have done when I was less fit, such as climb mountains!

THE ELEMENTS OF SUCCESSFUL BEHAVIOR CHANGE

Changing behavior is about the hardest task under the sun, whether it's giving up smoking, exercising more, following a healthy diet, stopping drug or alcohol abuse, or managing stress. This section is designed to help make the task of behavior change easier. Many women's efforts to improve their health fail because of a mismatch between their individual readiness to change and the intervention program they choose to follow. The plans and programs offered in this section are designed to match your individual needs and identify and reinforce the small steps that lead to success.

Two things are critical to successful behavior change: first, believing in your own ability to bring about change, a concept known as self-efficacy; and second, determining your readiness for change.

SELF-EFFICACY

Your sense of self-efficacy strongly influences every phase of your effort to make change. It affects how much effort you expend in a task, how you persist in the face of obstacles, and how you feel about your progress. A robust sense of self-efficacy will help you persevere despite barriers, frustrations, and setbacks.

We tend to motivate ourselves and guide our actions by visualizing our future. People with a well-developed sense of self-efficacy can easily visualize scenarios of success that guide them and support their efforts at change. Those who question their self-efficacy tend to dwell on failures and what may go wrong and often end up sabotaging their own efforts.

Self-efficacy is not something you're born with, but something you learn. It is developed by mastering tasks, sometimes with the help of coaches and friends, and by seeing people like yourself successfully manage similar challenges.

You may need help from someone to build your self-efficacy. For example, if you're setting your sights on regular strength training, you may need a personal trainer or community program to help you feel comfortable with the way you're doing the exercises and reinforce your ability to succeed.

As you gain knowledge and skills needed to accomplish a course of action, your self-efficacy will increase. You will gain confidence in your ability to make change and to maintain it. In other words, it becomes an upward spiral. The more confident you are in your ability to master a task, the more apt you are to do it. The following chapters will give you concrete ways of building your skills, broken down into easily mastered steps.

In starting out, it's helpful to know where you are on the self-efficacy scale. Take a moment to go back to the self-efficacy test you took in the Smart Woman's Health Assessment to see where you fall on the spectrum. You may be in a different place now than you were when you took the assessment: Just reading this book should help you feel more confident and strengthen your self-efficacy. Ask yourself how confident you are that you can make the change. Focus on your past successes. What other difficult things have you accomplished? How can you apply what you learned from those challenges to conquering this one? For instance, if you've been trying to build regular exercise into your days and you managed to do so for a few weeks, ask yourself what made that work.

The test used in the Smart Woman's Health Assessment focuses on nutrition, physical activity, and general health promotion. Its questions do not address every health behavior. To understand your ability to change the specific behavior you wish to change—for example, substance abuse or unsafe sexual habits—you have to ask yourself similar questions about that behavior. I encourage you to develop your own self-efficacy scale focused on the particular behavior that you would like to modify. This will help you see where you are and what you need to do to get where you want to go.

READINESS FOR CHANGE

Are you ready to change your behavior? What has spurred you on? Often, it's some kind of trigger or catalyst, from something as simple as a comment by a colleague or friend (as in my case with exercise) or as momentous as a calamitous health event such as a heart attack. The trigger casts your life in a new light and crystallizes your understanding of the need for change. You can also find or invent your own catalyst, or "switch," that will get you going.

Among the most inspiring stories I know of successful behavior change belongs to my friend Deanne. At age 33, Deanne weighed 268 pounds. She was beset by migraines, high blood pressure, and high cholesterol. She was profoundly unhappy. She had tried diet after diet, but nothing stuck. Deanne told me that she remembers two triggering events that finally spurred her to make a commitment to weight loss and fitness.

"I was at an amusement park with my nephew," she recalls. "We had settled ourselves on a ride. But when they tried to lower the safety bar, it wouldn't close over me. Finally, the attendant came over and asked me to get off the ride. I was horrified. I thought, *I've got to do something!* But then I put it off. That winter, in the hospital I work at, we had several patients who were so heavy that we had to get five or six people to help every time we moved them. They weren't getting any better because their health problems were just made worse by their weight. I thought, *This could easily be me in 20 years, and I don't want that. It's time to do something.*"

Deanne flipped her switch. A few years later, by age 39, Deanne had lost 120 pounds, run the Boston Marathon, and discovered a deep sense of mental and physical well-being.

The bottom line here is that each person needs to find her own "switch" and turn it on. That means setting your mind on the change you wish to make.

THE FIVE STAGES OF CHANGE

Effective self-change like Deanne's depends on doing the right thing at the right time and believing in your ability to succeed. You can do it!

Making permanent behavior change doesn't happen overnight. It often takes 3 to 6 months—sometimes even years—to modify an entrenched behavior. For most people, the change occurs gradually, as part of a five-stage process: precontemplation, contemplation, preparation, action, and maintenance. Different people progress through the stages at different rates, and most move back and forth between the stages or cycle back around before finally attaining their goal.

Before you begin, it's important to understand which stage you're in. For instance, if you're in denial about your own overweight and the accompanying risk of chronic disease, it may be too much to expect yourself to leap into a new set of eating and exercise habits. Ask yourself how ready you are to make a change in your behavior. Are you not yet prepared to make change? Already changing? Somewhere in the middle?

Once you evaluate which stage you're in, then you can form a strategy best suited to that stage.

1. **Precontemplation.** Not yet ready for change. This is the earliest stage, when it hasn't really registered that you actually need to make a change. Try to identify the trigger or key issue that will spur you to make change.
2. **Contemplation.** You're thinking about making a change in the next 6 months or so, but you haven't actually begun to implement it. You're aware of the pros and cons of changing, but not yet sure you want to make a full commitment. This ambivalence can keep you stuck in this stage for long

periods of time. Often, it's a triggering event that tips you into the next stage. Consider what life would be like if you make this change—and if you don't. Contemplate the benefits of the change and the potential barriers that might keep you from it.

3. **Preparation.** You have decided that it's definitely time for a change and are looking into how best to make it within the next month or so. Clarify your goals and write a realistic action plan.

4. **Action.** You have begun to implement your action plan for change and are engaging in the healthy behavior consistently. Identify the toxic cues that might sabotage your success and figure out how to replace them with healthy cues. Surround yourself with friends and relatives or professionals who will support compliance with your behavior change.

5. **Maintenance.** You have been engaging in the behavior consistently for 6 months or longer. Reward yourself for your successes.

RELAPSE

At any stage along the way, relapse may occur. Perhaps you've been faithfully executing your plan but then something derails you—a holiday or life event. You may have to cycle back to the contemplation or preparation phase to get back on track. Most people go forward and backward in the five-stage process. Consider what you learned about yourself from the relapse and about the process of changing behavior. Make the necessary modifications and keep moving forward. The key is not letting your setbacks get you down. Just figure out when and how you can get going again.

RECOGNIZE THAT CHANGE IS HARD

I speak from experience when I say that bringing about permanent behavior change is very, very difficult. For some of my own behavior-change goals, I'm still in the early phases. It's important to recognize that we're not after perfection. We have to prioritize, pick our most urgent issues, and have realistic expectations. Don't punish yourself for setbacks; guilt has no place here, and it's not useful!

My friend Deanne achieved her tremendous success of losing weight by restructuring her personal environment in small, concrete ways. She started walking a half hour each day on a treadmill or outside. She went to Weight Watchers meetings and got a good idea of what and how much she should be eating and found the support she needed. She started strength training and eventually joined a gym. Understand that changing your behavior in small ways can completely revolutionize your life.

QUITTING SMOKING

Talk about hard change. Most smokers are well aware that the habit is bad for their health. But giving up smoking is one of the most difficult changes in life. It takes most smokers eight to ten attempts before they actually quit. This is because nicotine is a powerfully addictive drug—according to some experts, harder to give up than drugs such as heroin or cocaine. It actually alters the brain in the same way that other addicting drugs do, by affecting its pleasure pathways. Withdrawal can make you may feel irritable, depressed, and restless, and because of this, it's common for people to fall off the wagon.

Quitting is also challenging because the habit of smoking is part of a daily routine, something you do when you're on the phone, drinking morning coffee, or driving. You may turn to a cigarette when you're bored or stressed during the day. Giving up the habit means altering your routine.

Fortunately, there are more ways than ever for you to stop smoking and a much better understanding of how you can be successful. Remember that millions of people have kicked the habit for good, and you can, too.

Among the strategies for kicking the habit are do-it-yourself and assisted-quit methods, such as quit-smoking programs, nicotine replacement, and prescription drugs. Research shows that the hardest route is do-it-yourself, and that smokers generally have more success when they combine two or more methods. Whichever strategy you choose, it's a good idea to discuss it with your doctor.

According to the American Cancer Society, all methods of quitting have a higher success rate when they're accompanied by some kind of counseling support program. To find a program in your area, ask your doctor or consult the local chapter of the American Cancer Society or the American Lung Association. Or you can try a quitline. These are free counseling programs offered over the telephone in all 50 states. A quitline will team you up with a trained counselor to assist your efforts to stop smoking. The National Cancer Institute offers a Smoking Quitline at 1-877-44U-Quit (1-877-448-7848) and a National Quitline at 1-800-QUITNOW (1-800-784-8669).

CHANGING YOUR
PERSONAL ENVIRONMENT

Changing behavior is hard in part because we are products of our environment—how we were brought up, our education and knowledge, the friends we keep, our work and family schedules, and our food and physical activity surroundings. I can't emphasize this enough. Environmental influences shape how we live our lives, what we eat, and how much we move around. Some of these cues and factors are under our control; others are not.

Consider the environment created by the jobs many of us have—like mine—where we sit for 40-plus hours a week and have no real opportunity to be active. Or think of the kinds of food available in your grocery store or cafeteria or served at home by loved ones. Consider the pressures of modern life, its fast pace, long work hours, and endless commutes, which ratchet up our stress levels; prevent us from having regular family meals, exercising habitually, and getting sufficient sleep; and tempt us to overeat and overdrink.

In short, unhealthy cues in our modern environment conspire to make our *default* behavior unhealthy. The secret to successful change is reducing your exposure to these toxic cues by creating your own, more wholesome microenvironment, complete with healthy cues, nutritious foods, plenty of built-in physical activity, and a supportive community of family, friends, and other positive influences. This will make it easier and more natural to do the things that enhance your well-being and avoid the things that sabotage it. Self-monitoring is an important tool for figuring out what you need to change and sticking to your plan.

THE IMPORTANCE OF SELF-MONITORING

Research has shown that monitoring your own health behaviors in a log or journal may be the single most important thing you can do to improve your self-efficacy and achieve your goals for health-related behavior change. For instance, studies show that people who keep a food journal lose twice as much weight as those who don't.

On pages 335-336 you will find two examples of logs that can help you monitor your daily physical activity and nutrition. If you feel you need to make changes to your lifestyle, I strongly encourage you to keep these logs. You can copy the pages that follow and put them in a notebook or just jot down the information on a notepad.

If you have other health issues that need to be addressed, such as quitting smoking or substance abuse, you can modify these logs to suit your particular goals.

Keep the logs as a baseline for a week. Then analyze them by asking yourself the following questions.

For the food log:

- How many fruits and vegetables did I eat each day?
- How many daily servings of whole grains did I eat today?
- Did I eat three low-fat dairy servings?
- Did I eat fish twice a week?
- Did I have too many junk-food snacks or other nonnutritious foods?
- Did I eat too many refined grains?
- Did I drink more than one alcoholic beverage a day?
- Did I eat three times a day?
- Did I have breakfast?
- Were my eating routines wholesome—that is, did I eat at a table with family and friends rather than in the car or at my desk?
- Did I get sufficient sleep?

For the activity log:

- Was I active?
- Did I get planned physical activity at least three times a week?
- Did I break a sweat at least once a week?
- What was the most positive aspect of my physical activity this week?
- Did I get at least 10,000 steps a day?

Note: If you are using unplanned daily activity to fulfill your physical activity requirements, I would encourage you to wear a pedometer.

FOOD LOG

Write down everything you eat and drink. It's also helpful to include portion sizes.

Note the time and place you eat or drink. Also, record your quality of sleep each night and your body weight each week.

	Time	Place	Food and Drink
Monday (date):			
Tuesday (date):			
Wednesday (date):			
Thursday (date):			

	Time	Place	Food and Drink
Friday (date):			
Saturday (date):			
Sunday (date):			

Record Weekly:

Body weight _____

Quality of sleep: ☐ Poor ☐ Marginal ☐ Good ☐ Excellent

Comments:

_____

_____

_____

_____

ANY PHYSICAL ACTIVITY

Sports, yoga, leisure, commuting, errands on foot or bike, climbing stairs, physical play, work around the house or garden

Goal: as often as you can

DAY	ACTIVITY	DURATION

PLANNED AEROBIC EXERCISE

Goal: 3 to 6 times per week, at least 30 minutes per session

DAY	ACTIVITY	DURATION

STRENGTH TRAINING

Goal: 2 or 3 times per week

Strength Exercise	DAY	DAY	DAY

Steps per day

Monday	Tuesday	Wednesday	Thursday	Friday	Saturday	Sunday

SUN SALUTATION

This sequence of yoga postures is a mini total workout, stretching and strengthening the whole body and reducing stress. Breathing is an important element in yoga. At the start, try coordinating each posture with a full breath cycle, inhaling and exhaling. Then you can move on to holding each posture for three to five breaths. Perform the sequence twice, the first time with the right leg in the first lunge, and the second time with the left leg. If you really enjoy this routine, there are longer versions of the Sun Salutation. I encourage you to look them up online.

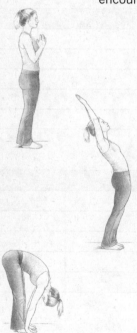

1. Mountain
Begin with feet about hip-width apart, hands in prayer position. Breathe in and out.

2. Hands Up
Sweep your arms up overhead and gently arch your back as far as it feels comfortable. Do not overstrain.

3. Head to Knees
Bend forward to let your hands rest beside your feet. If necessary, bend your knees.

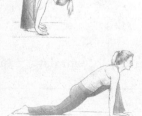

4. Lunge
Stretch the right leg behind you, with hands on either side of your left foot.

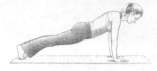

5. Plank
Stretch your left leg back into the plank position.

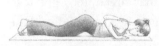

6. Stick
Slowly lower yourself as if coming down from a pushup. Only your hands, chest, knees, and feet should touch the floor.

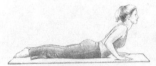

7. Upward Dog
Stretch forward and up, bending at the waist. Use your arms to lift your torso, but only bend back as far as feels comfortable.

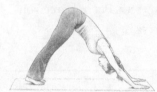

8. Downward Dog
Lift from the tailbone and hips, and push back up into a standing position.

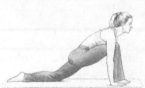

9. Lunge
Step the right foot forward into the lunge position.

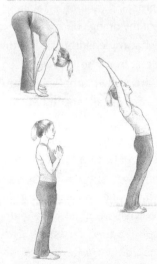

10. Head to Knees
Step forward with your left foot and lift your tailbone into the air. Bend forward to let your hands rest beside your feet. Bend your knees if necessary.

11. Hands Up
Return to standing. Sweep your arms up and gently arch your back (see opposite page).

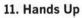

12. Mountain
In a slow, sweeping motion, lower your arms back into the prayer position.

A SIMPLE BEHAVIOR SWITCH: DAILY RITUALS

You probably already have morning and evening rituals that include a number of healthy behaviors, such as brushing your teeth, washing up, etc. But here I suggest that you make these little rituals a bit more deliberate. The morning and evening rituals outlined below take only a few minutes each day. Some you may already incorporate in your days; others may be new. As an experiment in behavior change, try building these more formalized healthy rituals into your daily life.

MORNING RITUAL

You may complete the following in any order you wish:

1. **Cleanse and cream.** Wash your face and brush your teeth. Put sunscreen on your face or use a favorite face cream with sun protection.

THE JOY OF JOURNALING

I'm convinced that journaling is an important part of staying healthy in body and mind. Since I was a child, I have been a journal writer. Although I have not necessarily written every day of every year, I have kept up a steady stream of daily scribbling and have found the process endlessly enlightening (and entertaining). My journals are reflective: I jot down a brief chronicle of my doings during the day and my thoughts, struggles, worries, and delights; what my children are up to; what I feel are the blessings in my life; and observations from the first crocuses of spring to the last leaves of autumn. I always learn from my journals. I love to look back at them to see where I've been and to linger over pages recently written to reflect on my current thoughts and what I hold important.

I encourage you to try the habit. The book itself can be anything you want it to be, from a tiny spiral notebook packed with jotted lists to a thick leather journal filled with formal writing.

My mother-in-law, Nancy, who recently passed away at age 86, kept a journal most of her adult life. When she died, we found her journals from her teen years to her old age. Some were little books; others were spiral-bound cardstock. The journals from her middle years abounded with notes about her garden, when things were planted and when they came up, the first and last frost. But later,

2. **Think positive thoughts.** Look in the mirror, smile, and think two or three positive thoughts, such as affirming your own unique beauty, inside and out, or what you intend to accomplish during the day in any realm—work, family, pleasure. So many of us look in the mirror and see only our flaws. Try to shift this negative train of thought so that you greet the mirror with "Hey, Beautiful!" This positive mind-set will boost your self-efficacy in the coming day.

3. **Greet the day.** The classic yoga Sun Salutation, practiced by millions around the world, takes only a couple of minutes but is a wonderful way to awaken the mind and body. (See pages 338–339.) It focuses your energy for the start of the day and builds core flexibility and strength. In the beginning, try it on weekends, and then see whether you can work it into your daily schedule.

4. **Sit down and eat breakfast.** Try not to eat standing or rush through your first meal of the day. As mothers have said for years: Breakfast really is the most important meal of the day.

---

when my sister-in-law Elizabeth was ill with terminal cancer, Nancy's journal turned to notes of Elizabeth and her family. The balance of Nancy's life went from gardening to caring for Elizabeth, and her journal reflected that shift.

Fast-forward a decade and a half. In her eighties, Nancy kept a wall calendar as a journal. Every night before she went to bed, she filled the day's box on the calendar with the seasons, what was happening to her plants and flowers, when her children and grandchildren came to visit, and other life events.

The last year of Nancy's life she had leukemia. Alongside the blooming forsythia in those calendar boxes were brief notes about transfusions and one doctor's appointment after another. Then, on a Tuesday, this simple note in her husband's handwriting: "Nancy died at 5:30 p.m."

I can't tell you how beautiful it was for our family to find this chronicling of Nancy's life. She was very disciplined and thoughtful about writing every day and wrote on that calendar until a couple of days before she died. Or, as she would probably say, it was the other way around. Her writing made her more disciplined and thoughtful.

Maybe you find the idea of keeping a journal every day daunting. But if you start with writing for only a minute or two and keep your goals simple, the practice will become an easy habit.

EVENING RITUAL

Closing the day with a calm, orderly sequence of steps can help you shed the hectic tensions of the day and prepare for a good night's sleep. You can do the following evening ritual anytime after dinner and before bed:

1. **Cleanse and floss.** Wash your face, brush your teeth, and floss.
2. **Take a moment to reflect.** Briefly reflect on the positive aspects of your day, as well as the struggles, and what you may have learned from them. Try to think of several joyful things, or aspects of life for which you're thankful.

   Note: You may already have your own reflective evening ritual that works well for you. By all means, keep it up. Many people find that evening prayer is a wonderful way of calming the mind and reminding themselves of their place in a larger world.
3. **Write for a few minutes in your journal.** I highly recommend writing regularly in a journal to keep track of your thoughts and activities during the day and, if you want, to monitor your health behaviors. (See the box The Joy of Journaling on pages 340–341.)
4. **Calm your mind.** Do some deep breathing, meditation, or even a yoga posture or two from the Sun Salutation.

. . . Then go to bed.

25

Managing Stress and Sleeping Well

When I ask my women friends what they consider their primary health concern, it's amazing how many times I get the same answer: stress. Stress about work, balancing job and family, money, caring for children or aging parents, and not having enough time to do all of life's tasks and do them well.

Surveys suggest that most women in this country believe they are living with higher-than-healthy levels of stress. More than 75 percent say that in the past month, they have experienced some kind of negative physical symptom related to stress, from headache and fatigue to upset stomach, muscle tension, and teeth grinding. Almost as many report psychological symptoms as a result of stress, such as irritability, nervousness, depression, or just feeling the desperate need to take a break from life's merry-go-round. Half of women surveyed say they lie awake at night because of anxious worries. This leads to a vicious cycle: Stress begets poor sleep, and poor sleep begets more stress. In fact, stress and our response to it are the most common causes of fatigue, which is the number one reason people visit their primary care physician.

Stress and fatigue, twin enemies, can wreak havoc with our lives, affecting everything from job performance and work and family relationships to sleep patterns, eating habits, disease, and our overall sense of well-being. That's why it's vital to address them as part of a plan for total health. The good news is that you can learn to moderate your response to stress with a variety of proven strategies, from relaxation techniques to cognitive restructuring.

WHAT IS STRESS?

The term is so overused that its meaning is often lost. Technically speaking, it's anything that challenges the body, disrupting its homeostasis, or equilibrium.

As most of us know, stress is a natural part of life, and always has been. Fortunately, our bodies have evolved an ingenious system for coping. Known as the stress response or the "fight/flight reaction," the system is a brilliant set of adaptations for dealing with physical dangers and other temporary crises, energizing your body to fight or to flee a source of danger.

In simple terms, here's how it works: In response to a threat, the brain releases neurotransmitters and hormones that trigger the adrenal glands—small almond-shaped glands atop your kidneys—to release a flood of cortisol, adrenaline, and other stress hormones. These in turn boost your heart rate and energy supplies and heighten your alertness by sending messages to the brain regions that control fear and motivation. Cortisol also dampens the activity of body functions not necessary for immediate action, such as immune activity, digestion, reproduction, and growth. All of this activity helps the body mobilize in the face of physical challenges.

The problem is that modern life throws at us a host of stresses that may not be physical in nature and certainly are not short term—worries about work, relationships, finances, or a sick parent or child. The adaptations our bodies possess are not as effective at dealing with these kinds of challenges, especially if they're relentless. The mechanisms that work so well to help us face an imminent threat may turn on us if they're constantly activated by the daily stresses of our lives. Chronic exposure to too much cortisol and other stress hormones can harm your body in myriad ways, boosting the risk of heart disease, depression, digestive issues, osteoporosis, obesity, and other health problems.

The point is that a little stress can be a good thing; prolonged, excessive, or unmanageable stress is not.

My friend and colleague Dr. Alice Domar defines this sort of stress as "the sensation one has when one's resources cannot meet the demands of life." Ali is executive director of the Domar Center for Mind/Body Health in Waltham, Massachusetts, and a world-renowned expert on stress and its effect on women's health. I've known Ali for many years and have always admired her wisdom and insights on this important health topic.

In any area of life, says Ali, we have resources such as time, money, and social support. If we feel these resources aren't equal to the demands in our lives, then we feel stress. She likes to give the example of two boys facing the task of calling a girl for a prom date. One boy has the phone number of one girl; the other boy has numbers for five girls. The boy with five numbers is going to feel less stressed about calling than the boy who has only one option.

"With adequate resources, most of us can handle extraordinary pressures in one area at a time," explains Ali. "The problem for many women is that they are trying to control a dozen different domains at once—job, childcare, cooking, cleaning, volunteer work, etc." The demands overwhelm their ability to cope.

I know this from my own experience. I can handle big challenges in one domain—say, work or family—but when crises collide in more than one arena, and my resources are stretched beyond their limits, I get stressed.

THE PERFECTION PROBLEM

As Ali points out, the problem is made worse by our efforts to strive for perfection in all areas of life. Many of us want to be the model employee, mother, wife, cook, home keeper, friend, sister, or volunteer—and, of course, we think we should also be slender and wrinkle free.

"It's fine to want to be really excellent in some piece of your life," says Ali. "However, to aspire to perfection in all domains is unreasonable and leads inevitably to stress and anxiety. There's no question that we want our surgeon to be a stickler in her work. But we really don't care how good she is at balancing her checkbook or setting an elegant dinner table or making brownies from scratch."

It's a matter of adjusting expectations.

I was interested to learn of an international survey of happiness among the world's nations conducted by a group of scientists not long ago. The results suggest that the happiest people are the Danes. What was the secret to Danish contentment? Modest expectations. By having reasonable and realistic expectations of the world and of ourselves, we are less disappointed with life, less stressed, and generally happier.

WHAT STRESS DOES TO YOUR BODY AND MIND

Some women are very aware of the effects of stress on body and mind; others experience its physical symptoms but don't recognize them as such. Each of us responds to stress in our own way, based on our own life experience and our physiological and psychological "wiring." Women who feel stressed-out a lot don't necessarily have more stress in their lives than other women, but they may be more sensitive to its effects. For instance, some people have more of what Ali calls "cardiac reactivity;" that is, their heart rate accelerates more in response to a stressful event.

It's important to be aware of the role stress plays in your life and how you react to it. We believe that too much stress is an increasing problem for many women in this country. "This is a real cause for concern because chronic or excessive stress can have a serious impact on so many aspects of our health," Ali warns. It speeds the effects of aging. It exacerbates a range of health conditions from diabetes to heart disease. It can lead to depression. And it can alter the normal functioning of the immune system.

Because the immune system is so vital in defending the body against infection and malignant disease, any change in its ability to perform normally can increase the severity of illness or cause greater risk of death from infection. Studies show that people who report persistent stress have a weaker immune response to vaccines; they have more outbreaks of genital herpes, more reactivation of latent viruses such as cytomegalovirus and Epstein-Barr virus, and slower wound healing. They also have greater production of immune chemicals that boost inflammation, which is linked with a variety of diseases, including arthritis, heart disease, type 2 diabetes, periodontal disease, osteoporosis, and certain cancers. When researchers studied long-term caregivers—people charged with caregiving for a spouse with dementia—they found that they produced more than four times as much of a pro-inflammatory chemical known as IL-6. The net effect of this excess is to prematurely age the immune response and accelerate the risk of a host of age-related diseases.

WARNING SIGNS OF CHRONIC OR EXCESSIVE STRESS

Too much stress can cause a range of physical, psychological, and behavioral symptoms. Among the physical symptoms are:

- Insomnia
- Headaches
- Neck or back pain
- Fatigue
- Palpitations or shortness of breath
- Gastrointestinal distress, including constipation, diarrhea, cramping, indigestion, and heartburn
- Weight loss or gain
- Teeth grinding
- Fainting or feeling lightheaded or dizzy

Psychological symptoms include:

- Irritability
- Difficulty concentrating
- Restlessness

- Sadness
- Depression

Some behavioral symptoms are:

- Gum chewing
- Alcohol or drug abuse
- Binge eating or eating unhealthy foods

- Sleep difficulties
- Frequent crying

Too often we respond to these symptoms in just the wrong way: by engaging in unhealthy behaviors that make things worse. When Ali and her colleagues conducted a survey of 12,000 people just after the terrorist attacks of September 11, 2001, they found that both women and men reported unhealthy behavior changes resulting from the stress. The men reported drinking more alcohol and watching more TV; women reported exercising less and eating more junk food. When we're "stressed-out," we don't pause to ask why we're feeling anxious or exhausted or have a pounding headache. Instead, if we're overworked, we skip our exercise class or stay up later to catch up, losing valuable sleep. We compensate for low energy by eating junk food. Some 43 percent of Americans say they manage stress by overeating or eating sweets and salty snack foods. If we feel tired, we head to Starbucks and drink a huge cup of coffee. If we have a headache, we pop a pill. To try to relax, we smoke, drink, or take prescription drugs.

There are definitely better ways to manage stress.

OUTSMARTING STRESS

Take a moment to think about how you experience stress. How do you feel when you're stressed? How does your behavior change? What situations or events trigger stressful feelings? Is your stress most often job-related? Is it rooted in relationship conflicts? In juggling work and family? The best way to reduce stress is to change the situation that's causing it. If it's unavoidable, however, there are excellent strategies for managing it. Ali recommends both physical and psychological methods.

PHYSICAL METHODS

1. **Exercise, exercise, exercise.** Physical activity is among the most effective ways of reducing stress. Exercise steps up your body's production of endorphins, neurotransmitters involved in modulating mood. It also helps clear your mind by focusing on movement rather than daily irritations and worries. In one 2008 study, researchers found that high levels of physical activity resulted in significantly lower levels of perceived stress, especially among postmenopausal women. What is important to realize, though, is that the exercise doesn't have to be overly vigorous or planned. Any type of physical activity helps.

2. **Relaxation techniques.** These are techniques designed to induce the relaxation response—the physiological opposite of the fight/flight response—so as to return the body to homeostasis. They modify your response to stress by slowing your breathing, reducing your heart rate and blood pressure, diminishing muscle tension, and boosting bloodflow. A new study suggests that the relaxation response actually alters the expression of genes involved in stress-associated changes in the body. The Sun Salutation that I outlined in the previous chapter is a good relaxation routine. So are these techniques:

   - **Meditation.** The classic transcendental variety of meditation involves repeating a word or phrase in synchrony with breathing: While inhaling, repeat the phrase "breathing in peace and calm"; while exhaling, "breathing out tension and anxiety." It is best if you can find a quiet place to meditate, but with practice, meditation can be done anywhere.

   - **Progressive muscle relaxation.** This technique involves lying down on your back in a comfortable position, then focusing on individual muscle groups and slowly and systematically tensing them, then relaxing them. You can work from your toes, moving up your legs to your torso, arms, and hands, and finally, to your head and neck. Hold the tension for about 5 seconds, then relax for 30 seconds, and repeat.

   - **Autogenic training.** With this method, you repeat to yourself suggestive statements to help you relax and release muscle tension, such as "my arm is feeling warm and heavy; my hand is feeling relaxed."

   - **Hatha yoga.** Among the many types of yoga, hatha is one of the most effective for stress reduction. It focuses on physical poses coordinated with controlled breathing.

These techniques work well in part because they put you in the moment, focusing on the task at hand while clearing your mind of worries and preoccupation. For some people, visualization achieves the same effect. In this technique, you imagine being in a peaceful place, such as a beach, and concentrate on evoking the sensory feelings in that place, the smell of the salt air or the feel of the warm sun on your skin.

Visualization doesn't make it to Ali's list of the top four antistress techniques because imagery is a very individual thing. I regularly use the image of a beautiful mountain scene to help calm me. For Ali, imagining a scene at the beach, with the waves washing over her feet, "is about as good as it gets for inducing the relaxation response," she ways. But this vision of sand and surf doesn't work for everyone. For some people, the ocean evokes fear, so the image is counterproductive. Choose what works for you.

PSYCHOLOGICAL METHODS

- **Cognitive restructuring.** This technique of changing your attitude and responses to stress is very effective for many women. "The vast majority of thoughts women have about themselves are negative," explains Ali. "We see the cup as half empty rather than half full. We beat up on ourselves. We are fat, stupid slobs, and everyone hates us. The vast majority of these thoughts are not true." Maybe one friend failed to call you, but that does not mean everyone hates you. Maybe you're carrying a few extra pounds; maybe you made a mistake at work. That does not mean you're fat and stupid. "Often the tape playing in our heads is born of fear or reflects something we've heard someone say in the past," explains Ali. "Often, it's patently false."

  The point of cognitive restructuring is to change that mental tape so that it's more in line with the truth, which is often far nicer.

  The key is to ask yourself: Does this thought contribute to my stress? Where did I learn to think it? Is it logical? Is it true? Once you've pinned down its nature in this way, you are free to create a new thought that is more positive or at least neutral, that is, in fact, true!

- **Social support.** Most of us know that it helps to have social support in stressful situations, and it's commonly thought that the more friends you have, the better off you are. However, not all friends are positive social supports; some are "takers," constantly demanding support for themselves and rarely offering much in return. It's important for your relationships to be a two-way street. Ask yourself, *Can I really count on this friend?* Can I confide in him or her? Evaluate your friendships and make sure that you have a circle of friends who don't drain your social energy but genuinely offer support and positive energy.

DE-STRESSING TIME

Many of us complain about feeling stressed because we have too little time. At my Strong Women summits, Ali and I ask women to create a pie chart showing how they use their time and energy. We also ask them to make a list of the 20 things in life that give them joy. Then we suggest that they look for overlap between their "time pie" and their "joy list."

Try this three-step exercise yourself:

1. For the "time pie," draw a circle on a sheet of paper. Assume that the entire circle equals 24 hours. How much time do you sleep? Block out that wedge of the pie. How much time do you usually spend at work? Volunteer work? Driving children to and from school and other activities? Caring for elderly parents? Household chores? Commuting? Try to figure out your entire typical day.

24-Hour Time Pie

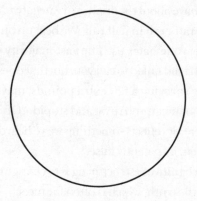

2. For the joy list, spend 1 minute writing down at least 20 different things that bring you happiness and joy. Reading? Walking? Gardening? Sex? Watching movies with your children? Count up how many items are on your list.

_____

_____

_____

_____

_____

3. Now look at your 24-hour time pie and see how many of the things that bring you joy are in your daily routine.

I hope you had a lot of items on your joy list. I was so pleased with myself when I first did this exercise and came up with about 25 things that brought me joy—from playing with my very silly cat, Chucky, to going hiking in the mountains. I had listed things I do every day, such as sitting down to a meal with my family, and also things I do rarely, such as spending time with my best friend, Isabelle, who lives far away.

When we do this exercise at our Strong Women summits, I'm shocked at how many women have only a few things on their joy list. And often, none of them are included in their time pie. There's a real disconnect between the activities that give them joy and the way they spend their time. It's not because there are too few hours in the day. "It's not that we don't have enough time to be an adequate employee, an adequate mother, an adequate volunteer," Ali says. "It's that we don't want to be just adequate. We want to do everything on our list well or perfectly." If we can let go of this notion, we often find that our obligations take less time and we have more hours for the things that bring us joy.

In a typical woman's time pie, work takes up 8 hours a day and sleep takes up 7 hours. The other chunk of 9 hours is consumed with commuting, shuttling children, doing loads of laundry, grocery shopping, helping with homework, doing bills, getting dinner on the table, and watching television. (I'm amazed at the amount of television most people watch—an average of 3 hours a day.)

The trick is to try to expand your wedge of remaining free time and use it in ways that give you joy and satisfaction, that rejuvenate you and bring pleasure and humor. It may be something as simple as buying fresh flowers every week or eating a little bit of chocolate after lunch. It may be taking the dog for a walk, reading, gardening, or listening to music. Spending time with friends does wonders for reducing stress. So does watching a funny movie or reading a funny book. In 2008, researchers found that even anticipating laughter reduces levels of cortisol, epinephrine, and other stress hormones.

Think hard about all the things that bring you joy; then figure out how to build them into your life on a daily, or at least weekly, basis.

GENERAL TIPS FOR REDUCING STRESS
- **Manage your time.** Organize and prioritize your work and home tasks on a daily basis. Create a "to do" list and arrange it in order of importance.
- **Create realistic expectations.** Set small goals for yourself, and feel good when you accomplish them. Divide large, burdensome tasks into smaller increments and do a little at a time.
- **Learn to say no** to nonessential work tasks or unwanted social invitations that you might be tempted to accept out of a sense of obligation or guilt.

- **When you start to feel stressed,** take a moment to ask yourself, *What do I need right now?* If you can muster your resources, you may be able to better cope with whatever challenges you face.

LORETTA'S LIST

Over the years, I've had the good fortune to work with many fantastic health experts. Among my favorites is Loretta LaRoche, a humorist who has done a lot of collaborative work with health researchers on humor and stress reduction. When I was writing this section, I asked Loretta to put together her list of the 10 ways to become a more positive, joyful person. Here is her list:

1. Give up your seat on the martyr train. Going to extremes to help others only creates feelings of helplessness and enables others to be selfish.
2. Stop trying to control everything and everyone. It makes sense if you're an air traffic controller; otherwise, it's exhausting and makes people around you want to run away from you.
3. Don't assume someone will rescue you from your life. No one's coming.
4. Take care of your physical, mental, and spiritual health because you deserve to feel good. Nothing feels as good as feeling good.
5. Spend time with friends who are happy and healthy. Their energy will energize you.
6. Don't assume being tired is to how you're supposed to feel. Get a good night's sleep, set priorities, exercise, and eat well, and your fatigue will fade away.
7. Spend time dancing to your favorite tunes alone or with your children, significant other, or friends. It will make your spirits soar.
8. Don't buy into media messages that focus on negative images of how a woman should look and feel. Tap into your inner wisdom; it will tell you the truth. Or ask your grandmother.
9. Live authentically and with passion. Nothing feels worse than not being yourself.
10. Laugh often, especially at yourself, and don't wait to have fun. Become the fun you're seeking.

- **Take time off from work.** During the workday, give yourself breaks to take a short walk, stretch, and get your body moving. Occasionally take a day off for mental health—a "duvet day," as the British call it. Go somewhere refreshing for a long weekend. Try to take regular vacations.

- **Evaluate the importance of household tasks.** Remember that a sink full of dirty dishes or a little dog hair on the rug will not significantly affect your quality of life. My husband has trained me well in this area. I used to always need to get the kitchen cleaned up before I could do anything after dinner. Now I don't mind occasionally leaving the dishes overnight if there is something better to do.

- **Consider reducing the amount of television you watch** and use the time you would have spent in front of the tube doing something that gives you real satisfaction and pleasure.

- **Distinguish between the things you can control and those you can't,** and let go of what you can't control.

- **Put YOU on your to-do list.** Get plenty of exercise and eat well. Plan to do one thing each day to nurture yourself—read, do some hatha yoga (or your Sun Salutations), take a long bath, spend time with a supportive friend, walk, or work out.

- **Get sufficient sleep.** When it comes to managing stress, a good night's sleep is not a luxury but a necessity.

Being at peace with yourself and successfully managing life's stresses will allow you to lead a healthier and happier life.

SLEEP

Another common concern I hear from women I meet is about getting too little sleep. Sometimes it's a matter of having trouble falling asleep or staying asleep or waking up too early. By some estimates, insomnia and other sleep issues occur almost twice as often in women as in men.

This is a potentially serious problem. Too little sleep has been linked with several chronic diseases, including diabetes, heart disease, depression, and obesity. In addition, drowsiness from too little sleep puts you at risk for accidents on the road and in the workplace. The National Highway Traffic Safety Administration estimates that drowsy driving causes some 100,000 accidents every year and 1,500 fatalities.

WHY DO WE NEED TO SLEEP?

Science is still working to understand why we sleep for about a third of our hours. We know that sleep is vital for physical and mental health. It appears to play an important role in keeping our nervous system healthy. We know that too little sleep impairs our judgment, our reaction time, and our ability to learn and remember. It makes us irritable. We have trouble concentrating and are apt to make errors.

We now know that sleep deprivation also has serious effects on health. It suppresses the immune response, slows wound healing, and impairs the body's ability to control its own blood sugar. It also appears to reduce our supply of leptin, a hormone that signals when we've eaten enough. When we don't sleep, we feel hungrier, especially for calorie-rich carbohydrates such as cake or bread, which can lead to dangerous weight gain. In fact, a study by the Centers for Disease Control and Prevention (CDC) found that people who got fewer than 6 hours of sleep a night were more likely to be obese. And one 2007 study of sleep patterns in new mothers by Harvard Medical School and Kaiser Permanente found that moms who slept only 5 hours a night had triple the risk of carrying roughly 11 extra pounds a year after the baby's birth than those who slept 7 hours.

We also know that getting deep sleep is vital. During this kind of sleep, growth hormone is released and the body's cells make more proteins—the building blocks that cells use to grow and to repair themselves from damage due to factors such as ultraviolet rays and stress. In this sense, deep sleep may in fact be beauty sleep.

HOW MUCH SLEEP IS ENOUGH?

Despite what you hear, sleep needs vary a great deal from person to person. Some people can get by on 5 or 6 hours, though they're in the minority. Teenagers need about 9 hours on average. Women in the first trimester of pregnancy often need more sleep than usual. Most adults function well on about 7 or 7½ hours. (It's a fallacy that we need more than 8 hours of sleep to be healthy. In fact, a CDC study suggests that sleeping more than 9 hours a night is as closely tied to poor health patterns as sleeping too little is.) Unfortunately, about a third of us are sleeping 6 or fewer hours each night, shorting ourselves by an hour or so. This may not seem like much of a deficit, but sleep debt is cumulative. It catches up with us.

Just as important as quantity of sleep is quality of sleep. A good night's sleep consists of both rapid eye movement (REM) sleep and non-REM, or quiet, sleep, which includes deep sleep—the most important kind of sleep for restoring the body's energy.

To judge whether you're getting sufficient good-quality sleep, ask yourself whether you feel rested when you rise. If you wake up 5 minutes before your alarm goes off and you feel reasonably refreshed, you're doing fine. But if your alarm wakes you out of a deep sleep and you feel exhausted, you're probably not getting enough shut-eye.

HOW AGE AFFECTS SLEEP

In general, as we age, we tend to sleep more lightly and for shorter periods of time; however, there's no evidence to suggest that we need less sleep as we age. Roughly half of all people over age 65 have sleeping problems, such as insomnia. This may be a result of normal aging or may come about because of other medical problems common in older people.

Disrupted sleep is a frequent issue for women entering or in the middle of menopause, when hot flashes and sweating can disturb deep slumber. Sometimes, these sleep troubles may lead to other problems, such as daytime drowsiness. If you're having trouble sleeping because of hot flashes, try wearing loose clothing to bed and keeping your bedroom cool and well ventilated. If these measures are not helping you get sufficient sleep and you're feeling exhausted from sleep loss, you might consider short-term use of hormone therapy. In the past year or so I have managed to continue to get a good night's sleep despite frequent nighttime hot flashes. I do find that I sleep without covers most of the night, but I've grown used to that!

HOW TO GET A GOOD NIGHT'S SLEEP

Here are tips for good sleep hygiene:

- **Stick to a schedule.** Try to go to sleep and wake up at roughly the same time.
- **Avoid caffeine, nicotine, and alcohol in the evening.** Both caffeine and nicotine are stimulants. Alcohol boosts the body's blood levels of the stress hormone epinephrine, which can cause middle-of-the-night awakenings.
- **Establish a consistent bedtime routine.**
- **Get regular exercise.** Physical activity during the day increases deep sleep at night.
- **Set a relaxing tone before bedtime.** Take a warm bath, meditate, or play quiet music.
- **Don't watch TV or use other electronic devices before you go to sleep.** Watching TV and working or playing games on a laptop or other device has a stimulant effect and makes it harder to fall asleep.
- **Make sure that your bedroom is dark, quiet, and cool.**
- **Move your clock.** Set your alarm and then put your clock in a place where you can't see it, so you're not tempted to check it every 10 minutes.
- **Let go of your worries.** Keep a pad and pencil by your bed and write down your concerns to help get them off your mind.

- **Practice the mind-calming routines outlined earlier in the chapter.**
- **Try a "white noise" device.** A sound machine, fan, or air cleaner can help.
- **If you can't fall asleep, get out of bed and do something relaxing.**
- **Use sleeping pills only after consulting a physician and use them sparingly.** Make sure that you don't mix sleeping medications with alcohol.

NAPPING

Napping is an excellent way to make up for lost sleep at night or just to boost your energy and productivity during the day. Most of us experience a dip in the early afternoon, when both mind and body flag. This is a good time to close your eyes, if you can, for 10 or 20 minutes—even if it means just putting your head on your desk. Studies show that a midday doze benefits mental acuity and overall health, and enhances alertness, mood, and efficiency in the later afternoon and evening.

WHEN TO SEEK HELP

Nearly all of us experience mild insomnia now and again. But if you have trouble sleeping more than 3 nights a week for more than a few weeks at a time and you have tried the sleep hygiene strategies outlined above without success, you should consult with your doctor. You may have an underlying medical condition such as depression or heart trouble. Or you may have a sleep disorder, such as sleep apnea (a disorder of interrupted breathing during sleep) or restless legs syndrome (which causes unpleasant prickling or tingling sensations in the legs and feet and an urge to move them for relief).

For short-term insomnia, your doctor may suggest an over-the-counter sleep aid containing antihistamines, which make you drowsy, or a dietary supplement such as melatonin (most useful with insomnia related to jet lag). These sleep aids are intended to be used for only a few nights at a time. For more persistent insomnia, your doctor may prescribe sleeping pills—after making sure that the pills do not interact with any other medications you may be taking. If you are prescribed sleeping pills, ask about interactions with other drugs and side effects. Some sleeping pills cause dizziness, weakness, confusion, high blood pressure, amnesia, or grogginess the day after they're taken. They may also cause a form of sleepwalking behavior that involves binge eating or even driving at night without any recollection of the behavior.

Try to wean yourself off sleep medications as soon as you can by practicing good sleep habits. If used nightly, most sleeping pills are effective only for several weeks. Many sleeping pills are habit forming, and long-term use can actually interfere with normal sleeping patterns.

26

Shifting Your Food Environment

Wholesome food can be a source of great pleasure in life. Good nutrition keeps your body and mind sound while you're young; it can also lower your risk for medical problems that often crop up in later years, including weight gain, high blood pressure, type 2 diabetes, heart disease, osteoporosis, cancer, and other disorders.

Most of us are aware of these benefits. So why do so many of us have unhealthy eating patterns? I believe it's because our environment makes it hard for us to eat well. The way we live and work, the food that surrounds us, the eating habits we've acquired for the sake of convenience and economy, government policies, and other environmental factors all conspire to create unhealthy dietary choices and patterns of eating.

In the past 5 decades, our food supply has changed radically, surrounding us with food choices based largely on expedience and cost. At the same time, our lifestyle has shifted to include more convenience eating in general and less physical activity. We eat more fast food, more meals on the run, more "desk-fasts"—breakfasts and other meals quickly consumed at our desks or in our cars. We consume far more high-calorie drinks, sometimes known as "liquid candy."

The key to eating well, then, lies in rethinking *how* we eat. Women in our society face a barrage of mixed messages about specific foods that we should or should not consume. Mention the word *diet*, and we all think of plans that contain prescriptions for or against this food or that food, whether carbohydrates or sugar or fat. This chapter takes a different tack. It offers a philosophy of eating and focuses on helping you create patterns of eating that will boost your overall health.

THE PROBLEM IN A NUTSHELL

Our bodies evolved in a world where food was hard to come by. Our Paleolithic hunter-gatherer ancestors had to work hard to feed themselves. Natural selection shaped their genes in ways that favored maintaining hearty appetites to make sure the body's basic needs were met, and then holding on to those hard-earned calories. We were programmed to eat, eat, and eat some more when food was available (especially fatty foods, which we didn't get often) and hardwired to hold the extra calories in fat reserves.

Now, in the 21st century, our bodies are not so different from those of our ancient forebears. They still feature big appetites; they still have ingenious ways of hanging on to calories through fat storage. But our environment has changed. We now have a steady supply of cheap, convenient food that we can easily secure without expending much energy. People in this country consume more food and hundreds more calories per day than did our counterparts even just 50 years ago, and fewer of us have jobs that demand physical labor. In short, our modern environment pressures us to eat more (and exercise less), while our Paleolithic bodies still work hard to maintain appetite and hold on to calories by storing them as fat. No wonder we gain weight and experience a host of attendant health problems.

WHAT WE EAT

If you look at food consumption trends, it's clear that Americans are consuming more calories today than we did 3 decades ago. In the 1970s, women ate about 1,500 calories per day; after the year 2000, that jumped to more than 1,800 calories. Where do those extra calories come from? In general, we are eating:

- **More meat.** We are a nation of carnivores. Americans eat close to 200 pounds of meat, poultry, and fish per person each year—an increase of 50 pounds per person from a half century ago. That's about 6½ ounces a day, some 16 percent above the recommended amount. Every 3½-ounce serving of beef and 1-ounce serving of cheese raises our intake of saturated fat by 12 grams (in excess of one-half the RDA).
- **Less milk but more cheese.** We drink only about 60 percent of the milk we drank 50 years ago, but we eat nearly four times as much cheese, up from about 7½ pounds per person per year to almost 30 pounds. This is probably not the result of eating more good-quality cheeses, but of consuming more convenience foods

and prepared foods, such as pizza, fast-food sandwiches, nachos, burritos, bagel spreads, and prepackaged cheese products.

- **More fruits and vegetables.** There are some positives here. Americans are eating about 20 percent more fruits and vegetables than we did in the 1970s. But we still don't eat enough of these healthy foods. The average fruit and vegetable consumption for women is just under two servings of vegetables and one serving of fruit per day, about half the recommended amounts. Also, we tend not to seek variety. Much of the rise in consumption for fruits is limited to apples, bananas, and grapes; the rise in vegetable consumption is limited to tomatoes, onions, and leafy lettuces. Potatoes still dominate our vegetable consumption and orange juice, our fruit consumption. Although I count a good old-fashioned baked potato as a vegetable, the majority of potatoes that we eat these days come in the form of fries or chips or as part of a processed meal. And unfortunately, some 80 percent of total tomato consumption comes from processed tomato products such as sauces, canned tomatoes, tomato paste, and ketchup.

- **Far too much refined grain and too little whole grain.** The single biggest group of foods that contributes to our calorie intake is refined grains—cookies, cakes, bagels, and other dessert foods. Between 1970 and 2003, total per capita consumption of grains rose by 43 percent. It's fine to eat whole grains in abundance, because these grains are digested slowly, satisfy hunger for longer periods of time, and provide protein, fiber, and other nutrients. However, of the 8 ounces of grains consumed per person per day in this country, less than 1 ounce is whole grains; the rest is refined grains, which have a higher starch and lower fiber content than whole grains have and are largely devoid of nutritional value, with the exception of some B vitamins. They also have lower concentrations of minerals, essential fatty acids, and phytochemicals that are vital to health.

- **More added fats and oils.** In the past 30 years, total consumption of added fats and oils rose by 63 percent. These added fats and oils account for 49 percent of the 300-calorie-per-day increase since 1970. In and of itself, this is not necessarily a problem. The latest research shows that a range of total fat consumption is healthy, from very low to very high. Certain kinds of fats are an important part of a healthful diet, such as the monounsaturated and polyunsaturated fats found in fish, nuts, and vegetables. However, much of the boost in fat consumption over the past few decades comes from saturated and trans fats, which are linked with high cholesterol and coronary heart disease. These added fats and oils are found in cooking oils and such processed food products as french fries, snacks, and baked goods.

- **Pounds and pounds of sweeteners.** Sugar and sweetener consumption has risen by 19 percent in the past 30 years. Statistics from 2005 suggest that each of us consumes about 103 pounds of sweeteners each year, including 46 pounds of refined sugar and about 56 pounds of corn sweeteners. (The higher consumption of corn sweeteners has been propelled mostly by the increased use of high-fructose corn syrup in soft drinks, processed foods, and baked goods.) That comes out to about 30 teaspoons per person per day of added sweeteners—equivalent to about 477 calories, and more than triple what is recommended by the US Dietary Guidelines.

- **A boatload of sweetened beverages.** A major source of the increased sugar intake comes from beverages. According to the US Department of Agriculture, the amount of carbonated soft drinks made by companies each year went from 18.7 gallons per person in 1966 to more than 52 gallons today. That's the equivalent of 557 12-ounce cans for each person. Sweetened beverages are the single biggest source of calories in our diet, providing about 300 to 400 calories every day for many women.

THE WAY WE EAT

There have also been radical changes in the *way* we eat.

Fifty years ago, most of us ate family meals sitting down at a table, with no TV in sight. Now we eat on the run, at fast-food counters, in our cars, at our desks, and in front of the tube. Too rarely do we eat at the dinner table with family and friends. Studies show that families who do not dine together do not eat as healthfully, consuming more fried foods and soda than families who share meals.

Our new way of eating includes:

- **Larger portions of calorie-dense foods.** Over the past few decades, the portion sizes of meats, pizzas, baked goods, sweetened beverages, and other calorie-rich foods have grown considerably. Many foods and beverages are now served in portions that are at least twice as large as the standard serving size defined by the US Guidelines. Twenty years ago, a slice of pizza delivered about 250 calories; today, it's more like 425. The average bagel was about 3 inches in diameter and contained 140 calories; now bagels are closer to 4 or 5 inches and deliver a hefty 350 calories. The average portion size of meat served in a restaurant has doubled or tripled. The original Burger King's meal of burger, fries, and soft drink contained about 600 calories. Today's supersize portion of the same meal holds more than 1,500 calories. We Americans love a bargain. If a 12-ounce drink is 99 cents and a 20-ounce drink is only 25 cents more, we're apt to go for the bigger size to get more bang from our buck despite the cost to our waistlines.

Even the sizes of our plates, bowls, and cups have increased—another hazard to our health. Studies show that people consume more food and more calories both when they're offered larger portions and when they eat from larger dining ware.

Be Careful of Portion Sizes

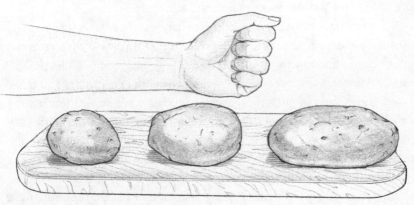

Potatoes are a healthy food. However, when it comes to calories, they more closely resemble a grain than a vegetable. A small serving of potatoes is defined as half a small potato. The potatoes pictured here, then, consist of 2 servings (small), 4 servings (medium), and 6 servings (large).

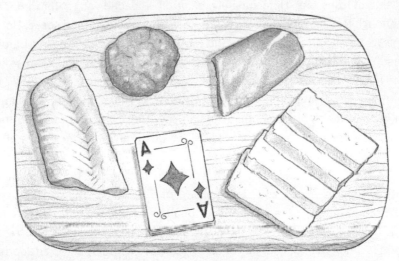

The secret to moderating food intake is small servings.

The illustration above shows standard portion sizes of equivalent calories (for scale, shown in relation to a deck of cards). Note that they are smaller than servings one might get in a restaurant or cook for oneself at home. For the same calorie count in a 4-ounce burger or chicken breast, one can eat a full 6-ounce serving of fish or 8 ounces of tofu.

TRANS FAT: NOT THE ONLY EVIL FAT

Trans fats, also known as trans fatty acids or partially hydrogenated oils, have recently earned the negative reputation they deserve. These fatty acids are formed by an industrial process called hydrogenation, which adds hydrogen to liquid vegetable fats. This changes the chemical structure of the fats, making them more solid and stable.

Trans fats have been popular in the food industry because they're inexpensive, are easy to use, and give foods a more desirable texture and a longer shelf life. They're frequently found in fried foods such as doughnuts and french fries; in cookies, crackers, biscuits, pie crusts, and other baked goods; and in stick margarines. Studies have shown that eating trans fats raises blood levels of "bad" (LDL) cholesterol and slightly lowers "good" (HDL) cholesterol, increasing the risk of developing heart disease and stroke. These fats also appear to boost the risk of metabolic syndrome and type 2 diabetes.

When the US government issued a regulation in 2006 requiring food manufacturers to label a product's content of trans fats, some companies replaced the hydrogenated oils in their products with palm oil and palm kernel oil. Now many packaged baked goods boast that they have zero grams of trans fats. Unfortunately, palm oil is loaded with saturated fat. Although less harmful than trans fats, it still promotes heart disease. Both the World Health Organization and the National Heart, Lung, and Blood Institute urge consumers to reduce their intake of palm oils because of the risk for heart disease and stroke.

Palm oils have another important drawback: The planting of oil palms in Indonesia and other Southeast Asian countries has contributed to the destruction of rainforest and wildlife, including endangered tigers, elephants, orangutans, and rhinoceroses.

More healthful and less environmentally damaging substitutes for trans fats include olive, soy, and canola oils.

Bottom line: For the sake of your health and the environment, try to minimize your intake of both trans fats and palm oils. Choose whole, fresh foods rather than packaged foods. If you have to buy packaged foods, read the labels carefully and avoid these fats.

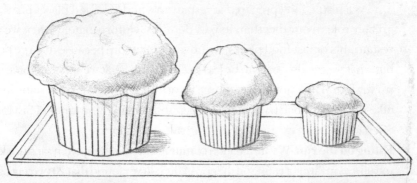

Muffins and other baked goods served these days are often much larger than they used to be. Note the calorie difference in the three sizes of muffin: very large (350 calories); medium (260 calories); and mini (110 calories): Typical muffins contain mostly sugar and few healthy ingredients.

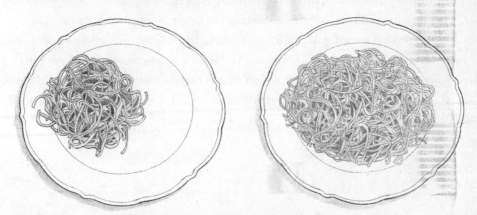

The plate on the left contains 1 cup of pasta; the one on the right, 2 cups. A small serving of pasta is defined as ½ cup—half the size of the plate on the left. One cup of pasta is actually considered a large portion, equivalent to two slices of bread.

- **More meals away from home.** In 1970, 26 percent of household food budgets in this country were spent on meals outside the home; by 2006, that share had risen to 46 percent. This number is expected to continue rising (24 percent between 2000 and 2020—18 percent for full-service restaurants and 6 percent for fast service).

  Just a few decades ago, we ate at cafeterias, restaurants, and fast-food places about twice a week; now we average one meal per day. A number of factors account for this increase: more women working outside the home, with busy lifestyles; more dual-income households resulting in higher overall income; longer commute times; and more affordable and convenient fast-food restaurants that advertise heavily.

As a result, food prepared at restaurants and fast-food places plays a much greater role in our diet than in past decades. Unfortunately, when we dine in restaurants or fast-food places, we not only eat more because of large portions, but what we eat also tends to be less healthy than what we serve at home. A 2005 survey found that women's top three favorite foods ordered in restaurants or for take-out were french fries, hamburgers, and pizza. These kinds of fast foods are often loaded with excess saturated fat, salt, and calories.

- **Eating on the run.** We are a nation of multitaskers, and we often sacrifice leisurely mealtimes in favor of eating on the go. A 2005 survey found that 20 percent of restaurant meals were purchased at drive-thru or curbside venues—up from 14 percent in 1998. (I am on a personal mission to get companies to do away with drive-thrus—as you can see, I haven't been very successful!) A 2006 survey by Nationwide Mutual Insurance found that almost half of young Americans and a third of baby boomers say they eat full meals in the car and an even larger number snack there.

- **Television viewing.** We watch far too much television, especially while we eat. After work and sleep, TV viewing is the most time-consuming activity in this country. Some 66 percent of Americans regularly watch TV during dinner. Unfortunately, people who watch television while eating are not able to properly monitor their own intake, which leads to overeating.

HOW CAN YOU EAT BETTER?

This is a good time to take a moment to review your eating habits by looking at the 24-hour food assessment you filled out in the Smart Woman's Health Assessment at the beginning of the book.

- How many times a day did you eat?
- Where did you eat?
- How many servings of whole grains did you have?
- How many servings of vegetables and fruits?
- How many servings of low-fat dairy products?
- How much junk food did you eat and under what circumstances?

Understanding where you are right now in your dietary patterns—the nature of your current eating habits—can be very helpful in addressing your need to eat more mindfully. Are you skipping breakfast? Are you eating a lot between meals? Consuming a lot of processed food?

There's a massive amount of advice offered about what constitutes a healthy diet. The vast majority of this advice suggests that you add or eliminate specific foods from your plate. Most of us have heard the dogma that around 30 percent of our calories should come from fat, about 10 to 15 percent from protein, and about 60 percent from carbohydrates. There are popular diets that espouse everything from combinations of high carbs and low protein, to low carbs and high fat/high protein. The reality is—and this may come as a shock—it doesn't matter what percentage of calories in your diet come from fat or carbohydrates, within reason. (See the box Healthy Eating Plans on pages 366–367.) A wide range of ratios works as long as you are getting a sensible amount of protein and the foods that contain the nutrients that you need, such as fruits, vegetables, whole grains, nuts, and legumes. The variety of good food choices is broad indeed. The real secret to healthy eating lies in following three simple rules. If you adhere to these basic rules, you will naturally adopt a more wholesome pattern of eating.

Rule 1. Eat real food. Whenever possible, stick with foods that are:

- Whole
- Fresh
- Locally grown
- Made with few ingredients and little processing and packaging

Real foods are delicious, nutrient-packed foods that are free of additives and other artificial ingredients, unrefined, and minimally processed. They include vegetables, fruits, legumes, whole grains, low-fat and fat-free dairy foods, fish, and lean meats.

The flip side of this tenet is minimizing the amount of junk food you eat. As I discussed at the beginning of this chapter, we eat far too much in the way of processed and refined foods. Try to stick to only one or two servings a day of foods such as white bread, white rice, pasta, or cookies.

Rule 2. Eat a little less (*hara hachi bu*). Women often ask me how many calories they should eat each day. There is no easy answer to this question; it depends on many factors. It's much better to ask: Do I weigh too much? Am I gaining weight? If you're putting on additional pounds or need to take off weight, you have to reduce your food intake. If you are maintaining a healthy body weight, then you are balancing your energy intake well.

Everyone knows what it means to eat less. But it's hard to do because our bodies are programmed to eat the same amount or more each day. When we consciously limit our calories by, say, eating a smaller lunch or dinner, our bodies scream for us to fill in those calories during the rest of the day, and we often succumb to that big bag of chips so easily secured from our pantry or that fast-food restaurant we pass on our way home from work. The secret is learning to override the body's hunger signals at every meal.

(continued on page 368)

HEALTHY EATING PLANS

There are numerous ways to eat a healthy diet. Every woman has a different set of culturally defined tastes and values that will determine what she prefers. Here I suggest two excellent dietary plans: the DASH diet (Dietary Approaches to Stop Hypertension), endorsed by the National Heart, Lung, and Blood Institute, and the Mediterranean Diet, promoted by a group called Oldways (and followed by millions of people who live near the Mediterranean). You will see that both of these dietary patterns focus on whole foods, with very few processed foods and very little sugar.

DASH Diet

For years, many of us in the nutrition community have been advocating a diet rich in whole foods, especially vegetables, fruits, whole grains, low-fat and fat-free dairy foods, legumes, nuts and seeds, and small amounts of animal proteins. This is a pattern of eating that maximizes the good ingredients in food (vitamins, minerals, phytochemicals, healthy proteins, the right oils, and fiber) and minimizes the negative ones (salt, saturated fats and trans fats, sugars, and unnecessary chemicals), while at the same time naturally keeping calories at a modest level. For the most part, this dietary pattern is quite modest in fat.

Recent research by the National Institutes of Health supports the benefits of just such a diet for heart health, the DASH diet. The early research on the benefits of the DASH diet focused solely on hypertension, a leading risk factor for heart disease and stroke. The results showed that the DASH diet reduces blood pressure in virtually everyone, male or female, young or old, people with high blood pressure and those with normal blood pressure. More recent research has shown that the diet also lowers the risk of heart attack and stroke and reduces body weight. I'm not surprised by these findings, because I've always been a firm believer in the benefits of eating the kinds of whole foods advocated by the DASH diet. But what is surprising to many people is the *amount* of food allowed in this diet. For example, take a look at the number of fruit and vegetable servings you can eat each day:

	1,600 CALORIE DIET SERVINGS	2,000 CALORIE DIET SERVINGS
Vegetables	3 or 4	4 or 5
Fruits	4	4 or 5
*Grains	6	7 or 8
Low-fat and fat-free dairy	2 or 3	2 or 3
*Lean proteins	1 or 2	2
Nuts, seeds, legumes	3 per week	4 or 5 per week
Fats, oils	Limited	Limited
Sugars and sweets	5 or fewer per week	5 or fewer per week

*More than half of your grains need to be whole grains. A protein serving equals 3 to 4 ounces. It's best to focus on fish and vegetarian options and only limited animal protein.

For more information on the DASH diet, go to Dashdiet.org or Nhlbi.nih.gov and type "DASH diet" in the search box.

Mediterranean Diet

Research demonstrates that eating in a food pattern followed by cultures living near the Mediterranean confers numerous health benefits. I love traveling to Italy and France, and I can say without a doubt that this is my favorite way to eat! This is not a low-fat diet, but it is low in saturated fat.

The basic foundation of the Mediterranean Diet is as follows:

- Use olive oil as your primary source of fat.

- Eat plenty of foods from plant sources such as fruits and vegetables, breads, grains, beans, nuts, and seeds.

- Eat low to moderate amounts of fish and small amounts of beef, pork, and poultry weekly.

- Eat low to moderate amounts of cheese and yogurt daily.

- Drink a moderate amount of wine (one or two glasses per day for men, one glass per day for women).

For more information and details of how to follow the Mediterranean Diet, see the Oldways Web site at Oldwayspt.org.

The Japanese have a marvelous concept known as *hara hachi bu*. It means, literally, "eight parts out of ten full." By eating until you feel 80 percent full at every meal, you will naturally consume 20 percent fewer calories. If you follow the *hara hachi bu* philosophy 5 days a week, it will give you a little leeway at other times to go ahead and have that piece of wedding cake or a few of those yummy appetizers at your office party.

It's a good idea to limit your portion size (and your plate size!). It also helps to take your time eating. The brain requires about 20 minutes to register that your stomach is full, so give your mind time to keep up with what you're taking in; otherwise, you may end up consuming more calories than you really want or need. If you eat mindfully, you will get pleasure from your eating.

Rule 3. Enjoy your meals. Eating is as much about satisfying your emotional and aesthetic needs as your nutritional ones. Be thankful for the good food before you and enjoy sharing it with family and friends. Create pleasant ceremonies around your meals, no matter how simple. Be conscious while you eat so that you can revel in the flavors and aromas of your meals. Focus on quality, not quantity. Savor each bite of the foods you love rather than eating for fullness. Be discerning: Eat only what you really like and not what you don't.

WHAT ABOUT VITAMINS AND MINERALS?

One of the most common questions women ask me is, "Which vitamins and minerals should I take?" The answer is not straightforward, because it depends on the individual. But research demonstrates that the most important aspect of your nutritional health is the *food* you eat. People tend to want a quick remedy or a pill to fix their nutritional woes. But no vitamin or mineral supplement can undo a poor diet. Eat well and you will get nearly all of the vitamins and minerals your body needs.

Having said this, there is strong evidence that women benefit from taking a vitamin D and calcium supplement for bone and immune system health. (For specific guidelines, see the box Vitamin D and Calcium on pages 164–165.)

As for other vitamins and minerals supplements, there is little evidence of benefit if you are in good health. In fact, taking a range of vitamins and minerals at high doses can have negative side effects. Moreover, many foods these days—cereals, dairy, grains, snacks—are fortified with vitamins and minerals. For these reasons, I don't advocate taking a multivitamin.

There are two exceptions to this rule: If you are pregnant or planning to get pregnant, you should take folate to prevent birth defects. Also, if you are at high risk for macular degeneration or cataracts (or already have these conditions), you may want to consider taking special vitamin preparations. (See Chapter 20.)

Remember, no vitamin preparation can enhance your health if you have a poor diet. The foods you eat matter the most.

HOW TO CREATE A HEALTHY PERSONAL FOOD ENVIRONMENT

Following the three basic rules of eating well is easier if you reshape your personal food environment with an eye to the *what, why, where, how,* and *when* of healthy eating. This involves replacing the "toxic" environmental cues that encourage overeating and consumption of unhealthy food with healthy environmental cues. It also includes taking stock of the *way* you eat and making changes to ensure healthy eating patterns.

WHAT

- **Cut out the crap!** Eliminate highly processed foods and sweetened beverages from your kitchen shelves, car, office, and grocery cart. Stick with healthy snacks such as fruit, yogurt, and small amounts of nuts and seeds; for beverages, drink fat-free milk, tea, coffee, and water (and a little alcohol if you like).
- **Think carefully about where and how you shop, and be careful about the foods you bring into the house.** You are most likely the gatekeeper to the foods available in your house. Because of the huge selection of foods now available to us and the long lists of additives and other ingredients in nutritional labels, shopping has become quite daunting. When possible, buy local and buy fresh. If you have a farmers' market nearby, support it. Go for variety: Expand your repertoire of fruits and vegetables. When I go to a big grocery store, I like to linger in the outer aisles, where the produce (and dairy items) are kept, scoping out what looks freshest and ripest among the fruits and vegetables. In general, I minimize my shopping in the middle aisles, which tend to contain highly processed, highly packaged foods. The reality is that you will eat the foods that you have in your kitchen. If good food is there, that is what you will eat; the same goes for unhealthy food. Be wise and make good choices.
- **Plan ahead.** We all have busy lives that make it a challenge to cook fresh meals from scratch every night. It helps to plan ahead so that you have ingredients on hand for wholesome and tasty dinners. I tend to shop on weekends and stock up on a combination of vegetables, including some that are perishable and some that will keep a bit longer, such as carrots, green beans, cabbage, celery, and

squash. By midweek, most of the perishables are gone, so for meals later in the week, I combine some of the other vegetables with nonperishables, such as canned beans and brown rice.

- **Eat a variety of foods and make sure they have plenty of flavor.** Make use of fresh herbs and spices, squeezes of citrus juice and zest, and spare drizzlings of olive oil instead of flavoring your food with a lot of added fat, salt, or sugar.

- **Limit your portion sizes of calorie-rich foods, at home and at restaurants.** Bigger servings of high-calorie foods are not better, even when they seem to offer great "value"; they boost our overall calorie intake and encourage overeating. A serving size of meat should be about 4 ounces, or no larger than the size of a deck of cards. A serving of tofu or fish can be 6 ounces. (See the illustration on portion sizes on page 361.) It's fine to eat large portions of vegetables, fruits, and whole grains.

- **Indulge occasionally in a special treat.** If you really crave a cookie or a small dish of ice cream, go ahead and have it, but limit your portion and really savor it. And don't do this several times a day!

WHY

- **Examine your routines for unhealthy habits.** How much food do you eat and under what circumstances? Do you eat when you're feeling bored or stressed? Understanding your eating patterns will help you make small changes in your environment that will help you eliminate unhealthy habits. For instance, do you walk or drive past the bakery or Starbucks and have trouble resisting the lure of a doughnut or a grande caffè latte? Try changing your route to avoid temptations. If you eat unhealthy snacks when you're bored, find other activities to fill the void, replace the food with healthy snacks such as carrots or celery sticks, or have a cup of herbal tea.

WHERE, HOW, AND WHEN

- **Establish good eating habits.** Eat three meals a day. Eat at a table, with utensils, and with people when possible. Eat slowly. Leave a meal feeling 80 percent full (remember *hara hachi bu*). Avoid eating in front of the TV or computer. This habit may be the most difficult to change, but it also may have the most impact on your caloric intake.

- **When you eat out, be selective.** Be choosy about where you eat and try to avoid chain restaurants. An hour or so before you go out, have a small healthy snack, such as an apple or a carrot and hummus, so that you aren't famished when you get to the restaurant and can resist the temptation to gobble up the contents of the bread basket. Order soup or a salad or a side dish of vegetables and eat this first; it will help fill you up before your more caloric main dish arrives. I usually order one entrée to split with my husband and double the side dishes of vegetables. I eat just the amount I want, and we save money.

- **Be vigilant about maintaining good eating habits during holidays.** For a long time we thought that most weight gain took place in slow increments over the course of the year. But it turns out that for many people the 3- to 5-pound annual gain often occurs between December and New Year's or other holidays. As much as you can, try to stick to your healthy patterns at these times.

27

Getting Active

Being physically active may be the most important thing you can do for your health. In fact, your life depends on it.

I've been in the thick of research on the benefits of exercise for a quarter of a century. I began my investigations with my colleagues on tightly controlled clinical trials looking at the impact of physical activity on bone density, arthritis, joint health, heart health, diabetes, and many other conditions. In trial after trial, the benefits of exercise were made clear. In recent years, a tsunami of evidence has confirmed that physical activity is good for virtually every system in the body. It affects not just your physical well-being but also your emotional and mental health. It's the closest thing we have to a magic bullet for taking care of our own bodies: We are built to move, and when our bodies move on a regular basis, they are healthy; when they don't, when we're largely sedentary, our bodies deteriorate.

Most of us know this. We know that exercise is good for us. And yet, despite this, our society has become more sedentary than ever: We spend more hours of the day sitting—working on our computers, surfing the Internet, playing computer games, watching TV. I sympathize with this tendency. I may be the queen of exercise research and advocacy, but I can all too easily sit at my desk for 10 hours a day.

Exercise doesn't have to be a boring chore. You just need to find an activity that you enjoy. If you don't like to exercise, try picking a form of physical activity that doesn't feel like exercise to you, such as walking, ballroom dancing, raking leaves, or taking a bike ride. To keep my workouts interesting, I plan my weekend physical activity around the seasons: In summer, I bike, swim, and hike. In fall and spring, I run and hike a little. In winter, it's cross-country skiing and climbing at our indoor rock gym. It doesn't matter what form of exercise you choose; the important thing is to be consistent about doing some kind of physical activity.

This chapter will help you build a physical activity plan. What you'll find here is a menu of choices, different ways to build regular physical activity into your days. Pick and choose what suits you. If you get bored with one activity, move on to something new. At the end of the chapter I provide a simple but effective strength-training program that you can do at home with minimal equipment. Whatever you do, get active. Remember: Your life depends on it!

NEW PHYSICAL ACTIVITY GUIDELINES FOR AMERICANS

Given all of the exciting new discoveries about the health benefits of exercise, in 2007 the US Department of Health and Human Services decided it was time to issue new guidelines for physical activity in this country. I was appointed vice chair of the scientific advisory committee charged with shaping the new *2008 Physical Activity Guidelines for Americans*. Our committee looked closely at the new scientific information on physical activity and health and then helped create science-based recommendations for the types and amounts of activity that provide the greatest benefits. Here are some of the general findings:

- Just about everyone benefits from physical activity—people of all ages, from children to older adults, pregnant and postpartum women, people with disabilities, and members of every racial and ethnic group.
- Even just a little physical activity is better than none.
- Physical activity improves health regardless of your body weight (healthy, overweight, obese).
- Both aerobic exercise and strength training improve health.
- More physical activity equals greater health benefits.
- There are many ways to be physically active, so choose what you like.

(More findings from our report can be found online at Fitness.gov.)

HOW MUCH DO I NEED TO EXERCISE?

According to the *2008 Physical Activity Guidelines for Americans*, the amount you should exercise depends on your age.

Children ages 6 and older should get 1 hour or more of physical activity every day, including mostly aerobic exercise, and at least some muscle-strengthening and bone-strengthening activity at least three times a week.

For adults, substantial health benefits can be gained if you:

- Do 2½ hours per week of moderate-intensity aerobic exercise, such as brisk walking.
    OR
- Do 1 hour and 15 minutes per week of vigorous-intensity aerobic exercise.
    OR
- Do some equivalent combination of moderate- and vigorous-intensity exercise each week.

You should perform aerobic activity in bouts of at least 10 minutes. Although it may be best to spread the activity throughout the week, it is just fine to get all of your activity over a couple of days on the weekend. It is also recommended that you do muscle strengthening involving all of the major muscle groups on two or more days a week.

For more extensive health benefits, you can:

- Increase your aerobic physical activity to 5 hours a week at moderate intensity.
    OR
- Do 2½ hours a week of vigorous-intensity aerobic physical activity.
    OR
- Do an equivalent combination of moderate- and vigorous-intensity activity.

Older adults should adhere to the guidelines for adults or be as physically active as their fitness level and condition allow. If they are at risk for falls, they should also do exercises to maintain or improve balance to avoid falls.

INCIDENTAL ACTIVITY: DOWN WITH THE SEDENTARY AND UP WITH THE ACTIVE!

The evidence is overwhelming that physical activity enhances our health and well-being and extends our life span. And yet, more than 60 percent of American women aren't active enough to meet the minimum requirements of 150 minutes of moderate activity a week. Twenty-five percent of American women engage in no physical activity at all.

The reasons for this are complicated and involve not just our own personal choices but also our built environment, where we live and work, and how we commute. Physical activity related to work, transportation, and household jobs have all declined, and desk-bound jobs have risen. For many of us, active leisure pursuits such as walking or working in the garden have been replaced by sedentary activities such as surfing the Internet or watching TV. All of this inactivity contributes to the incidence of obesity, breast cancer, colon cancer, diabetes, and heart disease—and to associated medical costs, to the tune of an estimated $75 billion a year in the United States.

Fortunately, there are plenty of opportunities for you to boost your physical activity and decrease your sedentary behavior on a daily basis. When we talk about physical activity, we tend to think only of structured exercise, but there are other ways to build movement into your day. Here are some examples of 10- to 30-minute sessions of daily activities:

1. **Do an errand or two on foot or bicycle.** Walk or bicycle to the post office to mail that package or to the corner convenience store for a half gallon of milk.
2. **If possible, walk or bike to work.** If this isn't convenient, take a 10- or 15-minute walk during your lunch break.
3. **Park at a distance,** or get off the bus or metro one stop early and walk the rest of the way to your destination.
4. **Use the free exercise equipment.** Shun the elevator and go for the stairs.
5. **Do your own yard work and snow shoveling.** Mow the lawn, rake leaves, weed the flower garden, and shovel your sidewalk. My favorite is stacking wood.
6. **Get outside and walk your dog or play with your kids.** A 125-pound woman can burn 142 calories in 30 minutes of outdoor play or walking.
7. **For indoor entertainment, shut off the TV, turn on the music, and dance.** If you're into video games, go for higher intensity activity games, such as Dance Dance Revolution!
8. **When talking on the phone or watching TV, be active.** Walk around, stretch, lift weights, or do situps or lunges.

AEROBIC EXERCISE, STRENGTH TRAINING, FLEXIBILITY, AND BALANCE

Building incidental physical activity into your day can go far to boost your overall movement. But to maximize the health benefits of physical activity, you want to have both aerobic activity and strength training. If you are older and at risk for falls, you also want to include balance activities. For years we have also included flexibility as part of the guidelines, but the reality is that there is very little evidence that flexibility is important for overall health. I still believe that stretching exercises are beneficial and will help make sure that you do not become inflexible. But your stretching routine can be quite short and follow your aerobic and strength-training activities.

Both aerobic and strength-training activities have three components:

- **Intensity:** How hard you work during the activity
- **Frequency:** How often you perform the activity
- **Duration:** How long you do the activity in a single session or how many repetitions you complete

Experts agree that the most important element in any physical activity program is the total amount of physical activity you get each week from a combination of moderate and vigorous activities.

AEROBIC EXERCISE

Aerobic exercise is the focus of just about any fitness program. This type of exercise works your cardiovascular system, making your heart beat faster than it does at rest, increasing cardiovascular health. In most forms of aerobic exercise, the body's muscles move rhythmically and persistently for a prolonged period of time, forcing the heart and lungs to work harder. Examples include jogging, running, brisk walking, jumping rope, rowing, hiking, dancing, playing basketball or soccer or other running sports, bicycling, and swimming.

Intensity levels for aerobic exercise depend on your current fitness level. A brisk walk may be moderate exercise for one person but vigorous for another person. In general, during moderate-intensity exercise, you are able to talk easily, but not sing, while performing the activity. Moderate activity for most people includes brisk walking, biking at less than 10 miles per hour, water aerobics, leisurely swimming, and doubles tennis.

Vigorous-intensity exercise increases your heart rate, and may make you feel winded so that saying more than a few words is hard. Examples include race-walking, jogging and running, singles tennis, biking at more than 10 miles per hour, jumping rope, swimming at a fast pace, and biking uphill.

How Much Total Aerobic Activity Should I Get Each Week?

To enjoy the health benefits of aerobic exercise, you should do at least 150 minutes of moderate-intensity aerobic activity each week *or* 75 minutes of vigorous activity *or* a combination of the two. I am pleased that the new guidelines allow for people to meet the recommendations with either moderate or vigorous activity or a combination of both. This allows for flexibility with your activity routine.

If you need to lose weight or have lost weight and want to keep it off, you may need more total activity than is suggested here.

How Many Days a Week Should I Perform the Activity?

It's best to distribute your aerobic activities over several days each week. This will help reduce your risk of injury and excessive fatigue. However, if you can only exercise on weekends, it's fine to squeeze in your 75 minutes of vigorous activity or 150 minutes of moderate activity into a couple of days.

For How Long Should I Exercise During Each Session?

You should do both moderate- and vigorous-intensity aerobic activities in sessions of at least 10 minutes. You can accumulate your activity throughout the week in short or long sessions.

STRENGTH TRAINING

An essential part of any physical activity program, strength training builds muscle and bone strength by causing the body's muscles to work against, or "resist," an applied force or weight. It often involves the use of free weights, elastic bands, weight machines, or your own body weight. Examples include training with weights or resistance bands; calisthenics such as pushups, pullups, and situps; and heavy physical work, such as digging or carrying heavy loads.

Regular strength training will make you feel and look better. Increasing your ankle, leg, and lower-body strength will give you better balance, mobility, and speed of movement, all of which will reduce your risk of falling if you lose your footing. Strength training also boosts your ability to perform everyday activities, such as carrying heavy grocery bags or climbing stairs. Finally, if you are trying to lose weight, strength training helps preserve your muscle and bone so that you lose mostly body fat.

How Much Total Strength-Training Activity Should I Get Each Week?

Each week, it is optimal to get at least two sessions of strength-training exercises that work all of the body's major muscle groups, including arms, shoulders, chest, abdomen, hips, and legs. Contrary to what you may think, you do not need to separate the sessions with a non-strength-training day unless you are working out at very high intensities.

For How Long and How Intensely Should I Strength Train?

The amount of time is less important than the number of repetitions and/or amount of weight. You should do your muscle-strengthening exercises to the point at which it would be difficult to complete another repetition. Generally, a good rule of thumb is one or two sets of 8 to 12 repetitions of each exercise. If you can lift more repetitions than 12, the weight is too light.

In strength training, intensity is measured by how much weight or force is used relative to how much you can lift. The physical activity guidelines recommend a moderate- to high-level intensity workout that involves all of the major muscle groups of the body. Over time, your muscles will develop strength and endurance. The key to improving strength is to increase the amount of weight you lift as you get stronger. There is no need to increase the number of repetitions beyond 12.

FLEXIBILITY AND BALANCE

As we age, our muscles tend to shorten and grow stiffer. Stretching and other flexibility exercises can counteract this propensity. Finishing your workout with a brief series of stretches is a great way to relax and maintain flexibility and good posture. The Sun Salutation outlined in Chapter 24 promotes flexibility and good posture.

If you are at risk for falls or have poor balance, consider adding some balance exercises to your routine. These include any activity that challenges your balance, such as a one-legged stand, tandem walk, and various tai chi poses. They are easy to build into the warmup part of any workout. The Sun Salutation outlined in Chapter 26 also helps with balance.

HOW CAN I MEET THE GUIDELINES?

The possibilities for meeting the recommendations are virtually limitless. There is no single "recipe" for the perfect physical fitness plan. In deciding how to meet them, you should think about your current level of fitness. How much physical activity are you already doing? What are your fitness goals, and how can you best achieve them within the framework of your work and family life? To help you devise your own plan, I have outlined four options below. These scenarios offer combinations of moderate- to vigorous-intensity aerobic activities and muscle-strengthening exercises that you can do over the course of a week to meet the guidelines.

1. I have the time and want to do it right.

If you can devote time throughout the week to being active, there are numerous ways to meet the guidelines. I suggest engaging in your favorite aerobic activity (walking, running, cycling, etc.) 5 days a week for 30 to 45 minutes. If possible, mix moderate- and vigorous-intensity activities that make you break a sweat to get the full cardiovascular benefits. Then, 2 or 3 days a week, do your strength training—following the program in this chapter, a community program, or one at a fitness center. Make sure that you target all of the major muscle groups in your body—arms, trunk (front and back), and legs.

2. I have more time on the weekends.

This describes me. I have very little time during the week to be active, but a lot more time on the weekends. So, yes, I become a weekend warrior—filling up my time with a lot of fun exercise—running, biking, rock climbing, and cross-country skiing. If you fit into this category, I encourage you to participate in your favorite vigorous-intensity aerobic activity on both Saturday and Sunday. Work toward getting at least 45 minutes of vigorous activity each weekend day. Then, during another portion of the weekend, try to get out and just be active in any way that you can—rake the leaves or go for a walk with your dog (or friend, or both). Basically, try your best to stay moving. Also, engage in a good strength-training workout, following either the program outlined here or one at a fitness center. Then if at all possible, try to work out at least once during the week. I do my best to squeeze in at least one run (aerobic) and one rock-climbing session (strength training) during the week.

3. I really don't have time to do any "planned" exercise.

Believe it or not, it is possible to build physical activity into your day so that you don't have to do much planned exercise. If you're creative, you can engineer plenty of incidental activity into your daily routine. When my life is really busy, and I just don't have time to exercise, this is how I stay active. The key is to figure out ways to be active within your daily routines. For instance, take public transportation and add a walk to and from the station. If I take the train to work, I have the option of either hopping on the subway from the train station to work, or walking 22 minutes. If I walk, it usually takes me only about 5 to 8 minutes longer than if I ride the subway because of the usual subway delays.

At work, take the stairs rather than the elevator. If you work on the 20th floor, get off at the 10th floor and walk up the last 10 flights. At lunch, walk to do some errands. At home, walk or ride your bike instead of driving to the store.

4. I want to do as little as possible to reap the health benefits.

If you are healthy now, you can get by with a minimal amount of exercise. However, if you have a chronic disease or need to lose weight, you should try to build more physical activity into your life. The minimum amount of exercise to meet the guidelines is 75 minutes per week of vigorous activity and two strength-training workouts. You can accomplish this by doing two 35- to 40-minute vigorous aerobic workouts and two strength-training workouts per week (20 minutes per session).

THE STRONG WOMEN'S TOTAL HEALTH STRENGTH-TRAINING PROGRAM

This strength-training program is basic but effective. It consists of 10 strength-training exercises that target all of the major muscle groups in your body. It will take you about 20 to 30 minutes to complete. The program starts out very easy. As you get stronger, you will need to either increase the amount of weight that you are lifting or work toward harder and harder modifications as described. For this program, you will need a mat or padded rug and dumbbells.

1. Wide-Leg Squat

This simple exercise will strengthen the muscles of the front, back, and inner thighs as well as the buttocks, which makes it especially important for the hip bones. It also helps improve balance and prevent falls.

Starting Position

Stand with your feet slightly greater than shoulder-width apart about 6 to 8 inches in front of a chair with your arms crossed in front of your chest, shoulders relaxed.

The Move

1. Leaning forward slightly at the hips, aim your buttocks into the chair and slowly lower yourself back to a seated position. Keep your chest lifted and your back, neck, and head in a straight line.

2. Pause for a breath in the seated position.

3. Leaning forward slightly, stand up slowly, making sure you keep your knees directly above your ankles. As you do this, push up from your heels through your lower legs, thighs, hips, and buttocks, which will help keep your knees from moving in front of your feet.

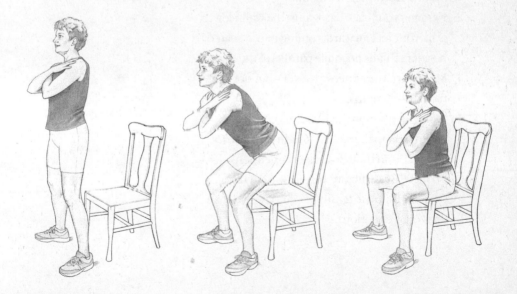

Reps and Sets

Complete 10 repetitions for one set, rest for a minute, and then do another 10 repetitions for the second set.

Where You Will Feel the Effort

In your thighs, buttocks, and lower back.

Notes: Keep chest lifted throughout the move, so that the body doesn't curl forward. Eyes should be looking straight ahead rather than down at the floor. If you experience any pain in your knees, make sure you're not letting your knees move forward past your toes during the move and that your lower leg stays perpendicular to the floor.

Make Sure You

- Lean just slightly forward when beginning the move.
- Don't allow knees to come in front of toes.
- Tighten abdominal muscles.
- Don't hold your breath.

To make this exercise more difficult, use dumbbells in each hand. Start with 3 pounds and then move up as you get stronger.

Modification
Wall Slide and Hold

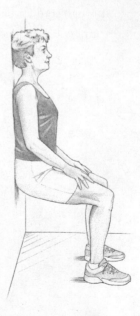

1. Stand leaning against a wall.
2. Keeping your back flat against the wall, slowly walk your feet forward, coming into a "seated" position, thighs not quite parallel to the floor.
3. Make sure your knees are over—but not in front of—your ankles.
4. Hold the position for 10 to 30 seconds.
5. Slide back up the wall to standing, pause for 30 seconds, and then do 2 more repetitions.
6. To increase difficulty, hold the "seated" position for up to 2 minutes, and repeat for a total of 5 repetitions.

2. *Biceps Curl with Rotation*

The muscles on the front of the arm, known as the biceps, are vital for many day-to-day activities, such as carrying, lifting, and doing household chores. This exercise will strengthen and tone these muscles and make many of these tasks easier.

Starting Position

Stand (or sit) with palms facing the outer thighs and a dumbbell in each hand.

The Move

1. Slowly bend your elbows and lift the dumbbells up toward your shoulders, keeping the upper arm firmly planted at your side (as if you were holding a newspaper under each arm). As you lift, rotate the dumbbells so that your palms face your shoulders.

2. Pause for a breath.

3. Slowly lower the dumbbells back to the starting position.

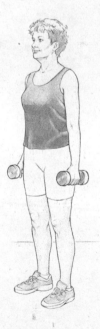 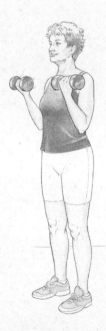

Reps and Sets

Complete 10 repetitions, rest for a minute, and then repeat.

Where You Will Feel the Effort

In your biceps and forearms.

Make Sure You

- Maintain a straight back with shoulders relaxed.
- Keep wrists straight through the entire lift.
- Keep shoulders pressed down and back.
- Don't hold your breath.

To make this exercise more difficult, increase the weight of each dumbbell. Start with 3 pounds, and then move up in weight as you get stronger.

3 and 4. Side Leg Raises: Hip Abduction and Adduction

The next two exercises are great exercises to strengthen the muscles and bones of the hip and thigh. Strengthening these muscles is important for agility and balance. If you want to increase the intensity of these exercises, either use an ankle weight or place your upper hand holding a dumbbell on your thigh.

3. Hip Abduction

Starting Position

Lie on the floor on your right side, legs straight and together, one on top of the other (ankle weights are optional and will increase intensity). Bend your right leg at the knee, keeping your hips and knees aligned, and use your right arm to support your head with your left hand planted on the floor for balance.

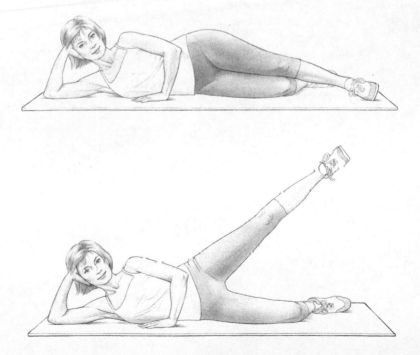

The Move

1. Keeping your leg straight, slowly lift your left leg with the foot flat and toes pointed straight ahead.

2. Pause for a breath.

3. Slowly lower the left leg back toward the floor so that it is resting on the right leg.

Reps and Sets

Complete 10 reps on each leg for one set, rest for a minute, and then do another 10 reps on each leg for the second set.

Where You Will Feel the Effort

In your outer thigh and hip of the moving leg.

Make Sure You

- Keep your body in a straight line.
- Keep your toes pointing forward, not up.
- Breathe throughout the exercise.

4. Hip Adduction

Starting Position

Lie on the floor on your right side, legs straight and together, one on top of the other (ankle weights are optional and will increase intensity). Bend your left leg and place your right foot behind your right knee for stability, and use your right arm to support your head with your left hand planted on the floor for balance.

The Move

1. Keeping your bottom (right) leg straight, slowly lift your right leg with the foot flat and toes pointed straight ahead.

2. Pause for a breath.

3. Slowly lower the right leg back toward the floor.

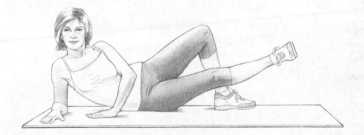

Reps and Sets

Complete 10 reps on each leg for one set, rest for a minute, and then do another 10 reps on each leg for the second set.

Where You Will Feel the Effort

In your inner thigh of the moving leg.

Make Sure You

- Keep your body in a straight line.
- Keep your toes pointing forward, not up.
- Breathe throughout the exercise.

5. One-Arm Bent-Over Row

I love this exercise because it focuses effort in the middle of the back, an area that is usually weak in women. Build greater strength in your shoulder and back by working one arm at a time.

Starting Position

> With a dumbbell in your right hand, stand several feet from the back of a chair or a counter. Expand your chest and squeeze your shoulder blades together. Bend over slowly from your hips, allowing the knees to bend as well. Reach out and rest the left hand on the back of the chair or the counter. Do not allow your back to change position as you lower from the standing position.

The Move

> 1. Pull your elbow to your side and raise the upper arm so that it is level with or slightly higher than your back.
>
> 2. Shift your shoulder back slightly and squeeze between your shoulder blades as you pause.
>
> 3. Lower your arm slowly.

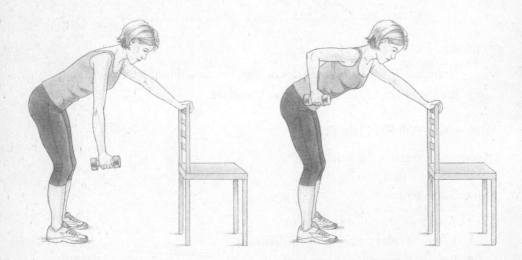

Reps and Sets

Complete 10 reps on each arm for one set, rest for a minute, and then do another 10 reps on each arm for the second set.

Where You Will Feel the Effort

In the mid-back, from the shoulder to the hip, in the backs of the shoulders, and throughout the muscles between and beneath the shoulder blades.

Make Sure You

- Take care to set up good form. Practice putting your body into the starting position.
- Use abdominal strength to maintain the body position while performing this exercise.
- Keep a flat back throughout the exercise and do not arch it. Hold a slightly diagonal angle from the hips instead of a straight line from hips to shoulders and head.
- Don't hold your breath.

To make this exercise more difficult, increase the weight of each dumbbell. Start with 3 pounds, and then move up in weight as you get stronger.

6. The Plank

Use this static posture to build core strength. This has become one of my favorite exercises. It looks easy, but it's not!

Starting Position

> Begin on hand and knees, with palms flat on the floor and hands positioned directly below the shoulders.

The Move

> 1. Extend your legs out straight behind you, positioning feet onto toes, with your back, buttocks, and legs all flat and in alignment.
>
> 2. Hold the position for a count of 10 to 30 seconds.
>
> 3. Come back to knees and relax; do 2 to 5 reps, and extend the holding time as core strength increases.

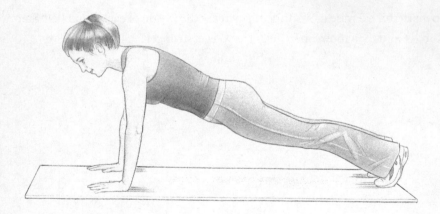

Where You Will Feel the Effort

Throughout your entire trunk, neck, back, hips, abdomen, thighs.

Make Sure You

- Use abdominal strength to maintain the position.
- Keep a flat back throughout the exercise. Hold a slightly diagonal angle from the hips instead of a straight line from hips to shoulders and head. *To keep your back safe, avoid arching the lower back.*
- Don't hold your breath.

Modification

To further increase intensity and greater core strengthening, modify the above-described move by positioning yourself on your elbows instead of palms. Hold and repeat as in the standard plank posture.

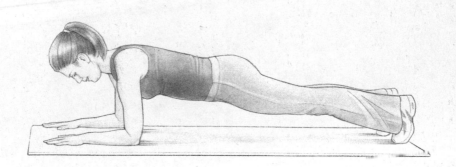

7. Pushups (Modified)

Pushups can be a daunting exercise. The modified pushup is a way to experience the benefits of the exercise without all of the intimidation or intensity of a classic pushup.

Starting Position

Get down on hands and knees, then inch the knees back until your torso is diagonal to the floor. Your hands should be directly underneath your shoulders. Point your fingers in the same direction as your head and spread the fingers out. Squeeze your shoulder blades together and unlock the elbows.

The Move

Bend the elbows to lower your entire body toward the floor. There will be a slight bend in your hips, but do not increase the bend or allow your back to arch.

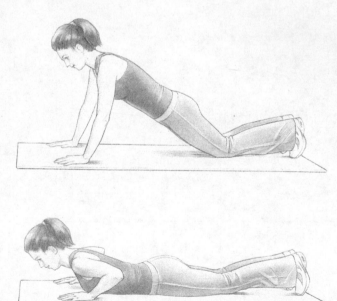

Reps and Sets

Do two sets of 10 repetitions each, with a minute rest between sets.

Where You Will Feel the Effort

In the chest, front of the shoulders, and back of the upper arms. You will feel the chest, abdominal, and back muscles tighten as you do this exercise.

Make Sure You

- Keep your abdominal muscles contracted for stability.
- Pause for a breath when your nose is near the floor.
- Press back to the starting position smoothly, and stop before your arms are completely straight.
- Control the pushing up and lowering down movements.
- Don't "scoop" your upper body toward the floor while pushing up.
- Don't arch your back.
- Don't hold your breath.

Modification

Classic pushup. You will experience a genuine sense of accomplishment with every set of pushups. This is a challenging exercise that builds strength and muscle tone in the chest, front of the shoulders, back of the arms, and between the ribs.

Starting Position

Get down on hands and knees, then walk your feet back until your body is parallel with the floor. Your hands should be directly underneath your shoulders. Point your fingers in the same direction as your head and spread the fingers out. Squeeze your shoulder blades together and unlock the elbows. Be sure to tighten your abdominal muscles so that your lower back does not sway.

The Move

1. Bend the elbows to lower your entire body toward the floor.

2. Keep your abdominal muscles contracted for stability.

3. Pause for a breath when your nose is 2 to 3 inches from the floor.

4. Press back to the starting position smoothly, and do not allow your back to arch or change position.

5. Stop before your arms are completely straight.

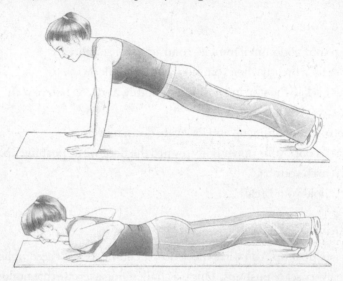

Reps and Sets

Do two sets of 10 repetitions, with a minute rest between sets.

Where You Will Feel the Effort

In the chest, front of the shoulders, and back of the upper arms. You will feel the abdominal and back muscles tighten as you do this exercise.

Make Sure You

- Can do two sets of modified pushups with excellent form before attempting this exercise.
- Keep your abdominal muscles contracted throughout the entire exercise.
- Don't bend at the hips—the low back should be in a straight line with the rest of the body throughout the entire movement.
- Don't "scoop" the upper body toward the floor as you push up. The body should maintain a straight line throughout the entire movement.
- Don't arch your back.
- Don't hold your breath.

8. Stepups

This dynamic exercise is most like the everyday activity of climbing stairs. It is beneficial for strengthening hip bones and improving balance and coordination.

Starting Position

Stand at the base of a sturdy staircase that has a hand railing. Place your hand on the railing for balance and support. Face the top of the staircase with your body, holding good posture and keeping eyes focused on a point in front of you.

The Move

1. Place your right foot on the first step; keep the toes pointed forward.

2. Push through your right foot, leg, and buttocks to raise your body.

3. Touch the first step lightly with your left foot and pause for a breath.

4. Slowly lower your left foot down to the starting position, supporting your body weight with the right leg.

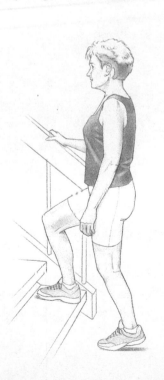
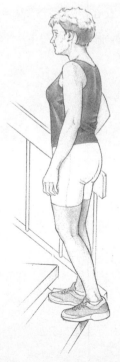

5. Keep your right foot on the first step and repeat until you have completed all repetitions for this leg.

6. Perform the same move with your left foot on the first step.

Reps and Sets

Complete 10 repetitions with the right leg forward, then repeat on the left side. Rest for a minute and repeat the set.

Where You Will Feel the Effort

The muscles in the front and back of the working leg will be challenged by the exercise. Stabilization in the feet, ankles, abdominal muscles, back, and torso will feel like sustained effort that is nonfatiguing.

Note: If you feel effort in your knees, try tightening the muscles in the back of your leg, your buttocks, and your core and pushing more forcefully through the front leg to step up. This should keep your knee directly above your ankle, instead of letting it jut over the toes. As you become stronger in this exercise, try stepping up with the front leg up on the second step instead of the first. Eventually, you can add more challenge by holding a light dumbbell in each hand while stepping up and down.

Make Sure You

- Don't hold your breath.

9. Front Lunge

The benefits of the front lunge exercise include improvement in your balance and coordination, as well as newfound strength in the muscles of the hips, legs, core, and back. Over time, lunging will strengthen the bones of the hip and spine.

Starting Position

Stand sideways behind the back of a chair. Place your feet hip-width apart and soften your knees, maintaining good posture in your upper body. Rest your hand on a counter or the back of the chair.

The Move

1. Step forward several feet with your right leg.

2. Land on your right heel and allow your foot to roll forward. Transfer your body weight to your right leg as the foot flattens.

3. Sink your hips slowly down into the lunge, allowing both knees to bend while maintaining erect posture with your upper body. Make sure you can see your toes throughout the entire move.

4. Build your strength to progress to a lunge depth where your upper leg is almost parallel to the floor, and the knee of your back leg is approaching the floor.

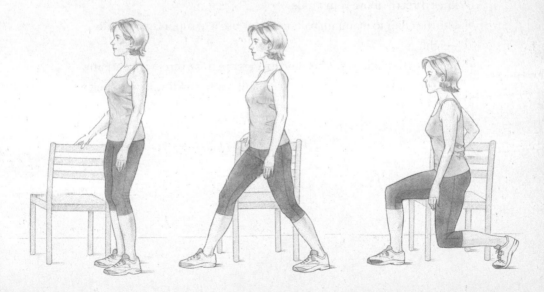

5. Lower the knee of your back leg toward the floor, and allow your back heel to come off the floor.

6. Find a balanced position where your weight is equally distributed between your front foot and the ball of your back foot.

7. Pause for a breath.

8. Push back through your front leg to return to the starting position.

Reps and Sets

Complete 10 repetitions with the right leg forward, then switch to your left leg forward and complete 10 more repetitions. The right leg and the left leg repetitions together make one set. Rest for a minute, and then complete a second set.

Where You Will Feel the Effort

Through your upper and lower legs, hips, buttocks, abdominals, and back muscles.

Make Sure You

- Keep the depth of the lunge to a level that you can strongly push back from. If you lunge too low before you have adequate strength, you will lose proper form and risk hurting yourself.
- Take a large enough step forward with your front leg to keep your knee directly above your ankle.
- Use the chair to maintain balance; don't use it to support your body weight.
- Remove the chair as you become stronger in this exercise. Eventually, you can make the exercise more challenging by holding a dumbbell in each hand.
- Don't hold your breath.

10. Tight Tummy

Many people have lost touch with their transverse abdominus, the muscles located below the belly button area. Realize that whenever you belly laugh or sneeze, these muscles contract involuntarily. The tight tummy exercise will help you contract these important muscles on cue.

Starting Position

Rest faceup on an exercise mat with knees bent and the soles of your feet on the floor. Place a hand on either side of the belly button with fingers pointing down so that you can monitor your abdominal contraction.

The Move

1. Gently press the small of your back against the floor, breathing out at the same time.

2. Begin to pull your belly button in, imagining you could flatten the tummy to touch the spine.

3. Hold this contracted position for 3 seconds, then relax.

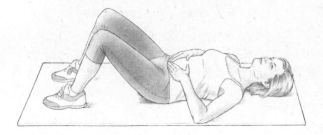

Reps and Sets

Repeat the hold 10 times, then rest for a minute and do a second set. For the intermediate move, each repetition consists of two leg movements.

Where You Will Feel the Effort

In the upper and lower abdominal muscles. When you perform the intermediate move, you will feel some effort through the hip and front of the leg as you raise and lower each leg. In the curl with tight tummy, focus on contracting the abdominals. You might also feel effort in your back, arms, and hips as you hold the position.

Make Sure You

- Don't hold your breath.

Modifications

Intermediate move. Once you can hold the contracted position for 3 seconds, try slowly lifting and lowering the right leg, followed by the left leg, while maintaining the abdominal contraction. Relax briefly after moving first one leg, then the other.

Curl with tight tummy. This is for those who have mastered the first and second variations of tight tummy. From a seated position, bend your knees and place your feet flat on the floor. Hold your arms out straight, next to your knees, and contract your abdominal muscles while lowering your upper body a few inches. Feel your tummy get tight and the small of your back round. Hold for 3 seconds, then pull back up to starting position.

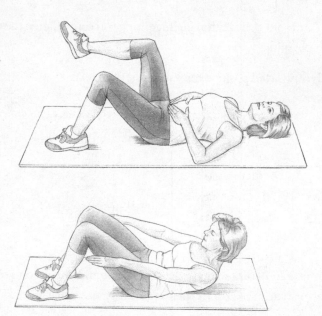

28

Screenings and Health Maintenance

A big part of taking care of yourself involves doing your best to maintain a healthy lifestyle—eating right, engaging in regular physical activity, managing stress, getting sufficient rest. But there is a second major component that is equally essential: making sure that you have excellent health care providers to care for you when you are ill and to give you the regular checkups, preventive screenings, and immunizations you need to stay healthy.

Most women need the following health care providers:

- Primary care provider
- Gynecologist (who may or may not also be your primary care provider)
- Dentist
- Eye care specialist

Depending on your own personal health issues, you may also require regular help from other medical experts, such as a dermatologist, an endocrinologist, a cardiologist, or a mental health specialist.

Although none of us relish the idea of getting regular checkups, screenings, and diagnostic tests, they are absolutely essential to good health. Nearly all are covered by insurance—and for good reason. Insurance companies understand the risk/benefit ratio of these preventive measures: If conditions are caught early, they are far easier and cheaper to treat, and the chances of cure are far greater.

However, many women are reluctant to see their doctors on a regular basis or get the screenings they need. My 81-year-old mother, for instance, has always had a fundamental problem with going to the doctor. "If I go," she says, "they'll find something!" In her mind, no news is good news; she feels almost as if going to the doctor actually causes her health troubles. However, her attitude changed recently when she found herself feeling fatigued all the time. At my urging, she finally went to her doctor and learned that she had iron-deficient anemia. The fix was fairly simple—dietary changes and supplements—and now her energy level is back where it should be.

Another woman I know is reluctant to visit her health care provider because she has gained a fair amount of weight over the years, and she fears being scolded for it. Her doctor recently refused to refill her prescription for medication she takes on a regular basis because he had not seen her for a checkup in years. Rather than go in for the much-needed medical visit, this woman just stopped taking her medications—a reckless act.

Your health care providers are there to help you. Seeing them regularly is a vital part of self-care, and neglecting to do so is careless. If you have a serious health problem and you need good medical care, but you haven't seen your doctors regularly or had proper screenings, they will be at a severe disadvantage: They won't know you or your medical history, how long you've had the problem, or whether there are other factors that may affect your current condition.

I'm lucky to have great health care providers. I admit that I have to push myself more than I'd like to make my appointments with them regularly, but I do it because I know it's essential to my overall well-being. A good health care provider is someone you can rely on to give you the finest available medical care and whom you can talk to openly without feeling inhibited or intimidated. To find one, ask someone you trust for a recommendation or call a university teaching hospital or a medical center or society and ask for the names of physicians. So, go ahead, make those appointments now—and keep them!

HOW TO TALK TO YOUR HEALTH CARE PROVIDER

You should be an active partner in your own health care by staying informed and engaging in the decisions that will affect you. Remember that no one knows your body the way you do. It's important to prepare for your visits so that you get the most out of them. Doctors' offices are often crowded and physicians feel rushed. Being prepared and knowing how to talk with your doctor comfortably and assertively will help you get the information you need. Here are some tips:

- **Before your appointment:**
  - Jot down any questions and concerns you might have. Bring the list with you to the office, along with a pen and paper to take notes on responses.
  - Make a list of any medications you may be taking to share with your doctor, including prescription drugs, over-the-counter medications, vitamins, and herbal supplements.
- **At your appointment:**
  - Refer to your list of questions and concerns.
  - If you're experiencing symptoms, describe them carefully, noting when they started, how often you experience them, what triggers them, and what you have done to address them.
  - Be candid about any lifestyle factors that affect your health, such as smoking, alcohol and drug use, diet, physical activity, and sexual activity.
  - Tell your doctor about medications you may be taking.
  - Describe any allergies you may have to drugs, foods, pet dander, or pollen.
  - Describe any current conditions that may affect your health, such as pregnancy or intention to become pregnant.
- **Tests.** If any tests are recommended, ask:
  - What is involved
  - What you need to do to prepare
  - Whether there are any dangers or side effects
  - When and how you will get the results
  - What the costs will be and whether these will be covered by health insurance
  - How the test will help determine your treatment plan
- **Diagnosis.** If you are diagnosed with a condition or an illness, ask:
  - What caused it
  - Whether it is temporary or permanent
  - How it can be treated
  - How you can manage symptoms
  - Whether it's recommended that you get a second opinion
  - Whether you should see a specialist
  - Whether you need a follow-up visit
- **Treatments.** If any treatments are recommended, ask:
  - All treatment options, including benefits and risks
  - Duration of treatment
  - Side effects
  - Costs and whether these will be covered by health insurance

- **Medications.** If medications are prescribed, ask:
  - Type
  - Length of time they should be taken
  - Purpose
  - Side effects
  - Whether there are generic versions
  - Whether there are interactions with any other drugs or supplements
  - Whether you should avoid any foods or activities while taking the medication
- **Ask questions.** Above all, if you don't understand something, be sure to ask questions. If you think it would help to have a family member or friend present, bring someone along. Take notes on the responses to your questions. Ask for written instructions. Follow up with the doctor's office if you need to.

SCREENINGS, TESTS, EXAMS, AND VACCINES

Getting regular screenings is among the most important things you can do to maintain good health. Below are general recommendations for screenings. (For more information on conditions that may require special screenings, see relevant sections on specific body systems, such as bones, heart, etc., in the earlier parts of this book.)

In general, women at average risk for most diseases should have the following screenings on a regular basis: blood pressure, fasting blood test for cholesterol and triglycerides, colon and rectal screening, mammogram and clinical breast exam, Pap test, bone density test, dental checkup, fasting blood glucose, and vision and glaucoma exam.

Depending on your ethnic background, family history, health history, environmental exposure, and other factors, you may be at greater risk for various conditions and should have extra screenings or more frequent screenings. For example, if you're African American, you may want to get genetic counseling to determine your risk of sickle cell anemia. Or if you're of Ashkenazi Jewish descent, you may want genetic counseling for Tay-Sachs disease (especially if you're considering getting pregnant) and for BRCA1 or BRCA2 mutation if you have a family history of breast or ovarian cancer.

On the opposite page is a schedule for standard screening tests for women by age group, drawn from several sources, including the Office of Women's Health (womenshealth.gov).

SCREENING TESTS	Ages 18–39	Ages 40–49	Ages 50–64	Ages 65 and Older
General health: Full checkup, height/weight	Discuss with your health care provider.	Discuss with your health care provider.	Discuss with your health care provider.	Discuss with your health care provider.
Thyroid test (TSH)	Start at age 35, then every 5 years	Every 5 years	Every 5 years	Every 5 years
HIV test	Get this at least once to find out your HIV status. Ask your health care provider whether and when you need the test again.	Get this at least once to find out your HIV status. Ask your health care provider whether and when you need the test again.	Get this at least once to find out your HIV status. Ask your health care provider whether and when you need the test again.	Discuss with your health care provider.
Heart health: Blood pressure test	At least every 2 years	At least every 2 years	At least every 2 years	At least every 2 years
Cholesterol test	Start at age 20; discuss with your health care provider.	Discuss with your health care provider.	Discuss with your health care provider.	Discuss with your health care provider.
Bone health: Bone mineral density test		Discuss with your health care provider.	Discuss with your health care provider.	Get at least once. Talk to your health care provider about repeat tests.
Diabetes: Blood glucose test	Discuss with your health care provider.	Start at age 45, then every 3 years	Every 3 years	Every 3 years
Breast health: Mammogram (x-ray of breast)		Discuss with your health care provider.	Every 2 years. Discuss with your health care provider.	Every 2 years. Discuss with your health care provider.

SCREENING TESTS	Ages 18–39	Ages 40–49	Ages 50–64	Ages 65 and Older
Clinical breast exam	Discuss with your health care provider.	Discuss with your health care provider.	Discuss with your health care provider.	Discuss with your health care provider.
Reproductive health: Pap test	Begin screening within 3 years of start of sexual activity or age 21, whichever comes first. Screen at least every 3 years.	Every 1–3 years	Every 1–3 years	Discuss with your health care provider.
Pelvic exam	Yearly	Yearly	Yearly	Yearly
Chlamydia test	Yearly until age 25 if sexually active. Older than age 25, get this test if you have new or multiple partners.	Get this test if you have new or multiple partners.	Get this test if you have new or multiple partners.	Get this test if you have new or multiple partners.
Sexually transmitted disease (STD) tests	Both partners should get tested for STDs, including HIV, before initiating sexual intercourse.	Both partners should get tested for STDs, including HIV, before initiating sexual intercourse.	Both partners should get tested for STDs, including HIV, before initiating sexual intercourse.	Both partners should get tested for STDs, including HIV, before initiating sexual intercourse.
Mental health screening	Discuss with your health care provider.	Discuss with your health care provider.	Discuss with your health care provider.	Discuss with your health care provider.

SCREENING TESTS	Ages 18–39	Ages 40–49	Ages 50–64	Ages 65 and Older
Colorectal health Use one of these three methods: fecal occult blood test; flexible sigmoidoscopy; colonoscopy			Yearly	Yearly. Older than 75, discuss with your health care provider.
Flexible sigmoidoscopy (with fecal occult blood test is preferred)			Every 5 years	Every 5 years. Older than age 75, discuss with your health care provider.
Colonoscopy			Every 10 years	Every 10 years. Older than age 75, discuss with your health care provider.
Eye and ear health: Complete eye exam	At least once from ages 20–29, at least twice from ages 30–39, or anytime that you have a problem.	Get an exam at age 40, then every 2–4 years or as your health care provider advises you.	Every 2–4 years or as your health care provider advises you.	Every 1–2 years
Hearing test	Starting at age 18, then every 10 years	Every 10 years	Every 3 years	Every 3 years

SCREENING TESTS	Ages 18–39	Ages 40–49	Ages 50–64	Ages 65 and Older
Skin health: Mole exam	Monthly mole self-exam; by your health care provider as part of a routine full checkup starting at age 20.	Monthly mole self-exam; by your health care provider as part of a routine full checkup.	Monthly mole self-exam; by your health care provider as part of a routine full checkup.	Monthly mole self-exam; by your health care provider as part of a routine full checkup.
Oral health: Dental exam	One or two times every year	One or two times every year	One or two times every year	One or two times every year
Immunizations: Influenza vaccine	Discuss with your your health care provider.	Discuss with your your health care provider.	Yearly	Yearly
Pneumococcal vaccine				One time only
Tetanus-diphtheria booster vaccine	Every 10 years	Every 10 years	Every 10 years	Every 10 years
Human papil-lomavirus vaccine (HPV)	Up to age 26, if not already completed vaccine series, discuss with your your health care provider.			
Meningococcal vaccine	Discuss with your health care provider if attending college.			

SCREENING TESTS	Ages 18–39	Ages 40–49	Ages 50–64	Ages 65 and Older
Herpes zoster vaccine (to prevent shingles)			Starting at age 60, one time only. Ask your health care provider if it is okay for you to get it.	Starting at age 60, one time only. Ask your health care provider if it is okay for you to get it.

Resources

I've written several other books on women's health that can provide you with additional information on specific health topics. They are listed below under the appropriate heading. I also maintain a Web site, Strongwomen.com, which offers a free monthly e-newsletter, online physical activity programs, and other resources. In addition, you can read my blogs and chat with me at BeWell.com, an online social network focused on women's health, featuring advice by experts around the country.

For information on my work at the John Hancock Research Center on Physical Activity, Nutrition, and Obesity Prevention at the Friedman School of Nutrition, Tufts University, please go to Jhrc.nutrition.tufts.edu. Finally, for more information on the not-for-profit StrongWomen community programs, please go to strongwomen.nutrition.tufts.edu.

Additional Sources

Ackerman, Jennifer. *Sex Sleep Eat Drink Dream: A Day in the Life of Your Body*. New York: Mariner, 2008.

Boston Women's Health Book Collective. *Our Bodies, Ourselves*. New York: Touchstone, 2005.

Carlson, Karen J., Stephanie A. Eisenstat, and Terra Ziporyn. *The New Harvard Guide to Women's Health*. Cambridge: Harvard University Press, 2004.

Legato, Marianne J. *Eve's Rib: The Groundbreaking Guide to Women's Health*. New York: Three Rivers Press, 2003.

Love, Susan M., and Alice D. Domar. *Live a Little: What the Research Really Says about Living a Pretty Healthy Life*. New York: Crown, 2009.

Organizations and Web Sites

Office on Women's Health, U.S. Dept. of Health and Human Services

    Womenshealth.gov

    Girlshealth.gov

National Women's Health Resource Center

    Healthywomen.org

Part I: Sex for Life: Reproductive and Sexual Well-Being

Books

Boston Women's Health Book Collective and Judy Norsigian. *Our Bodies, Ourselves: Pregnancy and Birth.* New York: Touchstone, 2008.

Boston Women's Health Book Collective, Judy Norsigian, and Vivian Pinn. *Our Bodies, Ourselves: Menopause.* New York: Touchstone, 2006.

Domar, Alice D., and Alice Lesch Kelly. *Conquering Infertility: Dr. Alice Domar's Mind/Body Guide to Enhancing Fertility and Coping with Infertility.* New York: Penguin, 2004.

Kagan, Leslee, Herbert Benson, and Bruce Kessel. *Mind Over Menopause: The Complete Mind/Body Approach to Coping with Menopause.* New York: Free Press, 2004.

Love, Susan M., and Karen Lindsey. *Menopause and Hormone Book: Making Informed Choices.* New York: Three Rivers Press, 2003.

Murkoff, Heidi, and Sharon Mazel. *What to Expect When You're Expecting,* 4th edition. New York: Workman, 2008.

Ricciotti, Hope. *I'm Pregnant, Now What Do I Eat?* New York: DK Publishing, 2007.

Schwartz, Pepper. *Prime: Adventures and Advice on Sex, Love, and the Sensual Years.* New York: Collins, 2007.

Stewart, Elizabeth G. *The V Book: A Doctor's Guide to Complete Vulvovaginal Health.* New York: Bantam, 2002.

Weschler, Toni. *Taking Charge of Your Fertility.* New York: Harper Paperbacks, 2006.

Organizations and Web Sites

Kaiser Family Foundation
Kff.org/womenshealth/repro.cfm

National Institutes of Health
Health.nih.gov/category/ReproductionandSexualHealth

United Nations: Development and Human Rights Section
UN.org/ecosocdev/geninfo/women/womrepro.htm

World Health Organization
Who.int/reproductivehealth

Additional Web Sites

American Association of Sex Education Counselors and Therapists (AASECT): Aasect.org

Centers for Disease Control and Prevention (for information on sexually transmitted diseases): CDC.gov/std

North American Menopause Society: Menopause.org

Pepper Schwartz: Drpepperschwartz.com

Planned Parenthood: PlannedParenthood.org

Part II: Beauty Inside and Out

Books

Taylor, Susan C. *Brown Skin: Dr. Susan Taylor's Prescription for Flawless Skin, Hair, and Nails.* New York: Amistad, 2003.

Organizations and Web Sites

American Academy of Dermatology
AAD.org

American Dental Association
ADA.org

Part III: Keeping in Balance
Books

Kessler, David. *The End of Overeating: Taking Control of the Insatiable American Appetite.* Emmaus, PA: Rodale, 2009.

Nelson, Miriam E., with Judy Knipe. *Strong Women Eat Well.* New York: Perigee Trade, 2002.

Nelson, Miriam E., with Sarah Wernick. *Strong Women Stay Slim.* New York: Bantam, 1999.

Nestle, Marion. *Food Politics: How the Food Industry Influences Nutrition and Health.* Berkeley: University of California Press, 2007.

Pollan, Michael. *The Omnivore's Dilemma: A Natural History of Four Meals.* New York: Penguin, 2007.

Wansink, Brian. *Mindless Eating: Why We Eat More Than We Think.* New York: Bantam, 2007.

Yoshida, Cynthia M. *No More Digestive Problems.* New York: Bantam, 2004.

Organizations and Web Sites

American Diabetes Association
Diabetes.org

American Dietetic Association
Eatright.org

Centers for Disease Control and Prevention
www.cdc.gov/healthyweight/

National Association for Continence
Nafc.org/bladder-bowel-health

National Institute of Diabetes and Digestive and Kidney Diseases (NIDDK)
Niddk.nih.gov

National Weight Control Registry
Nwcr.ws

Part IV: Standing Strong: Our Living Framework
Books

Nelson, Miriam E., Kristin R. Baker, and Ronenn Roubenoff with Lawrence Lindner. *Strong Women and Men Beat Arthritis.* New York: Penguin, 2003.

Nelson, Miriam E., with Lawrence Lindner. *Strong Women, Strong Backs.* New York: Putnam, 2006.

Nelson, Miriam E., with Sarah Wernick. *Strong Women Stay Young*. New York: Bantam, 2000.

Nelson, Miriam E., with Sarah Wernick. *Strong Women, Strong Bones*. New York: Perigee Trade, 2006.

Organizations and Web Sites

Arthritis Foundation

    Arthritis.org

National Osteoporosis Foundation

    Nof.org

Part V: Heart Smart and Breathing Easy

Books

Goldberg, Nieca. *Women Are Not Small Men: Life-Saving Strategies for Preventing and Healing Heart Disease in Women*. New York: Ballantine Books, 2003.

Legato, Marianne J. *The Female Heart: The Truth about Women and Heart Disease*. New York: Perennial Currents, 2000.

Nelson, Miriam E., and Alice H. Lichtenstein with Lawrence Lindner. *Strong Women, Strong Hearts*. New York: Penguin, 2006.

Organizations and Web Sites

American Heart Association National Center

    AmericanHeart.org

American Lung Association

    Lungusa.org

American Stroke Association National Center

    StrokeAssociation.org

DASH diet: For more information on the DASH diet, go to Dashdiet.org or Nhlbi.nih.gov and put "DASH diet" in the search box.

National Heart, Lung, and Blood Institute

    Nhlbi.nih.gov

Part VI: In Our Defense

Books

Henschke, Claudia I., Peggy McCarthy, and Sarah Wernick. *Lung Cancer: Myths, Facts, Choices–And Hope*. New York: W. W. Norton, 2003.

Love, Susan. *Dr. Susan Love's Breast Book*, 4th edition. New York: Da Capo Press, 2005.

Organizations and Web Sites

American Autoimmune Related Diseases Association

    Aarda.org

American Cancer Society
     Cancer.org

Dr. Susan Love Research Foundation
     www.dslrf.org
     Armyofwomen.org

Fred Hutchinson Cancer Research Center
     Fhcrc.org

National Cancer Institute
     Cancer.gov
     The NCI provides an online tool, the Breast Cancer Risk Assessment Tool, to help you determine your overall risk of breast cancer; see Cancer.gov/bcrisktool.

National Center for Preparedness, Detection, and Control of Infectious Diseases (NCPDCID)
Centers for Disease Control and Prevention (CDC)
     CDC.gov/ncpdcid
     HIV/AIDS resources at the CDC: You can locate a nearby testing location by calling 800-CDC-INFO (232-4636) 24 hours a day or by visiting the CDC HIV testing database at HIVtest.org.

Skin Cancer Foundation
     Skincancer.org

Part VII: Sensing: Staying in Touch with the World
Books

Harvard Medical School. *The Aging Eye*. New York: Free Press, 2001.

Organizations and Web Sites

American Optometric Association
     Aoa.org

National Association of the Deaf
     Nad.org

National Association for the Visually Handicapped
     Navh.org

National Institute on Deafness and Other Communication Disorders
     Nidcd.nih.gov

Part VIII: Headstrong: Minding Emotional and Mental Health
Books

Domar, Alice D. *Healing Mind, Healthy Woman: Using the Mind-Body Connection to Manage Stress and Take Control of Your Life*. New York: Delta, 1997.

Domar, Alice D., and Alice Lesch Kelly. *Be Happy Without Being Perfect: How to Break Free from the Perfection Deception*. New York: Crown, 2008.

Jamison, Kay Redfield. *Exuberance: The Passion for Life*. New York: Knopf, 2004.

Jamison, Kay Redfield. *An Unquiet Mind: A Memoir of Moods and Madness* New York: Knopf, 1995.

Jamison, Kay Redfield, and Frederick K. Goodwin. *Manic-Depressive Illness*, 2nd edition. New York: Oxford University Press, 2007.

Legato, Marianne J. *Why Men Never Remember and Women Never Forget*. Emmaus, PA: Rodale, 2006.

Solomon, Andrew. *Noonday Demon: An Atlas of Depression*. New York: Scribner, 2001.

Organizations and Web Sites

Alcoholics Anonymous
    AA.org

Alzheimer's Association National Office
    Alz.org

American Psychiatric Association
    Psych.org

American Psychological Association
    Apa.org

National Eating Disorders Association
    Nationaleatingdisorders.org

National Institute on Alcohol Abuse and Alcoholism (NIAAA)
    Niaaa.nih.gov
    The NIAAA has a new Web site tool, Rethinking Drinking, which offers a way to assess and change risky drinking habits; see RethinkingDrinking.niaaa.nih.gov.

National Institute on Drug Abuse
    Nida.nih.gov

National Institute of Mental Health (NIMH)
    Nimh.nih.gov

National Suicide Prevention Lifeline
    Telephone: 800-273-TALK (8255)
    Suicidepreventionlifeline.org

Rape, Abuse and Incest National Network
    Rainn.org

Sexual Assault Hotline: 800-656-HOPE (4673)

Something Fishy, an organization dedicated to helping people with eating disorders.
    Telephone: 866-690-7239
    SomethingFishy.org

Part IX: Flipping the Switch: An Action Plan for Health

Books

Benson, Herbert, and Miriam Z. Klipper. *The Relaxation Response*. New York: Harper, 2000.

Domar, Alice D. *Self-Nurture: Learning to Care for Yourself as Effectively as You Care for Everyone Else*. New York: Penguin, 2001.

Organizations and Web Sites

American Cancer Society

Cancer.org

The American Cancer Society's Web site offers a guide to quitting smoking.

DASH diet: For more information on the DASH diet, go to Dashdiet.org or Nhlbi.nih.gov and put "DASH diet" in the search box.

President's Council on Physical Fitness and Sports (PCPFS)

Fitness.gov

National Cancer Institute

Cancer.gov

The NCI's Quitlines provide information on quitting smoking.

Office on Women's Health

Womenshealth.gov

Acknowledgments

Jennifer and I would not have been able to write this book without the generous help of many people, including colleagues, friends, and family. We are deeply grateful for their abundant assistance and support.

I am very fortunate to work at Tufts University, a leading research institution that channels its many disciplines toward a unified mission of promoting citizenship and public service. It's an extraordinary experience to work in an environment that encourages and celebrates interdisciplinary approaches to solving national problems. Numerous colleagues from different fields at Tufts provided guidance on various chapters in the book. First and foremost was Dr. Rebecca Seguin, our research editor. Rebecca was instrumental first in helping us to frame the structure of the book and then, in seeking out and delivering the latest research in a number of areas. I also want to thank all of my other colleagues at the John Hancock Research Center on Physical Activity, Nutrition, and Obesity Prevention at the Friedman School of Nutrition Science and Policy for their assistance—in particular, Drs. Christina Economos, Sara Folta, Jennifer Sacheck, Ms. Mary Kennedy, and Ms. Eleanor Heidkamp-Young. Other colleagues at the Friedman School were gracious in their assistance—namely, Dr. Allen Taylor. A number of members of the larger Tufts community have consistently provided me with guidance, inspiration, and support over my years at the university, including President Lawrence Bacow and Provost Jamshed Bharucha, Eric Johnson, Jo Wellins, Donald Megerle, and most recently, Peter Dolan. I have been a part of this institution for more than two decades and can't imagine a better place to work.

Jennifer is also deeply grateful to the Jonathan M. Tisch College of Citizenship and Public Service at Tufts for her appointment as a Senior Fellow during the writing of this book.

Jennifer and I were fortunate to have colleagues at BeWell (formerly LLuminari), a consortium of nationally respected women's health specialists, willing to provide guidance on a range of topics, from mental health to sexuality. Special thanks to Drs. Alison Domar, Marianne Legato, Susan Love, Pepper Schwartz, Hope Ricciotti, Marcie Richardson, and Nancy Snyderman and Ms. Loretta LaRoche. Heartfelt appreciation goes to the leader of BeWell, Elizabeth Browning. Elizabeth not only provided intellectual guidance, but she and her husband, Paul, also provided us with a lovely house on the salt marshes of Delaware for a much needed writing retreat.

Other health experts around the country provided guidance in various chapters of the book. Deep thanks to Drs. Michael Holick, Stephanie Lee, Anna Magee, Jay McDermott, Ann McDermott, and Brian Wispelwey and to Ms. Megan Smith Watson. Ms. Catherine Buck and Ms. Helene Fuchs graciously provided helpful comments on the entire manuscript.

We consider Wendy Weil and Melanie Jackson the two best agents ever! At every step of the way, from the inception of the idea, to the publicity of the published book, we have relied on their abundant wisdom and expertise. Many thanks to them and to their very capable and efficient assistants, Emily Forland, Emma Patterson, and Anne Hays.

The entire team at Rodale has been a pleasure to work with. We are especially grateful to our keen-eyed editor, Julie Will, who offered sensitive, thoughtful, and intelligent input at every phase in the evolution of the book. Christina Gaugler provided wonderful leadership in the book's design.

We thank our two illustrators Lisa Clark and Karen Kuchar for their respective illustrations. The book is clearer and more beautiful for their artwork.

Several times during the two-year writing process, Jennifer and I came together for intensive writing retreats. These were some of the most rewarding times. Despite what our families think, we worked extremely hard during these times (and yes, we also enjoyed wholesome meals and long runs). One such retreat was on Elbow Mountain in Virginia. We thank Dan O'Neill for graciously providing his home to us for this writing retreat. The appearance of a mamma black bear and her two cubs made the week especially wonderful.

Finally, and most important, we thank Kin Earle and Karl Ackerman for being who they are—patient, loving, supportive husbands who are genuine champions of strong women. We also thank our children, Mason, Eliza, and Alexandra Earle and Zoë and Nell Ackerman, not only for supporting their mothers' work and for tolerating our frequent absence and distraction, but also, for contributing their own keen insights, observations, and experiences (and even, in Eliza's case, modeling for our illustrations!). We are truly blessed.

About the Authors

Miriam E. Nelson, PhD is director of the John Hancock Research Center on Physical Activity, Nutrition, and Obesity Prevention and associate professor of nutrition at the Friedman School of Nutrition Science and Policy at Tufts University. She is also a fellow of the American College of Sports Medicine, an honor reserved for those who have demonstrated leadership and research in the field of exercise. For the past 20 years, Dr. Nelson has been principal investigator of studies on exercise and nutrition, work supported by grants from the government and private foundations. From 2007 to 2008, Dr. Nelson served as the vice chair of the Physical Activity Guidelines Advisory Committee for US Department of Health and Human Services. The report was used to develop the inaugural Physical Activity Guidelines for Americans released in October of 2008. Most recently, she served on the 2010 Dietary Guidelines Advisory Committee for the US Department of Agriculture and US Department of Health and Human Services.

Dr. Nelson is the founder and director of the StrongWomen Program, a community-based exercise program for midlife and older women. This not-for-profit program is now running in communities in 40 states. Dr. Nelson has helped people learn how to stay younger, healthier, and stronger, and her research has revolutionized how people understand nutrition, exercise, and health. With colleagues, her current research is targeting obesity prevention.

Dr. Nelson is the author of the international best-sellers *Strong Women Stay Young; Strong Women Stay Slim; Strong Women Eat Well; Strong Women and Men Beat Arthritis; The Strong Women's Journal; Strong Women, Strong Hearts; Strong Women, Strong Bones;* and *Strong Women, Strong Backs.* These titles, published in 14 languages, have sold more than a million copies worldwide. *Strong Women, Strong Bones* received the esteemed Books for a Better Life Award for best wellness book of 2000 from the Multiple Sclerosis Society.

Dr. Nelson has appeared in her own PBS special entitled *Strong Women Live Well,* and she was the lead scientist for the PBS NOVA special entitled "Marathon." She has also been featured on other television and radio shows, including *The Oprah Winfrey Show, The Today Show, Good Morning America, ABC Nightly News,* CNN, *Fresh Air,* and the Discovery Channel.

Dr. Nelson lives in Concord, Massachusetts, with her husband and three children.

Please visit her Web site at **Strongwomen.com**

Jennifer Ackerman has been writing about health and science for the past two decades. She is the author of five books, including the forthcoming *Ah-choo! The Uncommon Life of Your Common Cold* (Twelve, 2011). Her most recent book, *Sex Sleep Eat Drink Dream: A Day in the Life of Your Body* (Houghton Mifflin, 2007), takes the reader through a typical day, from the arousal of the senses to hunger, fatigue, stress, sex, and the reverie of sleep and dreams, exploring the new science of what happens in the body. The book was selected as an "Editors' Choice" by the *New York Times* and a main selection by the *Scientific American* book club. It has been published in ten languages. Ackerman's book *Chance in the House of Fate: A Natural History of Heredity* (Houghton Mifflin, 2001) was named a *New York Times* "New and Noteworthy" paperback and was selected as a Library Journal Best Book of the Year in 2002. She is also the author of *Notes from the Shore* (1995), which describes the natural life of the mid-Atlantic region, and the editor of *The Curious Naturalist* (1991). A writer whose work has appeared in the *New York Times Magazine, National Geographic, Natural History,* and many science, nature, and women's magazines, Ackerman has written essays and articles on subjects ranging from the sexual habits of dragonflies to food safety. Her writing has been collected in several anthologies, among them *Best American Science Writing,* ed. Alan Lightman (Perennial, 2005). For seven years Ackerman was a staff writer and researcher for the book division of the National Geographic Society, where she contributed to *The Incredible Machine,* a book about the human body (1986, 1992).

Ackerman is currently a Senior Fellow at the Tisch College of Citizenship and Public Service at Tufts University. She is the recipient of numerous awards and fellowships in the past, including a 2004 NEA Literature Fellowship in Nonfiction, a fellowship from the Bunting Institute of Radcliffe College, and a grant from the Alfred P. Sloan Foundation.

Ackerman has been featured on many radio shows and has lectured at Harvard University, the Massachusetts Institute of Technology, the University of Virginia and its Medical Center, the American Association of University Women, and for numerous other groups and organizations.

Ackerman is married to novelist Karl Ackerman and has two daughters.

Please visit her Web site at **jenniferackerman.net**

Index

Boldface page references indicate illustrations. Underscored references indicate boxed text.